Comprehensive Clinical Nephrology

Comprehensive Clinical Nephrology

Edited by **Tanya Walker**

hayle
medical

New York

Published by Hayle Medical,
30 West, 37th Street, Suite 612,
New York, NY 10018, USA
www.haylemedical.com

Comprehensive Clinical Nephrology
Edited by Tanya Walker

© 2016 Hayle Medical

International Standard Book Number: 978-1-63241-427-4 (Hardback)

Printed in the United States of America.

Contents

Preface

The main aim of this book is to educate learners and enhance their research focus by presenting diverse topics covering this vast field. This is an advanced book which compiles significant studies by distinguished experts. This book addresses successive solutions to the challenges arising in the area of application, along with it; the book provides scope for future developments.

This book provides comprehensive insights into the field of clinical nephrology. The objective of this book is to give a general view of the different areas of nephrology and its applications. This discipline is mainly concerned with the diagnosis and treatment of diseases related to kidney. Nephrology includes providing cure for diseases such as kidney stones, chronic kidney disease, kidney failure, hypertension and disorders of electrolytes. This book provides significant information related to this field. It will help readers unravel the innovative aspects of nephrology by presenting path-breaking researches performed by experts across the globe. It aims to serve as a resource guide for students and experts alike and contribute to the growth of the field.

It was a great honour to edit this book, though there were challenges, as it involved a lot of communication and networking between me and the editorial team. However, the end result was this all-inclusive book covering diverse themes in the field.

Finally, it is important to acknowledge the efforts of the contributors for their excellent chapters, through which a wide variety of issues have been addressed. I would also like to thank my colleagues for their valuable feedback during the making of this book.

Editor

Qualitative Research and Narrative Sources in the Context of Critical and Renal Cares

José Siles-González, Carmen Solano-Ruiz

Nursing Department, University of Alicante, Alicante, Spain
Email: Jose.siles@ua.es, Carmen.solano@ua.es

Abstract

The objective of this study is to clarify the relevance of qualitative research in the context of critical care and renal dialysis requires using narrative sources. Also specific objectives are to identify the phases or cultural moments that are distinguished in these processes. Research Question: How can the narrative materials contribute to the study of the processes of critical care and/or qualitative research in nephrology? Method and Sources: There have been studies focusing on the narrative of patients who have written their experiences building a literature experience ill (Siles *et al.*, 1997, 1999, 2000). Sources have been used to extract testimony retrospective autobiographies written by people who have experienced the experiences of different diseases (Allué, 1996, 1997, Zorn, 1991, Gilbert, 1993; Comas, 2009; Gracia Armendáriz, 2010; Sampedro, 1996, Sacks, 2010). The analysis was developed by categorizing units of meaning, meaning families and networks. To identify the cultural moments we have followed the criteria established by Siles and Solano (2009): Multiculturalism, interculturalism and transculturalism. To identify rites of passage and liminality states have followed the principles outlined by Van Gennep (2013) and Turner (1990, 2008). Results: We identified cultural moments and characteristic states of liminality in critical care and kidney. Conclusions: narrative sources are effective for analyzing the meanings and experiences of patients in critical care and nephrology tool.

Keywords

Nursing, Narrative Anthropology of Care, Qualitative Research, Critical and Renal Cares

1. Introduction

Patients who live in the critical care unit and/or nephrology undergo a series of experiences that influence the way to tackle the disease and also influence their social, family and professional environment. The need to understand and describe the experiences of patients in critical care and/or nephrology is the first step for the professional care through reflection, and to find the corollary of meaning derived from such experiences. Through qualitative research in critical care and/or nephrology can come to understand and describe the experiences of patients and the meanings of the same, which is, first, an effective tool to adapt care to the "sensitivities" and personal, social and family characteristics of the patients, and, moreover, strengthens the vision and practice of humanism in care.

1.1. Objectives

-Clarify the relevance of qualitative research in the context of critical care and nephrology as a facilitator of the process of understanding, description and explanation of meanings involved in such care.
-Reflect on the appropriateness of the narrative materials in qualitative research.
-Identify cultural phases or moments that critical processes are distinguished and renal diseases requiring hemodialysis.
-Describe the situations of liminality that occur in the transition process health and disease.

1.2. Research Questions:

In what ways can the narrative materials contribute to the study of the processes of critical care and/or qualitative research in nephrology?

What cultural moments or phases can be identified in critical processes and renal diseases requiring hemodialysis?

2. State of the Question on Qualitative Research in Critical and Renal Cares

The variety of conceptual contributions that attempt to clarify the nature and scientific characteristics of qualitative research context and exceeds the limits of this study, but may give you some examples: interdisciplinary field, disciplinary and, in many cases, contradisciplinar. It crosses the humanities, social sciences and physica [1] [2]. Taylor and Bogdan [3] identified qualitative research as that which produces descriptive data: people's own words, spoken or written and observable behavior. Goetz and LeCompte [4] state that qualitative research has some essential features that can be summarized in the following points: a form of reality by inquiring descriptions from observations that take different forms (interviews, narratives, field notes, recordings, transcripts of audio, video, written records of all kinds, photographs, films, artifacts, etc.). Qualitative research involves a process in which data are presented in complex ways, as they really are, and to sort the researcher makes use of hermeneutics, understanding, sense through the experiences and subjective world. In this sense Szent-Györgyi [5] states: "If I go to nature, to the unknown, to the outskirts of knowledge, everything seems confusing and contradictory, illogical and incoherent. This is what makes qualitative research: lima contradiction and becomes simple, logical things". But qualitative research is not homogeneous, but its theoretical and methodological approaches depend on the starting paradigm: from the hermeneutic or interpretive paradigm and from the sociocritical paradigm, as the objective of either descriptive study of understanding and interpretation (hermeneutics), or, beyond that, the involvement and participation of the person and their environment (family, social, work) in solving their problems (sociocritical) [6]. In the second case, to encourage the participation of the individual and their environment, ideological stance based on democracy, freedom and awareness of the individual and the environment of the problem in question is adopted [7]. Ultimately, transdisciplinarity constitutes a challenge because in the conceptual richness of perspective and theoretical and methodological adoptions, the investigator must demonstrate their ability to work in research whose boundaries constitute genuine crossroads. It is what some authors denominate methodological and theoretical pertinence in qualitative research [8] [9]. It could carry a synthetic description of the characteristics of qualitative studies defining these as: Investigation of a particular phenomenon, conducted in depth and in a holistic manner through collecting narrative information and using a design flexible and transdisciplinary research.

Both critical and nephrological cares, can cause considerable disruption of perceptual capabilities that affect the patient-provider relationship, mainly in the processes of interaction and communication. Critical relationship between health problems and perception studied by Oliver Sacks from different perspectives in works such as: An Anthropologist on Mars, The Man Who Mistook His Wife for a Hat, and Musicophilia [10]-[12] (Sacks, 2004, 2006, 2009) or problems chronic diseases and sensory and perceptual disturbances. Sacks does not waive reflect on the phenomena of the mind from the complexity of it. This perspective allows you to discover the sensory and perceptual uncertainty in people who respond to your problems by building new existential landscapes in which experiences change color, shape, sound, touch, smell, etc.

In this context of the perceptual Maurice Merleauy Ponty fails to recognize that the body itself is more than one thing, something more than an object to be studied by science, since it is mainly a permanent form and necessary for the existence and opening interaction with reality through perceptions, but this perceptual openness involves more than relationship with reality, as constructed realities arising from the interpretation of perceptions. Consequently, the primacy of perception means the primacy of experience to the extent that perception has an active and constitutive dimension, for example, without perception of the health problem, there is no health problem and therefore there is no awareness Merleau Ponty himself [13].

Qualitative studies have been conducted in which the experiences of relatives of patients admitted in the intensive care unit [14] [17] are described. A considerable part of these experiences is the perception that family members have the critical patient. Uribe Muñoz and Restrepo [18] conducted a study analyzing the family perception of critically ill patients, especially their wives, considering the feelings and the impact on them of factors such as age, religion, morals, values, number of children, etc. Other authors emphasize the participation of patients [19]. Other studies focus on family care of critically ill patients [20], which, somehow, is a form of participation by the proximity of the care recipient. This involvement of families in the care of critically ill patients opens the way to studies in which the aim is to assess the needs of relatives in such complicated circumstances [15] [16] [21]-[24]; as a determining factor in a global context of professional-family interaction characterized by both the precariousness of professional training for such cases, and the difficulties arising from the situations (stressors themselves both for families and professionals). There are some researches that relate the stress experienced by families with critical with the emergence of anxiety problems and even depression patients [25].

3. Sources and Methods

Qualitative methodology focuses its focus on the opinion of the investigated biographical narrative [26]. In this sense Saltalamacchia [27] is expressed when endorses casuistry and subjectivism as two pillars of qualitative research that have been stigmatized by appealing to their unscientific character. The involvement of patients and families in the biographical narrative is essential to reinterpret reality in the light of new conditions of life that require adaptation efforts by both patients and family members. The narrative sources facilitate the study of the experiences of critical or chronic care in the time of receiving the diagnosis involves a radical change in the perception of the individual about himself and everything around him (family, work, leisure) [28]. In short, as Bruner [29] notes the biographical narrative facilitates the construction of new realities from the subjectivism of the subjects involved. There have been studies focusing on the narrative of patients who have written their experiences building a literature experience ill [30] [31] [32]. Several authors have addressed systematically the nature of narrative methods in the context of the experiences of patients [33]-[37]. Frank [38]-[40] (1995, 2001, 2002), meanwhile, profound questions (investigator suffering, the pain of the narrator and the dialogical ethics of narrative analysis processes) in qualitative research based on narrative accounts raises its various forms. Sources are considered suitable for this type of retrospective studies testimonials autobiographies written by the very people who have experienced the experiences of different diseases [41]-[48] account for the sense of isolation and the importance of the attitude of the professionals as the first step of that escape confinement: dialogues, nonverbal expression, touch, in short, some interaction sensory and emotional denoting a deal from person to person with a clear determination to enable some form of communication.

To identify cultural moments have followed the criteria established by Siles and Solano [49]. Also, to describe bonding and the parallels between the cultural moments and rites of passage or transition states of liminality and have followed the principles outlined by Van Gennep [50] and Turner [51] [52].

A qualitative design was used to study the liminal experiences of people with critical care and chronic renal disease. Constructivist perspective [53] was adopted because it is assumed that indi-viduals, groups and cultures create interpretations of realities and develop them through the stories they tell. Accepting that experience happens narratively [34], the stories narrated allow studying how people understand and make sense of what happens [54]. Connelly and Clandinin (2006) identified the three essential components of narrative inquiry: temporality, sociality, and the stage [37].

4. Results and Discussion

Relevance of qualitative research in the context of critical care and nephrology as a facilitator of the process of understanding, description and explanation of meaning: holism, complexity, mainstreaming person. The holism (derived from holos: all, entire, total) on the principle that all properties of a given system (biological, chemical, social, economic, mental, cultural) can not be determined by the component parts by alone, *i.e.*, the system-like "holos" whole-affects the behavior of the various component parts. Holism is summarized in the phrase "The whole is more than the sum of its parts", Aristotle coined in his "Metaphysics". When a system such as the human body is in a state of disease, determination or subject to certain limitations by it, the body, as holos, remains a disease that transcends all. Whereas the person is more than body art and it encompasses, it is logical that patients want to continue to be treated as people without the disease to become exclusively to surround the attention of health professionals. This may seem obvious, but as said Hurley [55] and Barthes [56], the obvious, too often, is as invisible as evident, leading to biased or obtuse interpretations of reality. Some autobiographical testimonies of kidney patients and critical care, describe situations in which, too often, they have to assert themselves as individuals and not just as a disease [57]. That is, in the stories described how patients in critical care units or hemodialysis machine steals limelight from the person while the nurse focuses on the machine. In the case of critical care due mainly to the deficit or apparent loss of perceptual abilities of patients, in the case of hemodialysis units to the need to care as much or more purifying machine (temporary repository of the soul or blood patient and, therefore, of his person). In both cases, patients expressed their need for care as. It also happens in something like Awakenings, where patients express stop being afraid to let its people awake state and return to a dormant irreversible [58]. Narrative inquiry is particularly suitable for the study of the experiences of disease where a diagnosis is often experienced as an interruption of one's life/story.

Personality: Etymologically, the term personality from the Greek "prosopon" (mask used by actors in the act of representing theatrical characters). Personality is, in that sense, what is perceived, what others are able to distinguish by observing each individual. The Latin etymology of the word "personare" (which resonates through) also refers to the way others perceive individuals. For authors like Gombrowicz [59], personality is the dialectical resulting from the need for social adaptation and the need to overcome the effect of such an adaptation that causes choking in absolute terms. Sontag [60] talks about the difficulty of speaking openly about cancer diseases (without rhetoric or the use of metaphors). These resources function as euphemisms and masks that keep the individual and those around him out of a reality shaped by the disease. The first types of personality we owe to the time of ancient Greece, as in this great compilation of the era is the "Corpus Hipocraticum" four varieties of personality that are related to the four elements (air, earth, fire, water) that formed the Cosmos. Hippocrates claimed that the microcosm of man was composed of these four elements transformed into moods and that the preponderance of any of them was as stumps types and other mood. The concept of person part of the consideration of the structural nature of it. The person considering this structure is as structurally character as an orderly whole according to their purposes and functions. Lain Entralgo gives the person is structural, since it is a unitary whole set, also executor of unit activities, including that of living as an individual [61]. The structure is the foundation unifying and holding points that walls, ceilings and other elements on which a building stands are located. The staff structure is a system that keeps a consistent and functional two primary subsystems: the psychological and organic. On the other hand, involves individuality human outstanding feature. Allport argues from a humanistic interpretation of social science that individuality is manifested in everyday life and on the social level when establishing relationships. In short, for Allport, individuality is the essential characteristic of human nature, while personality is "the only dynamic organization of psychophysical systems that determine a way of thinking and acting, in each subject in the process of adaptation environment" [62]. Other authors such as Huxley said that personality depends on three factors: heredity, circumstances and freedom. The only personality and individually manifested by perceptual capacity inherent to every human being: body awareness through the senses, historical memory, individual and collective consciousness, and so on. From other paradigms, such as the neo-positivist, he studied science from reductionist perspectives fragmenting the human being as a person and subject of research by reducing him to a mere object of study. The structural framework of the person is founded on a cultural basis on which four stand incidental spheres: law, religion, ethics and political system. These four spheres orbit and shape the circle in which different areas of personality develop: awareness of one's experience, myths, traditions and morals (**Figure 1**). In written sources autobiographical form, the authors reflect the relationship between your body and awareness by the same person.

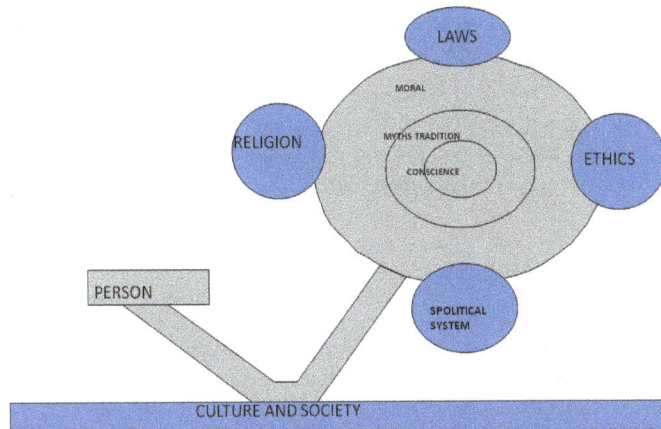

Figure 1. Structural framework of person. Source: Siles, J. & Solano, Mª C. (2009) [49] Siles, J. & Solano, C. (ed.) (2009) Antropología educativa de los cuidados. Una etnografía del aula y las prácticas clínicas. ICE. Universidad de Alicante, Alcoy, Alicante. Disponible en: http://rua.ua.es/dspace/handle/10045/20339.

It is a dynamic process of awareness as the body changes and new situations that will require re-interpretation processes of the body itself produce.

Temporality, sociality and scenarios:

Some examples of these meanings culled from the narratives are exemplified by Barthes (1986: 18) both the "ICU" and hemodialysis services: "(...) is the very pose of the character which leads to the reading of the meanings of connotation" [56] (Barthes, 1986: 18). They are situations where time takes on a totally different from everyday life dimension. Or not perceived (in the case of critical care in the ICU, or perceived in a distorted way in hemodialysis units sociability and personal interaction is limited to just touch sensation experienced by the patient to the technique that is being applied by the nurse. sometimes has totally altered or canceled their perceptual abilities, and their sociability is limited to the potential perceptual problem is that on many occasions the nurse knows the perceptual reality of his patient is a person who hears or feels as if I did (these situations are especially frustrating for patients in the ICU).

Scenarios have a great impact on the mood and perception of patients. In critical care or hemodialysis units are recharged the technology scenarios in which people appear prostrate, dependent, incommunicado (apparently at least), exiled from his family, cultural and plunged into a unifying environment on uniformity that objects have a pose that also invites interpret meanings that are part of this unifying homogeneity, since the item monitors where the constants of the people are green (go out of his body and exhibited in the object), oxygen masks that restrict vision partially hiding his face, hemodialysis machines to "walk" from the patient's blood inside your body to the "cleaner object" and, once the miracle wrought purification, the return again to be for it to continue. Of those felt by the patient before hemodialysis Gracia Armendáriz speaks connotations in his "Diary of a pale man": In this sense expresses Gracia Armendáriz [47]: "But sooner or later the day comes when the patient enters the circuit therapy, on the assumption of a routine in which you must get used to the scandal of the blood and fantaciencia of their vital fluids away from your body to circulate for four hours between the membranes and salt solutions of Machine". (Gracia Armendáriz, 2010:143). The analyzed materials present narrative situations transversely without sacrificing complexity. Describes ideas, facts, feelings, values, beliefs, etc. In all sources, which are linked to the process that is living. Based on the principles of holism in anthropology and complexity developed by Morin [63], Siles, Solano and Cibanal [8] point out the complexity anthropology seeks to address the fragmented and reductionist approaches to science, through a synthesis methodological, epistemological and bilogical. The human being is a complex system, therefore different types of subsystems that integrate biological, social, psychological, cultural, and the difficulty to analyze each of these subsystems from a holistic level.

4.1. Paradigms and Cultural Moments in Critical and Renal Cares

Paradigms are conceptual and methodological platforms consensus. Kuhn was the one who adapted the term from linguistics to science. For Kuhn paradigms serve, first, to identify the different disciplines have to investigate problems and, second, it is useful to guide scientists in adopting the theories, methods and techniques that have to adopt consistent and solid, what Siles called "methodological relevance" becomes a metaphor between poetry and research, as in any research process, the verses have to rhyme in assonance and consonant, what comes to signify the importance of epistemologically clarify both the nature of the research problem to know how to locate the paradigm with the theories, methods and techniques consistently for the research work do not waste your routine.

4.1.1. Hermeneutics
From this paradigm, which exceeds the purely technological level neopositivista-rational paradigm the research process is conceived as a subjective interval (both by the researcher subject and object-subject investigation). Theoretical knowledge is the result of the interaction that takes effect in practice of the given discipline (nursing, education, procedure). Since the approaches of this paradigm a nurse is considered a communicator and interpreter of reality of the patient agent. The characteristics of the interpretive paradigm within nursing have been studied by several authors [6] [9] [64]. To facilitate understand ding of the situations of critical care and nephrology type studies are performed mainly descriptive that analyze the meanings of the situations experienced by patients, families and professionals. Consequently, patients and their families have a voice, are listened to and what they say is collected through qualitative techniques such as life history, life stories, in-depth interviews, semi-structured, case studies, field notes, participant observation and nonparticipating narrative materials ranging from the story to the autobiographical novel in which life experiences are recounted, etc.. In short, paradigm, these approaches provide qualitative research in which people are cared for in critical care nephrology and they continue to be treated as such and not exclusively as carriers of disease. Although it is obvious that are more than a disease, too often they are treated as if they were locked in a category that eats them the status of a person leaving a look of pure disease is the absorbed the attention of professionals.

The sources consulted narratives share the characteristics of hermeneutics. The individual plays himself translating his experiences in a text which will then, in turn, to be interpreted by others. The transmission of knowledge, facts, beliefs, values, feelings that occurs by reading and inter-pretation of the autobiographical text facilitates another-distant geographical, cultural or temporarily-identifying the meanings experienced by the author.

4.1.2. Sociocritical Paradigm
The critical paradigm is characterized by the dialectical-critical nature of the process knowledge and taking into account the important role of ideology in the scientific process. The function and fundamental purpose of the budgets this platform are participatory emancipation and activities and tasks in the processes that occur in practice and are socially significant. The practice is critical and collaborative action. Habermas is the researcher who has contributed most to the development of critical paradigm.

The nurse is considered as an agent of socio change [6] [9]. One way to spray the isolation of patients by opening the living space critically their disease situations parallel facilitating any possible way of communication with the outside, the visits are their familiar social and professional network. Several studies have described the family visits as a tool to re-humanize the closed clinical context and also explain its benefits, but also, of course, the drawbacks that can lead [65]-[67]. For some authors, this insulation breakdown and isolation is a benefit not only for ethical reasons or humanists, but also for its worth as a positive influence on prognosis [68]. Also be considered as a relevant factor in this process of participatory involvement of the patient environment, the views and beliefs of professionals on the impact of visitors [68].

Qualitative methodology should focus on the opinion of the investigated biographical narrative [26]. In this sense Saltalamacchia [27] is expressed when endorses casuistry and subjectivism as two pillars of qualitative research that have been stigmatized by appealing to their unscientific character. The involvement of patients and families in the biographical narrative is essential to re-interpret reality in the light of new conditions of life that require adaptation efforts by both patients and relatives. In short, as Bruner [26] notes the biographical narrative facilitates the construction of new realities from the subjectivism of the subjects involved.

Participation in solving the problems is a form of freedom of the person as such and also the free-dom of his family, social and work environment [7] (López Parra, 2001) and, also, this position can only raise from ideological democratic and participatory schemes in which the person maintains at all times the condition is inherent in the mature and responsible citizen lifestyles. Freedom is not easy to take on and involves taking a compromising position with life. Is only true when it is conscious of its destiny, its mission, its fundamental questions, who am I? Where did I come from? and what for where I'm going? Is faced with the enigma of Oedipus before the Sphinx, which poses a fundamental dilemma. The Sphinx, in Greek mythology, monster with the head and breasts of a woman, body of a lion and wings of a bird. Squatting on a rock, addressed to all who would enter the city of Thebes by posing the following riddle: "What has four legs in the morning, two at noon and three at night ?" If challenged not solve the riddle, she killed them. When the hero Oedipus solved answered: "Man, who crawls shortly after birth, walks on two legs as an adult, and walks with a cane when he reaches old age," the Sphinx committed suicide [7] (López Parra, 2001). From this participatory perspective, the association is the highest expression of participation, since it involves groups of people who share similar problems due to a chronic process. In this sense, more associations of people with chronic diseases interactively collaborate on improving the quality of life there.

4.2. Moments Cultural Liminality in Chronic, Critical and Renal Cares

The changes in the different situations of health and illness experiences that cause different forms of interpretation of the phenomenon is derived. From the time of diagnosis of the disease to the patient's integration into the community of people who share with him the same problem a number of socialization processes loaded with symbolism, intercom and discoveries in the rites of passage that occur (Van Gennep, 2013, Turner, 2008) [50]-[52] that involve social changes. Through the transition made through rites of passage individuals leave situations of uncertainty and disorientation caused by not being part of the community of "sick" nor be part of the group and considered "healthy". Overcome situations of "liminality" (situations characterized by being authentic crossroads or limbs). The different phases are distinguished in these processes of change are called cultural moments [49]. Basically three phases which are called cultural moments and responding to different phases or sections within the situational process that occurs in all disease are distinguished. Liminality is especially true in multicultural times due to the lack of communication between the pre-diagnosis and the immediate post-diagnosis phase. The patient cannot find a way to tie these situations and reinterpret the new situation (**Figure 2**). Also in the transit of multiculturalism to interculturalism and transcultural situations of "liminality" characterized by the moments that have their times of uncertainty from one situation to another occur.

A) multicultural Moment (typical of the neo-positivist paradigm):

A1: From the perspective of the person who has been diagnosed with a disease, you can reply to the stage where there is a wall between lifestyle, expectations and prior to detection of the disease (**Figure 2**) culture. At this stage it is almost impossible reconciliation with the lifestyle required by the new situation demands produced by the new state of satisfaction of needs, or is struggling to implement compensatory mechanisms are not met. There is usually a feeling of rejection and hate for changing repudiating the new situation. In critical care the isolation is reinforced by the high technological level of critical care units. In nephrology care and periodic temporary dip keeps the patient in a position of strict dependence on the machine and that the "plug" it occurs.

A2: From the perspective of the professional-patient relationship is characterized by the lack of not strictly necessary for the performance of communication techniques and therapeutic compliance: The patient has no voice, only abides by the regulations and is subject to therapeutic procedures. This has been traditionally indoors and ICU services, but also in dialysis units and nephrology care services. In this phase all the scenery multicultural units or intensive care hemodialysis units represent anything into which the patient feels a stranger to monitors, hemodialysis ma-chines and other devices and people (professionals and other patients).

B) intercultural Moment (characteristic of hermeneutics):

B1: From the patient's perspective is a step forward, starting the process of recognition and recon-ciliation with the new state requirements. Reinterpreting the scale of values. Consequently gaps begin to occur in the wall (**Figure 3**) between before and after the diagnosis situation and the person talks to herself and is being recognized in the new situation, the disease until it finally comes to understand the new reality which is installed.

B2: particularly significant moments put the patient through their new reality through impact which is causing awareness of your body change as the previous fistula connected to the machine, the connection of the probe to a bag hanging on the side of bed or connecting to a monitor that unravels the secrets of her body showing them with lines undulating fluorescent green color or loud sounds. New evidence, fistula probe, connecting to a monitor, in short, show a certain state of dependence and contributes to the body's own reinterpretation of the patient

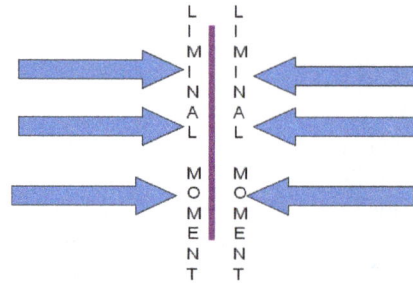

MULTICULTURALISM

Situation of solitary confinement with respect to their new reality.

(There is not a way to tie the two realities: pre and post diagnosis).

Figure 2. Cultural moments in critical and renal cares. Source: Siles, J. & Solano, C. (ed.) (2009) Antropología educativa de los cuidados. Una etnografía del aula y las prácticas clínicas. ICE. Universidad de Alicante, Alcoy, Alicante. Disponible en.

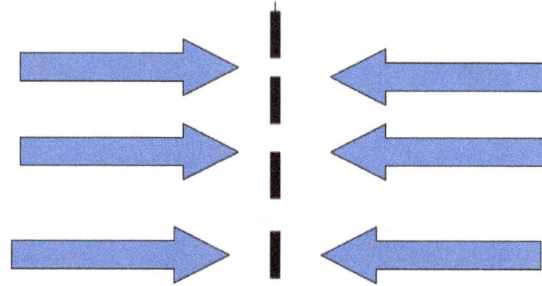

INTERCULTURALISM

Communication between the two realities and understanding of the new situation

Figure 3. Cultural moments in critical and renal cares. Source: Siles, J. & Solano, C. (ed.) (2009) Antropología educativa de los cuidados. Una etnografía del aula y las prácticas clínicas. ICE. Universidad de Alicante, Alcoy, Alicante. Disponible en: http://rua.ua.es/dspace/handle/10045/20339.

and through that rebuilding will start the new situation. From the perspective of the patient-professional rela-tion-ship, an interactive dialogue occurs between professional-patient resulting in more personalized care

C) Transcultural moment: (characteristic of Sociocritical paradigm)

C1: From the perspective of the patient in this period the patient's awareness that assumes its involvement in the process as a key factor in their care who actively participates together with their immediate environment (family, social occurs, professional). Accept the reliance on technology and seeks to lead as independent a life as possible (**Figure 4**).

C2: From the perspective of the patient relationship, professional collaborative interaction that affects the practice of care in which the patient and his environment have a voice and participation develops. Professional acts as an agent of socio change.

The Tool Musicophilia How Communication with Patients in Critical Care and Nephrology

How to enable some form of communication with critically ill patients when we are not sure of their perception

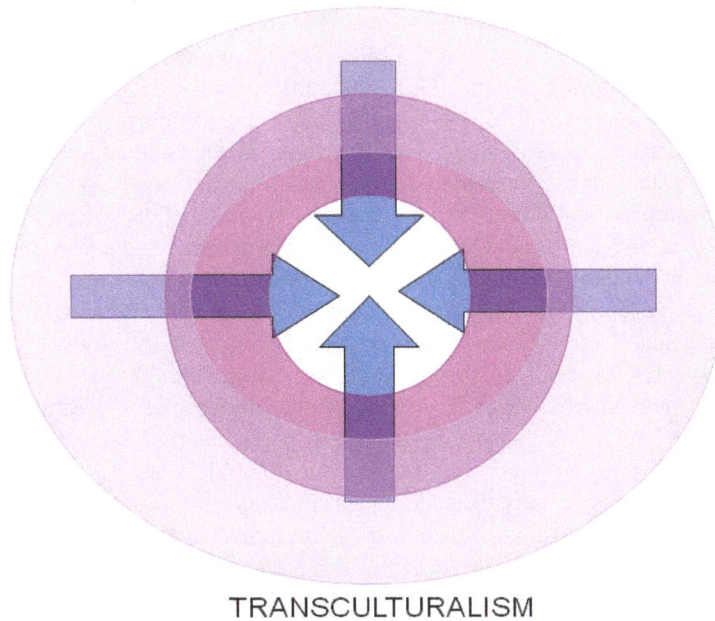

TRANSCULTURALISM

Figure 4. Cultural moments in critical and renal cares Source: Siles, J. & Solano, C. (ed.) (2009) Antropología educative de los cuidados. Una etnografía del aula y las prácticas clínicas. ICE. Universidad de Alicante, Alcoy, Alicante. Disponible en: http://rua.ua.es/dspace/handle/10045/20339.

to level ? Several studies have shown different effects of music critics and nephrology patients. Some studies have shown the usefulness of music for local produce sedation, anesthesia [66], in dental clinic and so on. In patients who are in critical care situations, music stimulates the feelings that still occupy some space in the brain that seem to relive the emotions in patients when they hear something that has to do, or not, with previous experience: music meaningful patient [67]. Oliver Sacks describes the use of music in patients with neurological problems and their potential to reorganize their perceptual and emotional systems [12].

4.3. The Narrative as a Source of Knowledge in Critical Care

Narrative materials describing the experiences of people living in nephrology or critical care are a source of knowledge from the principles of the hermeneutic and socio-critical paradigm, qualitative research methods and biographical and autobiographical narrative techniques. In short, this type of sources, theories and methods relevant for:

a) The descriptive study that reflected the facts, meanings and feelings on the part of that has lived, facilitating the understanding of the phenomenon holistically.

b) Tools that can contribute to the awareness of the new realities in which people and their environments (family, social and professional) in critical care situations or are nephrology. And consequently, enhance socialization of these people and their organization in groups and associations involved in improving their living conditions.

4.3.1. Narrative and Renal Cares

In any chronic condition affecting the body changes occur, but also the language to what is happening. Metaphors creatively to not bottom are used, often painful issue through metaphors, especially in situations such as cancer or AIDS, but metaphors are also used to refer to hemodialysis and ICU Sontag and Conelly and Clanding [54] [60] identified the three essential components of narrative inquiry: the person and time (time being and heideggerian), sociability, and space. In his view, the understanding of the people who are in these situations, build their reinterpretations of their new realities and problems considering primarily through personal time, social conditions, and the contexts in which the experiences take place. All this is essential for the design and analysis of rigorous narrative inquiry [35].

Kierans and Maynooth [69] explore the experiences of patients with chronic renal failure in the final state. They use in-depth interviews (77 cases) and 12 life histories applied as a source of data collection in hemodialysis units from different cities in Ireland. They found the cultural exchange of experiences from a natural event that affects the physiology of individuals. From the daily diagnostic needs are considered just or even trivialize as eating, drinking, urinating, having sex, social or labor participation and actions are not part of a response to everyday life. Now, in the new situation of dependence on the hemodialysis machine new ratings and sensations that affect the reinterpretation of the ranking values and priorities of the patient who needs to reinvent itself with a new self-image, an image that also has cultural components arise and social impact on one or sandwiched always linked with hemodialysis family, social and work experience. After a hemodialysis patient recounts how angry he was with his family when he returned home: "(...) I could hear the bubbling. I never imagined it would be this bad experience. When the anesthetic disappeared, the pain was terrible. Mentally I found most disturbing, I thought I had reached the end (...)" [69] (Kierans and Maynooth, 2001: 244). In general prevailing feeling of dependence on the hemodialysis machine and fistula nuclear occupies a place in the experiences of patients, because depending on how it evolves, adapting to family, social and professional life is more or less.

Anita E. Molzahn, Laurene Sheilds Anne and Bruce (2008) in her work: "Learning from stories of People with chronic kidney disease", study the panorama of patients who were being treated with hemodialysis Participants in this study were those who had the history of the heroes of the book: 100 stories of experiences with renal insufficiency (DTU, 2000). All were receiving treatment in Units Dialysis and Transplantation, Royal Victoria Hospital, McGill University Health Center in Montreal. The book includes stories of 100 people (62 men and 38 women). Their ages ranged from 21 to 88 years, and cover a wide range of treatment modalities and a wide range in the length of experience with the treatments. In Canada, in 2004, 18,827 people in Canada were being treated with hemodialysis for chronic renal failure overcome suffering. The survival rate at 5 years of this population is 40%. In this population, 34.6% had diabetes and 34.9% have heart disease, which significantly increase the risk of eventually become, for example, in a patient with renal cardiac critical care.

One of the recurring issues in these hemodialysis patients constitute travel from their villages to the cities where there hemodialysis service. The tour, periodically repeated, is itself the source of sensations and perceptions that lead to various family and employment difficulties in daily life. The search for flats near the cities where there hemodialysis machines, the impact the disease has on individuals and their families have been exposed in several works by Frank [38]-[40]. However, little is known about how people talk about these liminal experiences (right at the threshold of consciousness) that are sometimes beyond words and are complicated when externalize. This subliminal context fraught with uncertainty, is where the narrative materials reveal their potential to transmit both the facts (the behaviors, the obvious), such as feelings, beliefs, values that are affecting, at a given moment, the experiences of the patient or critical care nephrology. Francisco Herrera [71] on "Diseases of Sisyphus" described and demonstrated by accurate examples, the utility of narrative as a vehicle to understand the situations in which different types of diseases that are suffered by people who stubbornly remain so are a despite the stigma that has befallen them. Also the work of Gracia Armendáriz "Diary of a pale man" establishing an interesting comparative analysis with experienced authors who have racked their meat and their works the pain of the disease and/or the loss of a loved one being particularly significant allusion to Francisco Umbral and "Mortal y Rosa" [70]. Gracia Armendáriz, in his diary covering one hundred sixty-nine days recounting a process during which the protagonist is compelled to completely change their lifestyles, quit his job, accompanied by severe dieting take no less strong drugs. All this waiting for one hope: the transplant. Gracia Armendáriz [47] and Herrera [71] (to remind us of the process that went through his father) remind us of the existential characteristic landscape commas uremic produce stupor, disorientation and memory loss. Regarding the cult of technology prevailing at home in health centers, the author claims the humanization of care by way of empathy and patient - health professional interaction:

"A paranoid Phantasmagoria: are not machines that purify the blood of patients, but we, the pa-tients, who serve machines because without the support of our blood, with high levels of phosphorus and potassium, they cease instantly and the hidden and shameful gear they serve crumble, and with it all the health institution" [47] (Gracia Armendáriz, 2010: 143). "every physician should be subjected to the same treatments he administered to their patients" [47] (Gracia Armendáriz, 2010: 44). In relation to the concept of person, which remains despite all the sick, Gracia Armendáriz noted in relation to continue feeling that a person, not just a disease and demanding, therefore care that exceeded the boundaries of pathology to achieve the whole person:"Someone has a duty to remember the obvious" confirming reflections Hurley [55] and Barthes [56] on this issue.

4.3.2. Narrative and Critical Cares

In critical care we find autobiographical works in which, as in nephrology patients are holistically reflect the experiences of people who, despite their diagnosis status, they still have knowledge, history, beliefs, feelings, traditions, culture, etcetera. This is the case of José Comas, who being diagnosed with lymphoma, writes in a blog their experiences and send them to your friends. José Comas [46] written between December 2004 and February 2008, a day in which he describes his experiences as a person, journalist correspondent of the "Country" in Germany and lymphoma diagnosed "non-Hodgkin" at age 60. Try by all means to be an observer of himself, of his illness and tries to do so without losing the sarcasm and sense of humor: "I am a spectator of my own evil and I hope to maintain this position as far as necessary," but also echoes not particularly hopeful moments:"If everything goes wrong, I'll have to instruct the 'piper' to touch 'Asturias beloved country' and I prostitues to Sella" although even for the worst cases death, try to keep the ironic tone that characterized him:"the bone marrow transplant Stefan Morsch, who suffered from leukemia, was a success. The patient died of pneumonia" [46]. Marta Allué [41] [42], after an accident that nearly cost him his life and that gave significant sequelae in the form of burns, wrote about his experiences in "Losing l" and his work "Surviving in the ICU". The author makes an effort and try to recall over each time after his return to the perceptual activity when regains consciousness in an almost inhumane conditions: rescues of ostracism from the world of dreams those nightmares that alternated with episodes in which the hallucinations did nothing but increase the physical suffering caused by all kinds of processes which had to undergo during the cures. Later, tells the hard reality of the rehabilitation process. We talk about your values, your beliefs, but most of all, your feelings and your mood swings in which alternating phases too quickly for some hope with uncertainty and downright depressing vital reluctantly. The book begins with the same story of the time of the accident, and from here tells us his experience with the disease, the common thread being their way through various health institutions. From his time in the service of semi-consciousness ICU, in which memories are clouded and confused, until the "recovery" of their autonomy, to multiple surgical procedures (some of them in the US). History is not just a succession of events, but also the feelings and impressions of the author. Throughout the whole work, Marta Allué talks about her experiences in the patient role which is stripped of its status as a person. Ramón Sampedro (1996) wrote his "Letters from Hell" in a poetic prose in which he signified the pain he felt after being at twenty-five quadriplegic after an accident after jumping into the sea from the top of a rock. Rage, suffering, death wish. As a result of that sentimental corollary Sampedro in his attempt to convey the pain that burns his soul to the nurses leave comes as shocking and disturbing testimonies like this: "Guardians of complex dreams, all broken. Careers of eternal anguish with sacred fires. You, that you keep the miserable lives of agonizing bodies. Vestal that you keep the fire burning in this hell. Samaritans of balsamic smiles that give pain. Sensitive spirits contemplate smiling despair. Unknowingly you cease to hear the screams of the damned (...)." [43]. Almost all of the authors cited agree on one fact: qualitative research in general and employing sources, methods and narrative techniques in particular, have among their principles generalizing results. Nor, of course, the standardization of treatment based on the results. Consider this factor, especially when you consider the enormous variability of existential meanings and responses that lead to the experiences in critical care situations and/or nephrology. This variability may be due in large part to the diversity of belief, culture, values, family, social and work environment, etc., but above all, we must not forget, when it comes to people, each of them can be a world than to know. Consequently not all follow the same pattern or path, although you can set key points that are shared by the majority. Subjectivity is a source that works dialectic, in the sense that although conveys meanings that experiences have for people (accompanied by feelings, beliefs, values, etc..); however, does not provide clear-cut solutions for technical problems, procedural, etc. Therefore require further studies combining qualitative subjectivity is considered and valued, with quantitative research that the other dimensions of reality involved in care also have their place. In critical care combining narratives provided by the authors retrospectively (Allué, Sampedro, Grace Armendáriz, Comas, etc.), gives us an insight into the different experiences regarding the narratives collected "ad hoc" at the same time hemodialysis or interview relatives while their relatives are admitted to the ICU. While in the second, narratives diachronic lack that, in the first case a temporary overview where the longitudinal plane is present is provided. In nephrology care is much more common to find synchronous narratives in which the experience is transmitted in key this time.

4.4. The Narrative as a Source of Knowledge in Renal Care

Narrative materials describing the experiences of people living in nephrology or critical care are a source of knowledge from the principles of the hermeneutic and socio-critical paradigm, qualitative research methods and biographical and autobiographical narrative techniques. In short, this type of sources, theories and methods relevant for:

a) The descriptive study that reflected the facts, meanings and feelings on the part of that has lived, facilitating the understanding of the phenomenon holistically.

b) Tools that can contribute to the awareness of the new realities in which people and their environments (family, social and professional) in critical care situations or are nephrology. And consequently, enhance socialization of these people and their organization in groups and associations involved in improving their living conditions.

4.4.1. Narrative and Renal Cares

In any chronic condition affecting the body changes occur, but also the language to what is happening. Metaphors creatively to not bottom are used, often painful issue through metaphors, especially in situations such as cancer or AIDS, but metaphors are also used to refer to hemodialysis and ICU Sontag and Conelly and Clanding [54] [60] identified the three essential components of narrative inquiry: the person and time (time being and heideggerian), sociability, and space. In his view, the understanding of the people who are in these situations, build their reinterpretations of their new realities and problems considering primarily through personal time, social conditions, and the contexts in which the experiences take place. All this is essential for the design and analysis of rigorous narrative inquiry [35].

Kierans and Maynooth [69] explore the experiences of patients with chronic renal failure in the final state. They use in-depth interviews (77 cases) and 12 life histories applied as a source of data collection in hemodialysis units from different cities in Ireland. They found the cultural exchange of experiences from a natural event that affects the physiology of individuals. From the daily di-agnostic needs are considered just or even trivialize as eating, drinking, urinating, having sex, social or labor participation and actions are not part of a response to everyday life. Now, in the new situation of dependence on the hemodialysis machine new ratings and sensations that affect the reinterpretation of the ranking values and priorities of the patient who needs to reinvent itself with a new self-image, an image that also has cultural components arise and social impact on one or sandwiched always linked with hemodialysis family, social and work experience. After a hemodialysis patient recounts how angry he was with his family when he returned home: "(...) I could hear the bubbling. I never imagined it would be this bad experience. When the anesthetic disappeared, the pain was terrible. Mentally I found most disturbing, I thought I had reached the end (...)" [69] (Kierans and Maynooth, 2001: 244). In general prevailing feeling of dependence on the hemodialysis machine and fistula nuclear occupies a place in the experiences of patients, because depending on how it evolves, adapting to family, social and professional life is more or less.

Anita E. Molzahn, Laurene Sheilds Anne and Bruce (2008) in her work: "Learning from stories of People with chronic kidney disease", study the panorama of patients who were being treated with hemodialysis Participants in this study were those who had the history of the heroes of the book: 100 stories of experiences with renal insufficiency (DTU, 2000). All were receiving treatment in Units Dialysis and Transplantation, Royal Victoria Hospital, McGill University Health Center in Montreal. The book includes stories of 100 people (62 men and 38 women). Their ages ranged from 21 to 88 years, and cover a wide range of treatment modalities and a wide range in the length of experience with the treatments.

In Canada, in 2004, 18,827 people in Canada were being treated with hemodialysis for chronic renal failure overcome suffering. The survival rate at 5 years of this population is 40%. In this population, 34.6% had diabetes and 34.9% have heart disease, which significantly increase the risk of eventually become, for example, in a patient with renal cardiac critical care.

One of the recurring issues in these hemodialysis patients constitute travel from their villages to the cities where there hemodialysis service. The tour, periodically repeated, is itself the source of sensations and perceptions that lead to various family and employment difficulties in daily life. The search for flats near the cities where there hemodialysis machines, the impact the disease has on individuals and their families have been exposed in several works by Frank [38] [40]. However, little is known about how people talk about these liminal experiences (right at the threshold of consciousness) that are sometimes beyond words and are complicated when externalize. This subliminal context fraught with uncertainty, is where the narrative materials reveal their potential to transmit both the facts (the behaviors, the obvious), such as feelings, beliefs, values that are affecting, at a given moment, the experiences of the patient or critical care nephrology.

Francisco Herrera [71] on "Diseases of Sisyphus" described and demonstrated by accurate examples, the utility of narrative as a vehicle to understand the situations in which different types of diseases that are suffered by people who stubbornly remain so are a despite the stigma that has befallen them. Also the work of Gracia Armendáriz "Diary of a pale man" establishing an interesting comparative analysis with experienced authors who have racked their meat and their works the pain of the disease and/or the loss of a loved one being particularly significant allusion to Francisco Umbral and "Mortal y Rosa" [70]. Gracia Armendáriz, in his diary covering one hundred sixty-nine days recounting a process during which the protagonist is compelled to completely change their lifestyles, quit his job, accompanied by severe dieting take no less strong drugs. All this waiting for one hope: the transplant. Gracia Armendáriz [47] and Herrera [71] (to remind us of the process that went through his father) remind us of the existential characteristic landscape commas uremic produce stupor, disorientation and memory loss. Regarding the cult of technology prevailing at home in health centers, the author claims the humanization of care by way of empathy and patient-health professional interaction:

"A paranoid Phantasmagoria: are not machines that purify the blood of patients, but we, the patients, who serve machines because without the support of our blood, with high levels of phosphorus and potassium, they cease instantly and the hidden and shameful gear they serve crumble, and with it all the health institution" [47] (Gracia Armendáriz, 2010: 143). "Every physician should be subjected to the same treatments he administered to their patients" [47] (Gracia Armendáriz, 2010: 44). In relation to the concept of person, which remains despite all the sick, Gracia Armendáriz noted in relation to continue feeling that a person, not just a disease and demanding, therefore care that exceeded the boundaries of pathology to achieve the whole person: "Someone has a duty to remember the obvious" confirming reflections Hurley [55] and Barthes [56] on this issue.

4.4.2. Narrative and Critical Cares

In critical care we find autobiographical works in which, as in nephrology patients are holistically reflect the experiences of people who, despite their diagnosis status, they still have knowledge, history, beliefs, feelings, traditions, culture, etcetera. This is the case of José Comas, who being diagnosed with lymphoma, writes in a blog their experiences and send them to your friends. José Comas [46] written between December 2004 and February 2008, a day in which he describes his experiences as a person, journalist correspondent of the "Country" in Germany and lymphoma diagnosed "non-Hodgkin" at age 60. Try by all means to be an observer of himself, of his illness and tries to do so without losing the sarcasm and sense of humor: "I am a spectator of my own evil and I hope to maintain this position as far as necessary," but also echoes not particularly hopeful moments: "If everything goes wrong, I'll have to instruct the 'piper' to touch 'Asturias beloved country' and I prostitues to Sella" although even for the worst cases death, try to keep the ironic tone that characterized him: "the bone marrow transplant Stefan Morsch, who suffered from leukemia, was a success. The patient died of pneumonia" [46]. Marta Allué [41]-[42], after an accident that nearly cost him his life and that gave significant squeal in the form of burns, wrote about his experiences in "Losing l" and his work "Surviving in the ICU". The author makes an effort and try to recall over each time after his return to the perceptual activity when regains consciousness in an almost inhumane conditions: rescues of ostracism from the world of dreams those nightmares that alternated with episodes in which the hallucinations did nothing but increase the physical suffering caused by all kinds of processes which had to undergo during the cures. Later, tells the hard reality of the rehabilitation process. We talk about your values, your beliefs, but most of all, your feelings and your mood swings in which alternating phases too quickly for some hope with uncertainty and downright depressing vital reluctantly. The book begins with the same story of the time of the accident, and from here tells us his experience with the disease, the common thread being their way through various health institutions. From his time in the service of semi-consciousness ICU, in which memories are clouded and confused, until the "recovery" of their autonomy, to multiple surgical procedures (some of them in the U.S.). History is not just a succession of events, but also the feelings and impressions of the author. Throughout the whole work, Marta Allué talks about her experiences in the patient role which is stripped of its status as a person. Ramón Sampedro (1996) wrote his "Letters from Hell" in a poetic prose in which he signified the pain he felt after being at twenty-five quadriplegic after an accident after jumping into the sea from the top of a rock. Rage, suffering, death wish. As a result of that sentimental corollary Sampedro in his attempt to convey the pain that burns his soul to the nurses leave comes as shocking and disturbing testimonies like this: "Guardians of complex dreams, all broken. Careers of eternal anguish with sacred fires. You, that you keep the miserable lives of agonizing bodies. Vestal that you keep the fire burning in this hell. Samaritans of balsamic smiles that give pain. Sensitive spirits contemplate smiling despair. Unknowingly you cease to hear the screams of the damned (...)." [43].

Almost all of the authors cited agree on one fact: qualitative research in general and employing sources, methods and narrative techniques in particular, have among their principles generalizing results. Nor, of course, the standardization of treatment based on the results. Consider this factor, especially when you consider the enormous variability of existential meanings and responses that lead to the experiences in critical care situations and/or nephrology. This variability may be due in large part to the diversity of belief, culture, values, family, social and work environment, etc., but above all, we must not forget, when it comes to people, each of them can be a world than to know. Consequently not all follow the same pattern or path, although you can set key points that are shared by the majority. Subjectivity is a source that works dialectic, in the sense that although conveys meanings that experiences have for people (accompanied by feelings, beliefs, values, etc..); however, does not provide clear-cut solutions for technical problems, procedural, etc. Therefore require further studies combining qualitative subjectivity is considered and valued, with quantitative research that the other dimensions of reality involved in care also have their place. In critical care combining narratives provided by the authors retrospectively (Allué, Sampedro, Grace Armendáriz, Comas, etc.), gives us an insight into the different experiences regarding the narratives collected "ad hoc" at the same time hemodialysis or interview relatives while their relatives are admitted to the ICU. While in the second, narratives diachronic lack that, in the first case a temporary overview where the longitudinal plane is present is provided. In nephrology care is much more common to find synchronous narratives in which the experience is transmitted in key this time.

5. Conclusions

The relevance of qualitative research in the context of critical care and nephrology lies in its potential to clarify the meanings that experiences have for patients.

The study of the narrative sources identifies the incidence of experiences, feelings, beliefs and values in renal and critical care. It also promotes the humanistic perspective on this kind of care.

Pre-epistemological clarification, by reflecting on the paradigmatic location and consistent adoption of theories, methods and techniques in qualitative research is essential to the relevance and effectiveness of critical and renal cares. The narrative qualitative research materials are suitable for the study of experiences, meanings, feelings and ultimately, to maintain a holistic view of critical care and nephrology.

In this study we have identified three cultural moments: multicultural, intercultural and transcultural. These phases are loaded with symbolism and ritual components they involve social changes for the sake of community integration of kidney patients. Liminal moments occur especially in the multicultural moment due to the lack of communication between the pre-diagnostic and post-diagnostic phase, with the individual unable to reinterpret their new situation.

The preliminary step of any research must consider what kind of knowledge is sought (glob-al, partial, objective, subjective), according to the kind of knowledge to investigate some theories, methods and techniques adopted in the context of a particular scientific paradigm.

References

[1]   Denzin, N. and Lincoln, Y. (2000) Handbook of Qualitative Research. Sage, Thousand Oaks.

[2]   Denzin, N. (2001) Interpretive Interactionism. Sage, Thousand Oaks.

[3]   Taylor, S.J. and Bogdan, R. (2012) Introducción a los métodos cualitativos de investigación. Paidós, Barcleona.

[4]   Goetz, J.P. and Lecompte, M.D. (1988) Etnografía y diseño cualitativo en investigación educativa. Morata, Madrid.

[5]   Szent-Györgyi, A. (1980) Dionysians and Apollonians. In: Key, M.R., Ed., *The Relationship of Verbal and Non Verbal Communication*, Mouton, New York, 317-318.

[6]   Siles González, J. (1997) Epistemología y enfermería: por una fundamentación científica y profesional de la disciplina. *Enfermería Clínica*, **7**, 188-194.

[7]   López Parra, H.J. (2001) Investigación cualitativa y participativa un enfoque histórico-hermenéutico y crítico-social en psicología y educación ambiental. Escuela de Ciencias Sociales. Facultad: Facultad de Psicología Universidad Pontificia Bolivariana, Medellín.

[8]   Siles González, J., Solano Ruiz, C. and Cibanal, L. (2005) Holismo e investigación cualitativa en el marco de la antropología de la complejidad: una reflexión sobre la pertinencia metodológica en ciencias sociosanitarias y humanas. *Cultura de los Cuidados*, **9**, 68-81.

[9] Siles González, J. and García, E. (1995) Las características de los paradigmas y su adecuación a la investigación en enfermería. *Enfermería Científica*, **160/161**, 10-15.

[10] Sacks, O. (2006) Un antropólogo en marte. Anagrama, Madrid.

[11] Sacks, O. (2004) El hombre que confundió a su mujer con un sombrero. Anagrama, Madrid.

[12] Sacks, O. (2009) Musicofilia. Anagrama, Madrid.

[13] Merleau Ponty, M. (1985) Fenomenología de la percepción. Planeta Agostini, Barcelona.

[14] Bernat, R., López, J. and Fontseca, J. (2000) Vivencias de los familiares del enfermo ingresado en la unidad de cuidados intensivos. Un estudio cualitativo. Enferm Clin. 10/1:10:19

[15] Jamerson, P.A., *et al.* (1996) The Experience of Families with a Relative in the Intensive Care Unit. *Heart Lung*, **25**, 467-474. http://dx.doi.org/10.1016/S0147-9563(96)80049-5

[16] Wilkinson, P. (1995) A Qualitative Study to Establish a Self-Perceived Needs of Family Members of Patients in a General Intensive Care Units. *Intensive and Critical Care Nursing*, **11**, 77-86.

[17] Eggenberger, S.K. and Nelms, T.P. (2007) Family Interviews as a Method for Family Research. *Journal of Advanced Nursing*, **58**, 282-292. http://dx.doi.org/10.1111/j.1365-2648.2007.04238.x

[18] Escalante, M.T.U., Torres, C.M. and Ruiz, J.R. (2004) Percepción familiar del paciente crítico cardiovascular. *Investigación y educación en enfermería*, **22**, 50-61. http://aprendeenlinea.udea.edu.co/revistas/index.php/iee/article/view/2962/2669

[19] Torres, L. and Morales, J.M. (2004) Participación familiar en el cuidado del paciente crítico. Recomendaciones de la Sociedad Andaluza de Enfermería de Cuidados Críticos. *Tempos Vitalis. Revista Internacional para el Cuidado del Paciente Crítico*, **4**, 18-25.

[20] Henneman, E. and Cardin, S. (2002) Family-Centered Critical Care: A Practical Approach to Making It Happen. *Critical Care Nurse*, **22**, 12-19. http://www.ihi.org/resources/Pages/Publications/Familycenteredcriticalcareapracticalapproachtomakingithappen.aspx

[21] Abizanda, R. (2007) Sobre las necesidades reales de los familiares de pacientes de cuidados intensivos: percepción de los familiares y del profesional. *Medicina Intensiva*, **31**, 271-272.

[22] Molte, R.N.C. (1979) Needs of Relatives of Critically Ill Patient: A Descriptive Study. *Heart & Lung: The Journal of Acute and Critical Care*, **8**, 332-339.

[23] Maxwell, K.E., Stuenkel, D. and Saylor, C. (2007) Needs of Family Members of Critically Ill Patients: A Comparison of Nurse and Family Perceptions. *Heart & Lung: The Journal of Acute and Critical Care*, **36**, 367-376. http://dx.doi.org/10.1016/j.hrtlng.2007.02.005

[24] Santana, L., *et al.* (2007) Necesidades de los familiares de pacientes de cuidados intensivos: percepción de los familiares y del profesional. *Medicina Intensiva*, **31**, 273-280. http://dx.doi.org/10.1016/S0210-5691(07)74826-X

[25] Pochard, F., Azoulay, E., Chevret, S., Lemaire, F., Hubert, P., Canoui, P., Grassin, M., Zittoun, R., le Gall, J.R., Dhainaut, J.F. and Schlemmer, B. (2001) Symptoms of Anxiety and Depression in Family Members of Intensive Care Unit Patients: Ethical Hypothesis Regarding Decision-Making Capacity. *Critical Care Medicine*, **29**, 1893-1897. http://dx.doi.org/10.1097/00003246-200110000-00007

[26] Bolivar Botía, A. (2002) "¿De nobis ipsis silemus?": Epistemología de la investigación biográfico-narrativa en educación. *Revista Electrónica de Investigación Educativa*, **4**, 1-26. http://www.uvmnet.edu/investigacion/episteme/numero1-04/impresiones/resenas1.asp

[27] Saltalamacchia, H. (2008) Casuística y subjetivismo: Falsos estigmas de la investigación cualitativa. *Cinta de Moebio*, 109-126. http://www.moebio.uchile.cl/32/%20saltalamacchia.htm

[28] Gaydos, H.L. (2005) Understanding Personal Narratives: An Approach to Practice. *Journal of Advanced Nursing*, **49**, 254-259. http://dx.doi.org/10.1111/j.1365-2648.2004.03284.x

[29] Bruner, J. (1991) The Narrative Construction of Reality. *Critical Inquiry*, **18**, 1-21.

[30] González, J.S., Sánchez, P.F., Cañaveras, R.M.P. and Hernández, E.G. (1993) Las alteraciones en la vida cotidiana de los enfermos terminales a través del análisis de textos: Un modelo simulado para las prácticas con el proceso de enfermería. *Enfermería Científica*, 4-9.

[31] González, J.S., Bravo, E.M.G., Tolino, D.M., Frías, Y.G. and Hernández, E.G. (1997) Por una rentabilización pedagógica en la obra de Benedetti: Etnología narrativa y situaciones de vida-salud. *Cultura de los Cuidados*, **1**, 17-24. http://rua.ua.es/dspace/bitstream/10045/5309/1/CC_01_04.pdf

[32] Siles González, J. (2000) Antropología narrativa de los cuidados. CECOVA, Alicante.

[33] Clandinin, D.J. (2006) Handbook of Narrative Inquiry: Mapping a Methodology. Sage, Thousand Oaks.

[34] Clandinin, D.J. and Connelly, F.M. (2000) Narrative Inquiry: Experience and Story in Qualitative Research. Jossey-

Bass, San Francisco

[35] Clandinin, D.J., Pushor, D. and Orr, A.M. (2007) Navigating Sites for Narrative Inquiry. *Journal of Teacher Education*, **58**, 21-35. http://dx.doi.org/10.1177/0022487106296218

[36] Garro, L. (1994) Narrative Representations on Chronic Illness Experience. *Social Science and Medicine*, **38**, 775-788. http://www.sciencedirect.com/science/article/pii/0277953694901503

[37] Connelly, F.M. and Clandinin, D.J. (2006) Narrative Inquiry: A Methodology for Studying Lived Experience. *Research Studies in Music Education*, **27**, 44-54. http://dx.doi.org/10.1177/1321103X060270010301

[38] Frank, A.W. (1995) The Wounded Storyteller. University of Chicago Press, Chicago. http://dx.doi.org/10.7208/chicago/9780226260037.001.0001

[39] Frank, A.W. (2001) Can We Research Suffering? *Qualitative Health Research*, **11**, 353-362. http://dx.doi.org/10.1177/104973201129119154

[40] Frank, A.W. (2002) Why Study People's Stories? The Dialogical Ethics of Narrative Analysis. *International Journal of Qualitative Methods*, **1**. http://www.ualberta.ca/~iiqm/backissues/1_1Final/pdf/frankeng.pdf

[41] Allué, M. (1996) Perder la piel. Seix Barral, Barcelona.

[42] Allué, M. (1997) Sobrevivir en la UCI. *Enfermería Intensiva*, **6**, 29-34.

[43] Sampedro, R. (1996) Cartas desde el infierno. Planeta Barcelona.

[44] Gilbert, H. (1992) El protocolo compasivo. Tusquets, Barcelona.

[45] Zorn, F. (1991) Bajo el signo de Marte. Anagrama, Madrid.

[46] Comas, J. (2009) Crónicas del linfoma. Rey Lear, Madrid.

[47] Armendáriz, J.G. (2010) Diario del hombre pálido. Demipage, Madrid.

[48] Sacks, O. (2010) Despertares. Anagrama, Madrid.

[49] Siles, J. and Solano, C. (2009) Antropología educative de los cuidados. Una etnografía del aula y las prácticas clínicas. ICE, Universidad de Alicante, Alcoy, Alicante. http://rua.ua.es/dspace/handle/10045/20339

[50] Van Gennep, A. (2013) Los ritos de paso. Alianza, Madrid.

[51] Turner, V. (1990) Liminality and Community. In: Alexander, J.C. and Seidman, S., Eds., *Culture and Society: Contemporary Debates*, Cambridge University, Cambridge, 147-154.

[52] Turner, V. (2008) The Ritual Process: Structure and Anti-Structure. Transaction Publishers, Piscataway.

[53] Gergen, K. (2001) Social Construction in Context. Thousand. Sage, Thousand Oaks.

[54] Salkalys, J.A. (2003) Restoring the Patient's Voice. *Journal of Holistic Nursing*, **21**, 228-241. http://dx.doi.org/10.1177/0898010103256204

[55] Hurley, R.E. (1999) La investigación cualitativa y el profundo entendimiento de lo obvio. *Health Services Research*, **34**, 1119-1136.

[56] Benner, P. (1991) The Role of Narrative Experience and Community in Skilled Ethical Comportment. *Advances In Nursing Science*, **14**, 1-21. http://dx.doi.org/10.1097/00012272-199112000-00003

[57] Sacks, O. (2013) Alucinaciones. Anagrama, Madrid.

[58] Gombrowicz, W. (1983) Ferdydurke. Sudamericana, Buenos Aires.

[59] Sontag, S. (1985) La enfermedad y sus metáforas. Muchnik Editores, Barcelona.

[60] Entralgo, P.L. (1986) Antropología médica para clínicos. Salvat, Barcelona.

[61] Allport, G. (1985) La personalidad: su configuracion y desarrollo. Herder, Madrid

[62] Morin, E. (1994) Introduccion al pensamiento complejo. Gedisa, Barcelona.

[63] Medina, J.L. and Sandin, M.P. (1995) Epistemología y Enfermería: Paradigmas de la investigación en Enfermería. *Enfermería Clínica*, **5**, 32-44.

[64] Arricivita, A., Cabrera, J., Arias, M., Robayna, M.C. and Díaz, L. (2002) Características de la organización de las visitas en las unidades de cuidados críticos de la Comunidad Autónoma de Canarias. *Enfermería en cardiología: Revista científica e informativa de la Asociación Española de Enfermería en Cardiología*, 36-40.

[65] Padfield, A. (1976) Letter: Music as Sedation for Local Analgesia. *Anesthesia*, **31**, 300-301. http://dx.doi.org/10.1111/j.1365-2044.1976.tb11819.x

[66] Peretz, I. (2001) Listen to the Brain. A Biological Perspective on Musical Emotions. In: Juslin, P. and Sloboda, J., Eds., *Music and Emotion: Theory and Research*, Oxford University Press, New York, 105-134.

[67] Diaz, R. (2006) Régimen de visitas en la unidad coronaria y su influencia en el pronóstico. *Revista electrónica de Me-*

dicina Intensiva (*REMI*), **6**. http://remi.uninet.edu/2006/03/REMI0964.htm

[68] Margall, M.A. and Asiain, M.C. (2000) Creencias y actitudes de las enfermeras de cuidados intensivos sobre el efecto que la visita abierta produce en el paciente, familia y enfermeras. *Enfermería Intensiva*, **11**, 107-117.

[69] Kierans, C.M. and Maynooth, N.U.I. (2001) Sensory and Narrative Identity: The Narration of Illness Process among Chronic Renal Sufferers in Ireland. *Anthropology & Medicine*, 8, 237-253.

[70] Herrera, F. (2011) Las enfermedades de Sísifo. Imprenta Rimada, Cádiz.

[71] Herrera, F. (2011) Diario de un hombre pálido. *Cultura de los Cuidados*, **31**, 127-141. http://rua.ua.es/dspace/bitstream/10045/20579/1/CC_31_16.pdf

Acronimos

AIDS = Acquired immunodeficiency syndrome
ICU = Intensive Care Unit.

Effects of Darbepoetin-α on Oxidative Stress Marker in Patients with Chronic Renal Failure

Norio Nakamura[1*], Michiko Shimada[2], Ikuyo Narita[2], Yuko Shimaya[2], Takeshi Fujita[2], Reiichi Murakami[2], Hiroshi Osawa[3], Hideaki Yamabe[2], Ken Okumura[2]

[1]Community Medicine, Hirosaki University Graduate School of Medicine, Japan
[2]Department of Cardiology, Respiratory Medicine and Nephrology, Hirosaki University Graduate School of Medicine, Hirosaki, Japan
[3]Department of General Medicine, Hirosaki University Hospital, Hirosaki, Japan
Email: *nnakamur@r2.dion.ne.jp

Abstract

Objective: Long-acting darbepoetin-α (DA) has recently been used to treat renal anemia in patients with chronic renal failure. It is considered clinically useful because its duration of action is longer than that of conventional epoetin-α. In this study, we investigated changes in the levels of the oxidative stress marker malondialdehyde-modified low density lipoprotein (MDA-LDL), renal anemia, and renal function when patients were treated for chronic renal failure switched from epoetin-α to DA. Materials and Methods: The subjects included nine patients with chronic renal failure and renal anemia who were treated with epoetin-α on an outpatient basis at our department. Blood was sampled prior to the switch and at 3, 6, and 12 months after the switch. We then investigated changes in MDA-LDL, hemoglobin (Hb), and creatinine (Cr) levels. Results: There were no significant changes in MDA-LDL and Hb levels after switching to DA. A significant increase was observed in Cr levels after 12 months compared with those prior to switching. Conclusion: Once-a- month administration of DA did not result in an increase in oxidative stress, and therefore, DA is considered capable of controlling renal anemia.

Keywords

Chronic Renal Failure; Darbepoetin-α; Epoetin-α; Indoxyl Sulfate; MDA-LDL; Renal Anemia

---

*Corresponding author.

1. Introduction

Reports have stated that when treating renal anemia in patients with chronic renal failure, palliative care should be initiated for progression of renal failure in addition to treating anemia [1]. Furthermore, such treatment is reported to be extremely important for the prevention of cardiovascular disease [2]. From these perspectives, the importance of treating renal anemia in patients with chronic renal failure continues to increase.

Epoetin-α was released in the market in 1990 as a drug to treat renal anemia, but from 2005 onwards, darbepoetin-α (DA) began to be used in clinical practice. DA is a formulation with a modified epoetin-α molecular structure; therefore, the duration of its hematopoietic effects is longer than that of conventional epoetin-α, thereby allowing a prolonged administration interval [3]. In clinical practice, excellent results have been reported in patients undergoing dialysis and those who are in the conservative stage of renal failure [3].

Renal failure and uremia are known to cause oxidative stress [4]. This is believed to damage the kidneys and other organs [5]. Currently, although a few reports have investigated changes in the levels of oxidative stress markers due to DA administration, results have been inconsistent [6] [7].

For this reason, in this study, we investigated the changes in the levels of the oxidative stress marker malondialdehyde-modified low density lipoprotein (MDA-LDL), hemoglobin (Hb), and creatinine (Cr) inconservative-stage patients with chronic renal failure who were switched from epoetin-α to DA treatment.

2. Materials and Methods

The study population comprised nine patients with conservative-stage renal failure who were treated as outpatients at the Nephrology Department of the Hirosaki University Hospital. The patients' diseases were well- controlled by once-a-month administration of epoetin-α. After providing written consent, the subjects were enrolled into this trial.

Patients were switched to DA at an epoetin-α:DA ratio of 200:1. Laboratory examinations were conducted at the time of switching and at 3, 6, and 12 months after the switch. Changes in Hb, Cr, and MDA-LDL and indoxyl sulfate levels were measured. Serum MDA-LDL and serum indoxyl sulfate levels were measured by SRL Inc. (Tokyo, Japan).

According to the Japan Society for Dialysis Therapy for renal anemia treatment guidelines, patients with renal anemia should be administered iron supplements when the transferrin saturation ratio (TSAT) is ≤20% and/or when the serum ferritin level is ≤100 ng/mL, with the target Hb level of 11 g/dL.

Results were represented as mean ± SD. Scheffe's method was used for statistical analysis, and $p < 0.05$ was considered statistically significant.

3. Results

Patients' background is shown in **Table 1**. The underlying disease was determined by renal biopsy in one patient (focal segmental glomerulonephritis), five patients were suspected to have chronic glomerulonephritis, one patient had polycystic kidney disease, one patient was suspected to have benign nephrosclerosis, and one patient was suspected to have diabetic nephropathy. Epoetin-α was administered at the dose of 6000 units/month in one subject with comparatively well-preserved renal function, whereas all other patients were administered 12,000 units/month of epoetin-α.

Changes in serum MDA-LDL concentrations are shown in **Figure 1**. Increase in serum MDA-LDL was only observed in one patient at 6 months after administration, but there were no significant changes observed in any of the patients during the course of the investigation.

Changes in Hb levels are shown in **Figure 2**. No statistically significant changes were observed during the course of the investigation. After 12 months of administration, Hb level in one patient decreased to almost 6 g/dL, but this patient experienced abnormal vaginal bleeding due to a uterine tumor, which was thought to be the cause of the drop in Hb level.

Changes in serum Cr levels are shown in **Figure 3**. A tendency toward a gradual increase in Cr levels was observed in all subjects, and a significant difference was observed when the levels prior to administration were compared with those at 12 months after administration ($p < 0.05$).

Changes in serum in doxyl sulfate levels are shown in **Figure 4**. There was a wide variation in changes, but no significant changes were observed during the investigation period.

Table 1. Patients' background.

Case	Gender	Age	Cr (mg/dL)	Dose of epoetin (/month)	Cause of renal failure
S. K.	F	65	3.19	12,000	unknown
W. M.	F	47	4.07	12,000	unknown
S. O.	F	71	5.46	12,000	unknown
M. K.	F	39	4.33	12,000	FSGS
K. F.	M	85	1.76	6,000	unknown
Y. S.	M	83	3.93	12,000	unknown
A. S.	F	47	3.51	12,000	PKD
A. S.	F	60	1.83	12,000	unknown
T. S.	M	65	3.77	12,000	unknown

FSGS: Focal segmental glomerulonephritis, PKD: polycystic kidney disease.

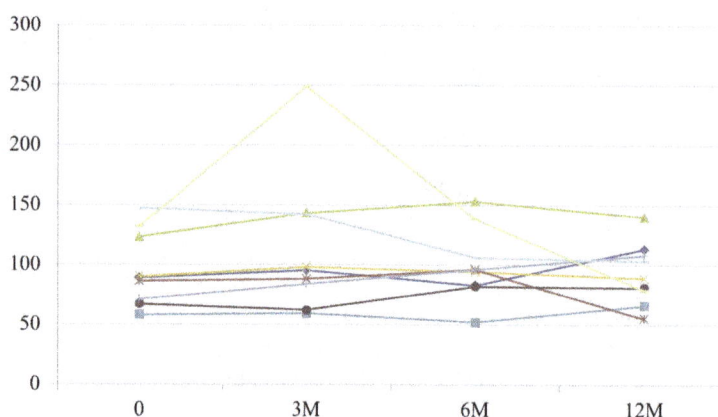

Figure 1. Changes in serum MDA-LDL levels (mg/dL) in patients with chronic renal failure.

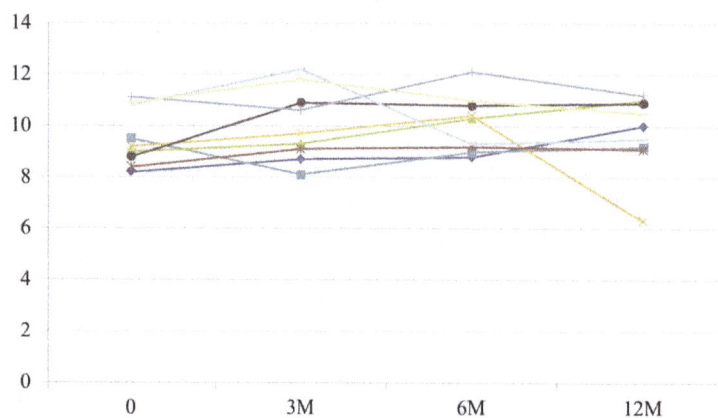

Figure 2. Changes in hemoglobin levels (g/dL) in patients with chronic renal failure.

Furthermore, no significant changes were observed in either systolic or diastolic blood pressure after the switch to DA (data not shown).

4. Discussion

In this study, we investigated serum MDA-LDL levels, Hb levels, and renal function in patients with conservative-stage renal failure who were switched from epoetin-α to DA treatment.

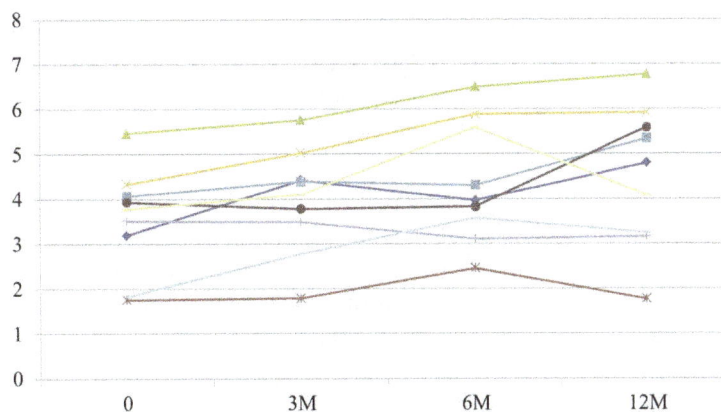

Figure 3. Changes in serum creatinine levels (mg/dL) in patients with chronic renal failure.

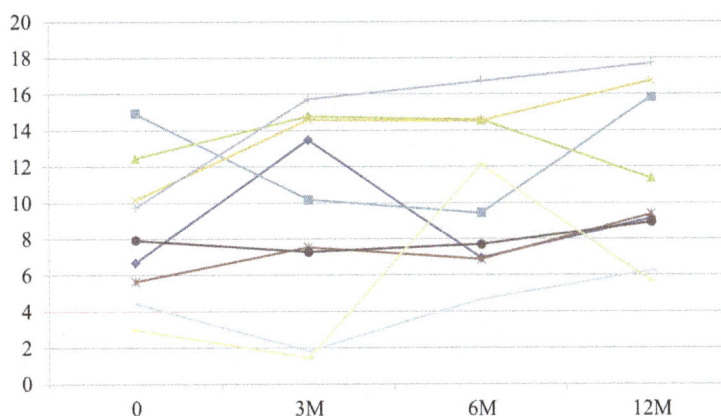

Figure 4. Changes in serum indoxyl sulfate levels (mg/mL) in patients with chronic renal failure.

During this study, when we investigated changes in the levels of MDA-LDL, an oxidative stress marker, no significant changes were observed after switching from epoetin-α to DA. MDA-LDL has recently received attention as a marker of oxidative stress and has also been suggested as being possibly related to cardiovascular events [8]. Although no obvious changes were observed in this study, serum Cr levels gradually increased. Practically, this increase may suppress the progressive oxidative stress associated with worsening renal failure.

Furthermore, Hb levels remained stable after the switch form epoetin-α to DA. After 12 months of administration, Hb level decreased in one patient, but the patient presented with abnormal vaginal bleeding due to a uterine tumor, which was thought to be the cause of the drop in Hb level. The subject received a transfusion, experienced no further problems, and was considered well-controlled.

In all cases, there was a tendency toward a gradual increase in serum Cr levels, and a significant difference was observed at 12 months after administration when compared with the level measured prior to administration. Some patients with advanced renal failure were included among the patients enrolled in this study, and thus, these subjects were believed to reflect the natural course of renal failure progression.

Moreover, there were no significant differences in the indoxyl sulfate levels. However, indoxyl sulfate is considered to promote renal failure and may act as an inhibitor of DA.

To date, few reports regarding DA and oxidative stress have been published; some of these reports have stated that oxidative stress is improved by DA administration [6], whereas other reports have stated that no significant changes are observed [7]; thus, no consensus has been reached yet. It is possible that these results were related to differences in the control groups and administration periods. In addition, *in vitro* reports have also been published, and according to Yang *et al.*, DA suppresses TNF-α-mediated production of endothelin-1 and acts to suppress atherosclerosis [9] in human aortic epithelial cells. These effects are stronger with DA than with epoetin-α. The underlying reason proposed by Yang *et al.* is that DA molecular structure contains more sialic acid than epoetin-α molecular structure. This theory, however, requires further investigations.

5. Conclusion

In this study, we investigated changes in MDA-LDL and indoxyl sulfate levels, anemia, and renal function in patients with conservative-stage renal failure who were switched from epoetin-α to DA. In our study, no increase in MDA-LDL or indoxyl sulfate levels was observed in response to the once-a-month administration of DA; therefore, DA could be used to control anemia. Thus, DA is believed to be a useful treatment for renal anemia in patients with conservative-stage renal failure.

References

[1]   Kuriyama, S., Tomonari, H., Yoshida, H., Hashimoto, T., Kawaguchi, Y. and Sakai, O. (1997) Reversal of Anemia by Erythropoietin Therapy Retards the Progression of Chronic Renal Failure, Especially in Nondiabetic Patients. *Nephron*, **77**, 176-185. http://dx.doi.org/10.1159/000190270

[2]   Hayashi, T., Suzuki, A., Shoji, T., Togawa, M., Okada, N., Tsubakihara, Y., Imai, E. and Hori, M. (2000) Cardiovascular Effect of Normalizing the Hematocrit Level during Erythropoietin Therapy in Predialysis Patients with Chronic Renal Failure. *American Journal of Kidney Diseases*, **35**, 250-256. http://dx.doi.org/10.1016/S0272-6386(00)70334-9

[3]   Kiss, Z., Elliott, S., Jedynasty, K., Tesar, V. and Szegedi, J. (2010) Discovery and Basic Pharmacology of Erythropoiesis-Stimulating Agents (ESAs), Including the Hyperglycosylated ESA, Darbepoetin Alfa: An Update of the Rationale and Clinical Impact. *European Journal of Clinical Pharmacology*, **66**, 331-340. http://dx.doi.org/10.1007/s00228-009-0780-y

[4]   Libetta, C., Sepe, V., Esposito, P., Galli, F. and Al Canton, D.A. (2011) Oxidative Stress and Inflammation: Implications in Uremia and Hemodialysis. *Clinical Biochemistry*, **44**, 1189-1198.

[5]   Sung, C.C., Hsu, Y.C., Chen, C.C., Lin, Y.F. and Wu, C.C. (2013) Oxidative Stress and Nucleic Acid Oxidation in Patients with Chronic Kidney Disease. *Oxidative Medicine and Cellular Longevity*, **2013**, Article ID: 301982.

[6]   Parissis, J.T., Kourea, K., Andreadou, I., Ikonomidis, I., Markantonis, S., Ioannidis, K., Paraskevaidis, I., Iliodromitis, E., Filippatos, G. and Kremastinos, D.T. (2009) Effects of *darbepoetin alfa* on Plasma Mediators of Oxidative and Nitrosative Stress in Anemic Patients with Chronic Heart Failure Secondary to Ischemic or Idiopathic Dilated Cardiomyopathy. *American Journal of Cardiology*, **103**, 1134-1138. http://dx.doi.org/10.1016/j.amjcard.2008.12.041

[7]   Malgorzewics, S., Lichodziejewska-Niemierko, M., Lizakowski, S., Liberek, T., Lysiak-Szydiowska, W. and Rutkowski, B. (2010) Oxidative Stress, Inflammation and Nutritional Status during Darbepoetin α-Treatment in Peritoneal Dialysis Patients. *Clinical Nephrology*, **73**, 210-215.

[8]   Lopes-Virella, W.F., Hunt, K.J., Baker, N.L., Virella, G., Moritz, T. and VADT Investigators (2012) The levels of MDA-LDL in circulating immune complexes predict myocardial infarction in the VADT study. *Atherosclerosis*, **224**, 526-531. http://dx.doi.org/10.1016/j.atherosclerosis.2012.08.006

[9]   Yang, W.S., Chang, J.W., Han, N.J. and Park, S.-K. (2011) Darbepoetinalfa Suppresses Tumor Necrosis Factor—An Induced Endothelin-1 Production through Antioxidant Action in Human Aortic Endothelial Cells: Role of Sialic Acid Residues. *Free Radical Biology & Medicine*, **50**, 1242-1251. http://dx.doi.org/10.1016/j.freeradbiomed.2011.02.005

3

Emphysematous Pyelonephritis in a Renal Transplant Patient

Kashif J. Piracha[1], Frank Darras[2], Edward P. Nord[1], Nand K. Wadhwa[1]

[1]Division of Nephrology, Department of Medicine, Stony Brook Medicine, Stony Brook, USA
[2]Transplantation Services, Stony Brook Medicine, Stony Brook, USA
Email: nand.wadhwa@stonybrookmedicine.edu

Abstract

Emphysematous pyelonephritis (EPN) is a necrotizing bacterial infection of the kidney that is caused by gas-forming organisms. We report a case of a 58-year-old man with a renal transplant who presented to the emergency room with nausea, vomiting and right lower quadrant abdominal pain. At the time of presentation, he was hemodynamically stable, and the abdominal examination was significant for tenderness over the allograft. Urinalysis was positive for large amounts of leukocyte esterase and white blood cells. He received empiric antibiotic coverage with piperacillin/tazobactam. Over the following 24 hours, the patient developed septic shock manifested by hemodynamic instability. A non-contrast CT scan of the abdomen and pelvis elucidated a heterogeneous gas containing collection in the allograft. Emergent transplant nephrectomy was performed. Postoperatively, the patient rapidly recovered and was subsequently discharged home to commence outpatient hemodialysis. A review of the literature suggests that early recognition of the severity of EPN as manifested by hemodynamic instability dictates emergent transplant nephrectomy as the treatment of choice.

Keywords

Emphysematous Pyelonephritis, Kidney Allograft, Transplant

1. Introduction

Emphysematous pyelonephritis (EPN) in the transplanted kidney is a rare, severe, often life-threatening condition that is characterized by acute necrotizing infection involving the renal parenchyma and surrounding tissues, caused by gas-forming organisms [1]. Risk factors include diabetes mellitus and urinary tract obstruction caused by calculi, tumors, and strictures [2]. Early recognition and prompt management is needed to obviate the high mortality associated with this diagnosis. We report a case of EPN in a renal transplant patient that was successfully treated with emergent nephrectomy. The indications for percutaneous drainage vs transplant nephrectomy are discussed.

2. Case Report

A 58-year-old man presented to the emergency room with a one week history of nausea, vomiting, decreased appetite, right lower quadrant abdominal pain and decreased urinary output. His past medical history was significant for end stage renal disease (ESRD) secondary to diabetic nephrosclerosis, and he was the recipient of a deceased donor renal allograft in July 2007. His serum creatinine had stabilized between 1.2 to 1.7 mg/dl (106.08 to 150.28 μmol/l). Immunosuppressive regimen comprised of tacrolimus 4 mg twice daily and mycophenolate-mofetil (MMF) 500 mg twice daily. In April 2010 serum creatinine increased to 2.7 mg/dl (238.68 μmol/l). Transplant kidney biopsy revealed acute T cell mediated rejection, acute tubular injury and transplant glomerulitis, and he received three doses of intravenous solumedrol. Serum creatinine remained stable at 2.6 mg/dl (229.84 μmol/l). However, in September 2010 serum creatinine increased to 3.16 mg/dl (279.34 μmol/l) and a second kidney biopsy was performed. On this occasion, histopathology showed interstitial fibrosis with no evidence of acute rejection. By December 2010, serum creatinine had risen to 5.6 mg/dl (495.04 μmol/l), and a third kidney biopsy was performed which revealed chronic allograft nephropathy. Following this biopsy, mycophenolic acid level was found to be <0.5 ug/ml so the dose of MMF was increased to 1000 mg twice daily. Tacrolimus dose had been maintained at 4 mg twice daily. The serum creatinine improved to 2.97 mg/dl (262.54 μmol/l) over a period of the next four months.

At the time of his current presentation, physical examination revealed a blood pressure of 139/69 mmHg, heart rate of 121 beats/min, temperature of 37.2°C, and oxygen saturation of 100% on room air. Abdominal examination revealed right lower quadrant tenderness over the renal allograft. The respiratory, cardiovascular and neurologic examinations were all unremarkable.

Laboratory data showed a white blood cell count of 7.5×10^3 cells/mm^3, hemoglobin 8.4 g/dl and platelet count of 49×10^3 cells/mm^3. The serum sodium was 126 mEq/l (126 mmol/l), potassium 5.4 mEq/l (5.4 mmol/l), chloride 102 mEq/l (102 mmol/l), and bicarbonate 13 mEq/l (13 mmol/l). Blood urea nitrogen was 121 mg/dl (43.19 mmol/l), serum creatinine was 7.8 mg/dl (689.52 μmol/l), and glucose 377 mg/dl (20.73 mmol/l). Urinalysis was positive for nitrite, large amounts of leukocyte esterase and >182 WBC/hpf. An ultrasound of the kidney allograft showed no evidence of hydronephrosis or perinephric fluid collection. The patient was started empirically on piperacillin/tazobactam 2.25 g intravenously every 6 hours for suspected acute pyelonephritis. He also received intravenous fluids with 0.45% NaCl with 75 meq/l (mmol/l) of sodium bicarbonate at 125 ml/hr.

Over the next 24 hours, he became febrile to 38.4°C, hypotensive with a blood pressure of 79/47 mmHg associated with acute respiratory distress. He was intubated and started on a norepinephrine drip. Physical examination was significant for marked tenderness over the transplanted kidney. Bowel sounds were intact. Repeat laboratory data revealed a white blood cell count of 13×10^3 cells/mm^3, hemoglobin 7.6 g/dl and platelet count dropped to 14×10^3 cells/mm^3. The serum sodium was 128 mEq/l (128 mmol/l), potassium 3.5 mEq/l (3.5 mmol/l), chloride 90 mEq/l (90 mmol/l) and bicarbonate 24 mEq/l (24 mmol/l). Blood urea nitrogen was 103 mg/dl (36.77 mmol/l), serum creatinine was 5.5 mg/dl (486.2 μmol/l), and glucose 254 mg/dl (13.97 mmol/l). Both urine and blood cultures grew Klebsiella pneumoniae. A noncontrast CT scan of the abdomen and pelvis revealed a heterogeneous gas containing collection in the surgical bed of the transplanted kidney, consistent with emphysematous pyelonephritis (**Figure 1(a)** and **Figure 1(b)**).

In the setting of persistent hypotension, emergent transplant nephrectomy was performed. Immunosuppression was discontinued. Postoperatively, blood pressure rapidly improved to 138/63 mm Hg and he was extubated. A tunneled subclavian catheter was placed and hemodialysis was initiated.

The gross pathological specimen revealed a friable, necrotic, gas filled kidney. The surface showed extensive hemorrhage with areas of yellow exudates (**Figure 2(a)**). Microscopic examination revealed acute severe pyelonephritis (**Figure 2(b)**). A two week course of antibiotics with piperacillin/tazobactam was completed. He was subsequently discharged home in stable condition and continued on outpatient maintenance hemodialysis.

3. Discussion

We report a case of emphysematous pyelonephritis (EPN) presenting with rapidly progressive multi-organ

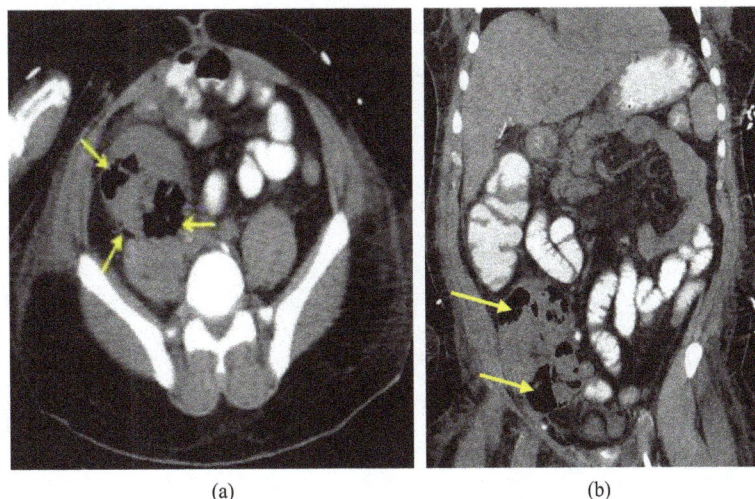

Figure 1. Axial (a), and sagittal (b) images of the abdomen and pelvis demonstrating an enlarged pelvic kidney with multiple bubbly and linear collections of gas within the renal parenchyma.

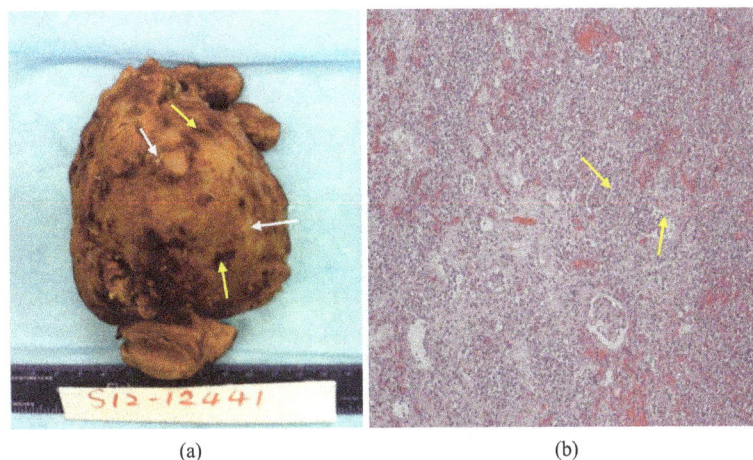

Figure 2. (a) Surface of the kidney shows areas of hemorrhage (yellow arrows) and exudates (white arrows); (b) Microscopy shows neutrophils within the tubular lumen which is an indication of acute pyelonephritis.

dysfunction and septic shock. The diagnosis of EPN was based primarily on the non-contrast CT scan of the abdomen (**Figure 1(a)** and **Figure 1(b)**) that showed a heterogeneous gas collection within the renal allograft. Emergent transplant nephrectomy was performed as a life-saving intervention. Post-operatively, the patient rapidly recovered and was subsequently discharged home on chronic maintenance hemodialysis.

Emphysematous pyelonephritis (EPN) is an acute necrotizing bacterial or fungal infection of the kidney associated with the presence of gas within the renal parenchyma, collecting system or perinephric tissue [1]. While EPN is well described in the native kidney, to the best of our knowledge, only 20 cases have been reported in the transplanted kidney. These data are summarized in **Table 1** and include our patient, making the total 21. In this population, mean age of presentation was 47 ± 15 years (range 12 - 76 years), and 14/21 patients (67%) were male. Of note, 19/21 patients (90%) were diabetic; of these 12/19 patients (63%) had diabetes mellitus prior to transplantation whereas 7/19 patients (37%) developed diabetes mellitus post transplantation. EPN developed as early as 4 days, and as late as 15 years after transplantation; in 6/21 patients (29%) EPN occurred in the first 3 months post transplantation. Deceased donor kidneys accounted for 13/21 (62%) of occurrences, while 5/21 (24%) occurred in living donor kidneys. The type of transplant was not stated in 3/21 patients (14%). The immunosuppressive regimen included prednisone 15/21 (71%), cyclosporine 10/21 (48%), azathioprine 6/21 (29%),

Table 1. Characteristics of renall allograft recipients with emphysematous pyelonephritis.

Case Reports, Year	Age	Gender	Septic Shock	Time after Transplant	Diabetes	Organisms	Treatment	Patient Outcome	Type of Transplant	Immunosuppression
Parameswaran et al. [9] 1977	53	F	Y	7 weeks	Y (post)	E. coli	Abx, TN	On HD	Deceased	Pred, Aza
Brenbridge et al. [10] 1979	33	M	N	2 weeks	Y (post)	E. coli	Abx, TN	On HD	Deceased	Pred, Aza
Balsara et al. [11] 1985	32	M	N	1.5 months	Y (post)	E. coli	Abx, PCD	Recovered	Deceased	Pred, Cyclo
Potter et al. [12] 1985	31	F	N	20 months	Y (pre)	E. coli	Abx, TN	On HD	Deceased	Did not mention
Potter et al. [12] 1985	39	M	Y	3 months	Y (pre)	E. coli	Abx, TN	Died	Deceased	Did not mention
O'Donnell et al. [13] 1986	27	M	N	5 years	Y (pre)	Enterobacter	Abx	Recovered	Living	Aza, Pred
Glen et al. [14]	66	F	N	not given	Y (pre)	E. coli	Abx, PCD	Recovered	Not given	Did not mention
Kalra et al. [15] 1993	35	M	Y	3 months	N	Klebsiella	Abx, TN	Died	Living	Cyclo, Pred
Akalin et al. [16] 1996	62	M	N	5 years	Y (pre)	Klebsiella	Abx	Recovered	Deceased	Pred, Aza, Cyclo
Cheng et al. [17] 2001	55	M	N	7 years	Y (post)	E. coli	Abx, PCD	Recovered	Deceased	Cyclo, Pred
Iqubal et al. [18] 2004	39	F	Y	2 years	Y (post)	E. coli	Abx, PCD	Recovered	Not given	Cyclo, Aza, Pred
Al-Makadma & Al-Akash [19] 2005	12	M	N	5 months	N	E. coli	Abx	Recovered	Living	Pred, MMF, Tacro
Fujita et al. [20] 2005	49	F	Y	15 months	Y (pre)	Salmonella	Abx, TN	On HD	Deceased	Cyclo, Pred
Arai et al. [21] 2006	61	M	Y	2 years	Y (pre)	E. coli	Abx, TN	Died	Not given	Pred, Cyclo, MMF
Baliga et al. [2] 2007	52	F	N	4 days	Y (pre)	E. coli	Abx	Recovered	Living	Cyclo, MMF, Pred
Chuang et al. [22] 2007	51	M	Y	15 years	Y (post)	E. coli	Abx, PCD	Recovered	Deceased	Pred, Tacro, MMF
Boltan et al. [23] 2008	76	M	N	10 years	Y (pre)	Klebsiella	Abx, TN	On HD	Deceased	Cyclo, MMF, Pred
Schmidt et al. [3] 2009	55	M	N	10 months	Y (pre)	E. coli	Abx, TN	On HD	Deceased	Did not mention
Al-Geizawi et al. [6] 2012	58	M	Y	15 months	Y (pre)	Klebsiella	Abx, PCD	Recovered	Deceased	Tacro, MMF
Alexander et al. [1] 2012	51	F	N	9.5 years	Y (post)	Klebsiella	Abx, PCD	Recovered	Living	Cyclo, Aza, Pred
Piracha et al. (current report) 2014	58	M	Y	5 years	Y (pre)	Klebsiella	Abx, TN	On HD	Deceased	MMF, Tacro

Key: Abx = antibiotics; TN = transplant nephrectomy; PCD = percutaneous catheter drainage; Pred = prednisone; Aza = azathioprine; Cyclo = cyclosporine; MMF = mycophenolatemofetil; Tacro = tacrolimus.

mycophenolate mofetil 7/21 (33%), and tacrolimus 3/21 (14%) in various combinations.

Fever, abdominal pain and dysuria were the presenting symptoms in 15/21 patients (71%), and 2/21 patients (10%) were asymptomatic with worsening renal function. Importantly, 9/21 patients (43%) developed multi-organ system dysfunction and septic shock during the hospitalization (**Table 1**). Escherichia coli and Klebsiella pneumoniae were reported in 13/21 (62%) and 6/21 (29%) patients respectively.

With regard the high incidence of EPN in diabetic patients, it has been suggested that the increased tissue and urine glucose levels may provide a favorable microenvironment for gas-forming bacteria [3].

A number of attempts have been made to classify EPN according to severity of clinical presentation, which in turn would guide therapy. In essence all of these classifications are reliant on CT scan results which depict the extent of gas formation [4] [5], and the early response to conservative therapy. Only one such classification exists which addresses EPN in renal allografts [6]. It should also be recognized that this approach was published in 2010, while much of the data summarized in **Table 1** pre-dates this classification. Interestingly, 18/21 patients (86%) had gas present in the renal parenchyma and collecting system whereas 3/21 patients (14%) had gas only in the renal collecting system.

Once recognized, EPN should be treated with aggressive medical management, primarily parenteral antibiotics, and aggressive optimization of hemodynamic status. Since gram negative bacilli account for the overwhelming number of infections (**Table 1**), initial empiric antibiotic coverage should take this observation into account. If hemodynamic stability can be attained, percutaneous catheter drainage of the renal pelvis should be undertaken [1] [7]. However, in the setting of multi-organ failure and uncontrolled sepsis, early transplant nephrectomy should be the approach of choice [3] [8]. As summarized in **Table 1**, 4/21 patients (19%) recovered with antibiotic therapy only, 7/21 patients (33%) underwent percutaneous catheter drainage and made a complete recovery, and 10/21 patients (48%) underwent transplant nephrectomy. Of the latter group, 3/21 of these patients died (mortality rate 14%).

4. Conclusion

In aggregate, EPN carries a high mortality in the diabetic, immunosuppressed renal transplant recipient. We submit that in such individuals who present with graft tenderness, a high index of suspicion is needed to diagnose this entity. For patients with stage 3 EPN [6], timely and judicious transplant nephrectomy may be a lifesaving modality.

References

[1] Alexander, S., *et al.* (2012) Extensive Emphysematous Pyelonephritis in a Renal Allograft Treated Conservatively: Case Report and Review of the Literature. *Transplant Infectious Disease*, **14**, E150-E155. http://dx.doi.org/10.1111/tid.12016

[2] Baliga, K.V., *et al.* (2007) Successful Medical Treatment of Emphysematous Pyelonephritis in a Renal Allograft Recipient. *Renal Failure*, **29**, 755-758. http://dx.doi.org/10.1080/08860220701460434

[3] Schmidt, S., *et al.* (2009) Emphysematous Pyelonephritis in a Kidney Allograft. *American Journal of Kidney Diseases*, **53**, 895-897. http://dx.doi.org/10.1053/j.ajkd.2008.12.032

[4] Huang, J.J. and C.C. Tseng (2000) Emphysematous Pyelonephritis: Clinicoradiological Classification, Management, Prognosis, and Pathogenesis. *Archives of Internal Medicine*, **160**, 797-805. http://dx.doi.org/10.1001/archinte.160.6.797

[5] Wan, Y.L., *et al.* (1996) Acute Gas-Producing Bacterial Renal Infection: Correlation between Imaging Findings and Clinical Outcome. *Radiology*, **198**, 433-438.

[6] Al-Geizawi, S.M., *et al.* (2010) Renal Allograft Failure Due to Emphysematous Pyelonephritis: Successful Non-Operative Management and Proposed New Classification Scheme Based on Literature Review. *Transplant Infectious Disease*, **12**, 543-550. http://dx.doi.org/10.1111/j.1399-3062.2010.00538.x

[7] Vivek, V., Panda, A. and Devasia, A. (2012) Emphysematous Pyelonephritis in a Renal Transplant Recipient—Is It Possible to Salvage the Graft? *Annals of Transplantation*, **17**, 138-141. http://dx.doi.org/10.12659/AOT.883469

[8] Baas, M.C., van Donselaar, K.A., van der Pant and Bemelman, F.J. (2009) Emphysematous Pyelonephritis in a Renal Transplant Patient. *The Netherlands Journal of Medicine*, **67**, 403-404.

[9] Parameswaran, R. and Feest, T. (1977) Gas Nephrogram: An Unusual Complication of Renal Transplantation. *British Journal of Radiology*, **50**, 438-440. http://dx.doi.org/10.1259/0007-1285-50-594-438

[10] Brenbridge, A.N., *et al.* (1979) Renal Emphysema of the Tranplanted Kidney: Sonographic Appearance. (*AJR*) *American Journal of Roentgenology*, **132**, 656-658. http://dx.doi.org/10.2214/ajr.132.4.656

[11] Balsara, V.J., Raval, B. and Maklad, N.F. (1985) Emphysematous Pyelonephritis in a Renal Transplant: Sonographic and Computed Tomographic Features. *Journal of Ultrasound in Medicine*, **4**, 97-99.

[12] Potter, J.L., *et al.* (1985) Emphysema in the Renal Allograft. *Radiology*, **155**, 51-52.

[13] O'Donnell, D., Rumbak, M. and Anderson, J. (1986) Emphysematous Pyelonephritis in a Transplanted Kidney. *Clinical Nephrology*, **25**, 52-53.

[14] Glen, D., Bayliss, A.P. and Robertson, E.M. (1989) Percutaneous Drainage in Emphysematous Pyelonephritis. *Clinical Radiology*, **40**, 434. http://dx.doi.org/10.1016/S0009-9260(89)80155-2

[15] Kalra, O.P., *et al.* (1993) Emphysematous Pyelonephritis and Cystitis in a Renal Transplant Recipient—Computed Tomographic Appearance. *The International Journal of Artificial Organs*, **16**, 41-44.

[16] Akalin, E., *et al.* (1996) Emphysematous Cystitis and Pyelitis in a Diabetic Renal Transplant Recipient. *Transplantation*, **62**, 1024-1026. http://dx.doi.org/10.1097/00007890-199610150-00023

[17] Cheng, Y.T., Wang, H.P. and Hsieh, H.H. (2001) Emphysematous Pyelonephritis in a Renal Allograft: Successful Treatment with Percutaneous Drainage and Nephrostomy. *Clinical Transplant*, **15**, 364-367. http://dx.doi.org/10.1034/j.1399-0012.2001.150511.x

[18] Iqubal, M., *et al.* (2004) Abdominal Gas Is Not Always Bowel Associated: Lessons from an Allograft Recipient. *Nephrology Dialysis Transplantation*, **19**, 503-504. http://dx.doi.org/10.1093/ndt/gfg465

[19] Al-Makadma, A.S. and Al-Akash, S.I. (2005) An Unusual Case of Pyelonephritis in a Pediatric Renal Transplant Recipient. *Pediatric Transplantation*, **9**, 258-260. http://dx.doi.org/10.1111/j.1399-3046.2004.00276.x

[20] Fujita, S., *et al.* (2005) Case of Emphysematous Pyelonephritis in a Renal Allograft. *Clinical Transplant*, **19**, 559-562. http://dx.doi.org/10.1111/j.1399-0012.2005.00264.x

[21] Arai, S., *et al.* (2006) A Case of Emphysematous Pyelonephritis in a Renal Allograft. *Transplantation*, **81**, 296-297. http://dx.doi.org/10.1097/01.tp.0000191623.83885.ee

[22] Chuang, Y.W., *et al.* (2007) Severe Emphysematous Pyelonephritis in a Renal Allograft: Successful Treatment with Percutaneous Drainage and Antibiotics. *Clinical Nephrology*, **68**, 42-46. http://dx.doi.org/10.5414/CNP68042

[23] Boltan, L.E., Randall, H. and Barri, Y.M. (2008) Iatrogenic Emphysematous Pyelonephritis in a Renal Transplant Patient. *Transplant Infectious Disease*, **10**, 409-412. http://dx.doi.org/10.1111/j.1399-3062.2008.00319.x

4

Effect of On-Line Hemodiafiltration on Dry Weight Adjustment in Intradialytic Hypotension-Prone Patients: Comparative Study of Conventional Hemodialysis and On-Line Hemodiafiltration

Sun Woo Kang[*]

Department of Nephrology, College of Medicine, Inje University, Busan, Korea
Email: *kswnephrology@hotmail.com

Abstract

Introduction: Correct adjustment of dry weight after hemodialysis (HD) with no signs of hypervolemia is important. Intradialytic hypotension (IDH) is the most common complication during HD. IDH occurs in 15% to 30% and possibly in up to 50% of dialysis sessions. IDH augments mortality essentially due to chronic overhydration and the inability to reach the proper dry weight. On-line hemodiafiltration (ol-HDF) has been reported to reduce the frequency of IDH. The aim of this study was to assess the effect of ol-HDF on hemodynamic stability and dry weight adjustment compared with low-flux HD. **Methods:** IDH-prone HD patients at our center were enrolled. This study was designed as a crossover trial with two phases (A arm: low-flux HD for 8 weeks followed by ol-HDF for 8 weeks *vs.* B arm: ol-HDF for 8 weeks followed by low-flux HD for 8 weeks) and two treatment arms (ol-HDF *vs.* low-flux HD), each phase lasting 8 weeks. We measured the proportion of body water using a body composition monitor (BCM). **Results:** In a comparison of the systolic blood pressure (SBP) and diastolic blood pressure (DBP) reductions from the baseline blood pressure between the HD and ol-HDF groups, statistically significant differences were observed only in the SBP of the B arm (SBP: HD *vs.* HDF, -9.83 ± 6.64 *vs.* -4.62 ± 1.61 mmHg, p = 0.036; DBP: HD *vs.* HDF, -3.29 ± 4.05 *vs.* -1.86 ± 1.49 mmHg, p = 0.261). Neither the mean of the interdialytic body weight gains nor the frequency of IDH was different between the A and B arms (p = 0.817 and p = 0.562, respectively). In terms of dialysis modality, there were no significant differences in the amount of overhydration between the conventional HD and ol-HDF groups during the two study phases, as measured by the BCM (A arm: p = 0.875, B arm: p = 0.655). **Conclusion:** Our study did not show a better benefit of ol-HDF to reach the dry weight compared with low-flux HD in IDH-

---

*Corresponding author.

prone patients.

Keywords

On-Line Hemodiafiltration; Hemodialysis; Intradialytic Hypotension; Body Composition Monitor; Dry Body Weight

1. Introduction

For hemodialysis (HD) patients, both hypervolemia and hypovolemia are associated with adverse outcomes and increased mortality. Several studies have shown that strict adjustment of dry weight after HD is associated with better outcomes and survival [1] [2], but others have shown increased morbidity and hospitalization [3] [4]. Hypervolemia may lead to pulmonary edema, uncontrolled hypertension, left ventricular hypertrophy, congestive heart failure, and even mortality. The recurrence of intradialytic hypotension (IDH) is the most common acute complication during conventional HD treatment and is a leading problem, especially in the elderly and patients with a compromised cardiovascular status. Because IDH may lead to chronic overhydration (OH) and fluctuations in volume status, IDH in HD patients is known to be associated with increased mortality [1] [2]. For physicians attempting to achieve a lean body weight in HD patients, IDH often impedes strict control.

Hemodiafiltration was first introduced in 1975, and it combined diffusion and convection to provide a wide range of solute removal according to the molecular weights of the solutes. Many observational studies have shown benefits of hemodiafiltration in terms of survival and other clinical parameters [5]-[8]. Other than efficacy, on-line hemodiafiltration (ol-HDF) has a beneficial effect on cardiovascular stability, reducing the frequency of IDH [9].

For proper control of the volume status of HD patients without IDH or hypervolemia events, assessment of the actual body fluid composition is thought to be essential. There are several noninvasive methods with which to assess the volume status. One such method is the recently introduced body composition monitor (BCM). Measurement using the BCM is a noninvasive, simple, and highly reproducible method for assessing excess body fluid.

The aim of our study was to establish the usefulness of ol-HDF for subtle adjustment of dry weight, which was conducted by using BCM measurement to estimate the exact volume status of IDH-prone patients.

2. Methods

2.1. Patients

We conducted a prospective, two-period, two-treatment, randomized, crossover trial at one outpatient HD center between April 2011 and December 2011. All patients signed written informed consent prior to randomization, and the study protocol was approved by the Institutional Review Board For Human Research of Inje University Busan Paik Hospital.

All patients on HD older than 20 years were screened for eligibility for the study. IDH was defined as a reduction in systolic blood pressure (SBP) by >20 mmHg or an SBP of <90 mmHg during dialysis treatment. Patients who experienced more than three episodes of IDH per month during the previous 3 months were considered IDH-prone patients and were eligible for registration. Exclusion criteria were cardiac or liver failure, active bleeding, peripheral vessel disease, deep venous thrombosis, a poorly functioning fistula, or a life expectancy <6 months due to non-renal disease. All patients were randomly assigned to either the A or B arm (**Figure 1**). Patients in the A arm underwent low-flux HD for 8 weeks followed by ol-HDF for 8 weeks, and patients in the B arm underwent ol-HDF for 8 weeks followed by low-flux HD for 8 weeks. There were no changes in dialysis prescriptions (flow rates, dialysate temperatures, dialysate composition, or anticoagulation) or patient position during the study period. The presence of associations between IDH and adverse symptoms during HD was determined by the investigator.

2.2. Baseline Data Collection

Age, gender, height, type of vascular access, type of dialysis, dialysis duration, and frequency of dialysis data

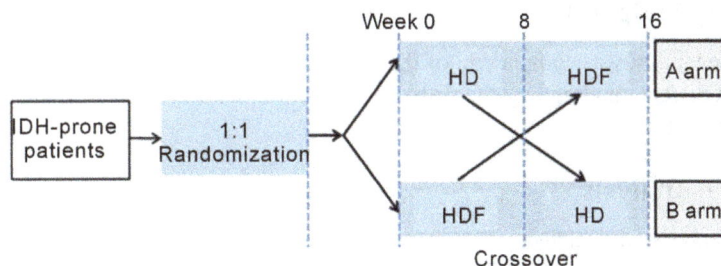

Figure 1. Crossover study design.

for each patient were recorded. For each dialysis session, the following patient data were collected: intradialytic symptoms (cramps, nausea, dizziness, headache, sweating, vomiting, etc.), IDH events, intradialytic weight loss, ultrafiltration volume, and postdialysis individual Kt/V. Blood pressure and heart rate during dialysis were measured every 30 min. Clinical parameters for volume overload such as dyspnea, pulmonary edema, and peripheral edema before dialysis were also observed. Predialysis and postdialysis body weights were recorded at each visit. Chest X-ray and biochemical parameters comprising serum BUN, creatinine, albumin, electrolytes, β2-microglobulin, and NT-proBNP level were measured at baseline.

2.3. Low-Flux HD and ol-HDF

The dialysis console used was the Fresenius 5008S (Fresenius Medical Care, Bad Homburg, Germany). The filters used were high-flux HF80S for HDF and low-flux F6HPS for HD (Fresenius Medical Care). The treatment modality was blinded to the patients by use of filter types unknown to the patients and not ordinarily used in the department. The tubing was mounted as in HDF in all sessions, and the indicators showing the treatment modality on the console were covered. All sessions in the study were 4 h in duration. The dialysate and infusate (substitution fluid) had an identical composition (mmol/L): sodium concentration close to patients' usual serum sodium concentration at the start of dialysis (138 ± 2); potassium, 2; chloride, 106; bicarbonate, 36; acetate, 3; magnesium, 0.5; glucose, 6; and calcium ion, 1.25. The ultrafiltration rate and sodium concentration were fixed during each session. The infusate was prepared online by the dialysis machine. The patients were instructed to achieve a predialysis weight close to 3% more than their usual end-of-dialysis weight (EDW) by fluid intake adjustments. The EDW was defined as the lowest weight a patient could tolerate without the development of hypotension or such suggestive symptoms as dizziness, faintness, nausea, or cramps. The ultrafiltration volume per study session was adjusted to reach the defined EDW. The effective dialyzer blood flow was individually adjusted to [1.3 × EDW (kg)] × (1000/270 mL/min) in all sessions with a maximum of 300 mL/min. The final substitution fluid volume was (mean ± SD) 1.20 ± 0.1 L/kg body weight/session (total volume, 67 ± 7 L/session). The infusate flow rate in the HDF sessions was equal to the dialyser blood flow rate. The dialysate flow was set to 500 mL/min on the console. The patients were not allowed to eat, drink, or sleep during the study sessions. All medications were continued and administered as usual throughout the study.

2.4. BCM Measurement

The body composition and fluid status were measured 30 min after dialysis using a portable whole-body multi-frequency BIA device (Body Composition Monitor – BCM®; Fresenius Medical Care). The BCM measures the impedance spectroscopy at 50 frequencies. Every mid-week day (Wednesday for a Monday-Wednesday-Friday schedule and Thursday for a Tuesday-Thursday-Saturday schedule), BCM measurement was performed 30 min after dialysis was finished. Based on the measurement of body resistance and reactance to an electrical current using the BCM monitor, the extracellular, intracellular, and total body water were determined using the approach described by Moissl *et al.* [10].

2.5. Primary Endpoint

The primary endpoint of this study was comparison of the OH status after dialysis between patients undergoing ol-HDF and low-flux HD. OH in liters was estimated with the BCM; OH of ≥1.1 L after dialysis was considered overhydrated, and OH of <−1.1 L was considered dehydrated [11] [12].

2.6. Secondary Endpoint

The secondary endpoint was comparison of the mean systolic blood pressure (SBP) and diastolic blood pressure (DBP) between patients undergoing the different dialysis modalities and other parameters representing fluctuations in fluid volume during the dialysis session.

2.7. Statistical Analysis

A descriptive analysis was carried out for variables identified for baseline characteristics. The statistical analysis for comparison of parameters within the low-flux HD or ol-HDF session in each arm was performed using the Wilcoxon signed-rank test. Comparison of parameters within the A and B arms was performed using the Mann–Whitney U test. All variables are reported as means ± standard deviation (SD). All analyses were performed on an intention-to-treat basis, and a p value of <0.05 was considered to indicate statistical significance. All statistical analyses were performed using the SPSS software (version 15.0.0; SPSS Inc., Chicago, IL, USA).

3. Results

A total of 20 patients were enrolled, and 19 patients completed the study. **Table 1** summarizes the baseline characteristics of the patient groups, and there were no statistically significant differences. Of the 20 patients who enrolled the study, 12 were allocated to the A arm and 8 were allocated to the B arm. A female patient of A arm did not complete the study because she died of a sudden cardiac death. The mean age of the study group was 54.47 ± 16.03 years. The patients comprised 4 (20%) male and 16 (80%) female patients. The mean baseline BMI was 23.82 ± 4.00 kg/m^2, and the mean OH was 0.117 ± 1.32 L.

3.1. Systolic and Diastolic Blood Pressure

The mean difference in blood pressure during dialysis was calculated for each patient. The degrees of reduction in the SBP and DBP during dialysis from baseline blood pressure were not different between the A and B arms (SBP: A vs. B arm, -8.85 ± 9.22 vs. -4.64 ± 4.13 mmHg, p = 0.757; DBP: A vs. B arm, -7.22 ± 3.64 vs. -2.57 ± 2.47 mmHg, p = 0.316). In a comparison of the SBP and DBP reductions from baseline blood pressure between the HD and ol-HDF groups, statistically significant differences were observed only in the SBP of the B arm (SBP: HD vs. HDF, -9.83 ± 6.64 vs. -4.62 ± 1.61 mmHg, p = 0.036; DBP: HD vs. HDF, -3.29 ± 4.05 vs. -1.86 ± 1.49 mmHg, p = 0.261) and not in the A arm (SBP: HD vs. HDF, -10.32 ± 11.2 vs. -7.37 ± 8.79 mmHg, p = 0.347; DBP: HD vs. HDF, -5.54 ± 5.21 vs. -3.74 ± 3.92 mmHg, p = 0.155).

3.2. Interdialytic Body Weight Gains and Ultrafiltration Volumes

Comparison of interdialytic body weight gains (HD vs. ol-HDF, 2.52 ± 0.6 vs. 2.57 ± 0.7 kg, p = 0.754 in the A arm; HD vs. ol-HDF, 2.53 ± 0.6 vs. 2.54 ± 0.5 kg, p = 0.889 in the B arm) (**Table 2**) and ultrafiltration volumes (HD vs. ol-HDF, 2.85 ± 0.6 vs. 2.93 ± 0.6 kg, p = 0.530 in the A arm; HD vs. ol-HDF, 2.92 ± 0.6 vs. 3.05 ± 0.6 kg, p = 0.263 in the B arm) (**Table 2**) between the low-flux HD and ol-HDF groups revealed no statistically significant differences. There was no significant difference between the study arms in intradialytic BW gain (A vs. B arm, 2.55 ± 0.6 vs. 2.54 ± 0.6 kg) or ultrafiltration volume (A vs. B arm, 2.90 ± 0.6 vs. 2.99 ± 0.6 kg, p = 0.877) (**Table 3**).

3.3. Frequency of IDH

The difference in the mean frequency of IDH between dialysis modalities in the A and B arms was also not statistically significant (A vs. B arm, 83.3 ± 30.7 vs. 71.5 ± 18.2 events among all sessions, p = 0.562) (**Table 3**). The same was true in the comparison of dialysis modalities in each group (HD vs. ol-HDF, 44.6 ± 17.0 vs. 38.6 ± 17.4 events among all sessions, p = 0.272 in the A arm; 42.8 ± 16.7 vs. 28.6 ± 7.9 events among all sessions, p = 0.093 in the B arm) (**Table 2**).

3.4. OH Status

Patients were considered normohydrated if OH was between -1.1 and 1.1 L. If the absolute OH value increased,

Table 1. Baseline characteristics.

	A arm (*n* = 12)	B arm (*n* = 8)	p-value
Age (years)	61.1 ± 12.6	48.1 ± 16.5	0.640
Sex (male, %)	8.3	25.0	0.537
Underlying disease (%)			
Diabetes	60	40	1.000
Hypertension	75	87.5	0.619
Heart disease	41.7	50.0	1.000
Systolic BP (mmHg)	125.0 ± 13.8	128.7 ± 29.9	0.50
Mean BP (mmHg)	66.6 ± 9.8	78.7 ± 16.4	0.62
Dialysis vintage (years)	6.5 ± 3.5	8.1 ± 8.8	0.532
Dry body weight (kg)	54.7 ± 10.8	57.6 ± 12.4	0.511
Laboratory test			
Hemoglobin (g/dl)	10.8 ± 0.9	10.6 ± 0.8	1.000
Hematocrit (%)	33.1 ± 3.2	32.0 ± 2.4	0.671
Serum protein (g/dl)	6.7 ± 1.0	6.9 ± 0.4	0.587
Serum albumin (g/dl)	4.1 ± 0.7	3.9 ± 0.2	0.560
Blood urea nitrogen (mg/dl)	72.8 ± 15.1	57.7 ± 12.3	0.032
Serum creatinine (mg/dl)	10.2 ± 1.31	9.9 ± 1.9	0.440
Dialysis dose (Kt/V)	1.6 ± 0.2	1.5 ± 0.2	0.280
Urea reduction rate (URR)	74.6 ± 4.3	72.5 ± 5.2	0.247

Table 2. Comparison of HD and on-line HDF in each arm with respect to volume status parameters.

		HD	On-line HDF	p-value
Interdialytic body weight gain (kg)	A arm	2.52 ± 0.6	2.57 ± 0.7	0.754
Interdialytic body weight gain (kg)	B arm	2.53 ± 0.6	2.54 ± 0.5	0.889
UF for each dialysis session (L)	A arm	2.85 ± 0.6	2.93 ± 0.6	0.53
UF for each dialysis session (L)	B arm	2.92 ± 0.6	3.05 ± 0.6	0.263
Frequency of IDH[†]	A arm	44.6 ± 17.0	38.6 ± 17.4	0.272
Frequency of IDH[†]	B arm	42.8 ± 16.7	28.6 ± 7.9	0.093
Absolute value of OH (L)	A arm	0.9 ± 0.5	0.9 ± 0.6	0.875
Absolute value of OH (L)	B arm	1.4 ± 1.5	1.3 ± 1.4	0.655
Frequency of hyper/hypovolemia[‡]	A arm	2.3 ± 2.9	3.0 ± 3.2	0.107
Frequency of hyper/hypovolemia[‡]	B arm	3.0 ± 3.6	4.0 ± 3.1	0.197

[†]Mean frequency of IDH during all sessions; [‡]Mean frequency of hyper/hypovolemia during all sessions.

Table 3. Comparison of the A and B arms in terms of volume status parameters.

	A arm	B arm	p-value
Interdialytic body weight gain (kg)	2.55 ± 0.6	2.54 ± 0.6	0.817
UF for each dialysis session (L)	2.90 ± 0.6	2.99 ± 0.6	0.877
Frequency of IDH[†]	83.3 ± 30.7	71.5 ± 18.2	0.562
Absolute value of OH (L)	0.9 ± 0.5	1.4 ± 1.5	0.847
Frequency of hyper/hypovolemia[‡]	5.3 ± 6.0	7.0 ± 6.5	0.509

[†]Mean frequency of IDH during all sessions; [‡]Mean frequency of hyper/hypovolemia during all sessions.

the patients became further diverted from a normovolemic status. Thus, we decided to estimate the effect of each dialysis modality on volume control using the absolute OH value. The frequency of failure to achieve a normovolemic status, shown here as the frequency of hyper/hypovolemia, was also estimated. There was no difference in the absolute OH value assessed by BCM measurement after dialysis or the frequency of hyper/hypovolemia between study arms (absolute value of OH: A *vs.* B arm, 0.9 ± 0.5 *vs.* 1.4 ± 1.5 L, p = 0.847; frequency of hyper/hypovolemia: A *vs.* B arm, 5.3 ± 6.0 *vs.* 7.0 ± 6.5, p = 0.509) (**Table 3**) or between the low-flux HD and ol-HDF group in each arm (absolute value of OH: HD *vs.* ol-HDF, 0.9 ± 0.5 *vs.* 0.9 ± 0.6 L, p = 0.875 in the A arm; 1.4 ± 1.5 *vs.* 1.3 ± 1.4 L, p = 0.655 in the B arm; frequency of hyper/hypovolemia: HD *vs.* ol-HDF, 2.3 ± 2.9 *vs.* 3.0 ± 3.2, p = 0.107 in the A arm; 3.0 ± 3.6 *vs.* 4.0 ± 3.1, p = 0.197 in the B arm) (**Table 2**).

4. Discussion

Among the various causes of IDH, including rapid reductions in blood volume, lack of vasoconstriction, and certain cardiovascular factors, the most common is thought to be the larger amount of fluid removal compared with the total body fluid volume.

Recent trials have shown the value of BCM measurement on fluid control in dialysis patients [1] [13] [14]. The BCM provides an objective assessment of normohydration that is clinically applicable. Guiding patients toward this target of normohydration by the BCM leads to better control of dry weight in overhydrated patients and less intradialytic adverse events in HD patients.

This was a prospective randomized study, and the primary reason for designing this study was to clarify whether ol-HDF is superior to low-flux HD in reaching an accurate dry body weight as measured by the BCM. The crossover design excluded the halo effect, which may be caused by the dialysis modality sequence. For example, there is a possibility that the results would be better with the ABAB sequence than with the BABA sequence. A certain carryover effect may exist, which means that the benefits in terms of IDH prevention are prolonged in period A even beyond the end of the preceding period B. This phenomenon also occurs with dialysis techniques that differ from traditional HD, such as hemodiafiltration, which maintains a certain degree of protection with regard to hypotensive phenomena when prolonged for a certain period of time [15]. Therefore, we originally considered the crossover design. To eliminate possible confounding factors, the dialysis dose and ultrafiltration volume were matched. We decided to employ predilution-HDF and not hemofiltration alone to ensure matching of the dialysis dose. At the same time, we utilized a dose of hemofiltration during the intervention session (1.20 L/kg/session) that would have been sufficient if used as predilution hemofiltration monotherapy. Interactions between the blood components and the filter material may theoretically interfere with the hemodynamic parameters. To minimize this effect, polysulfone filter material originating from the same manufacturer was used in both treatment modalities. The predilution mode is also reportedly advantageous based on the results of a prospective multicenter randomized study performed by Locatelli *et al.* [9], which showed a lower frequency of IDH in the predilution HF and predilution HDF groups than in the low-flux HD group.

Our study did not demonstrate a superior effect of ol-HDF over low-flux HD in controlling the volume status of IDH-prone patients in terms of the absolute OH value. It did, however, elucidate the degree of deviation from normovolemia and the frequency of failure to achieve normovolemia. This could be explained by the poor difference in the frequency of IDH and interdialytic body weight gains between the low-flux HD and ol-HDF groups. None of the parameters concerning the volume status of each group of patients was significantly different. Individuals at high risk for IDH should be kept within a safe range of the dialysis ultrafiltration rate (interdialytic weight gains of ≤3% of EDW). As a matter of fact, the mean interdialytic weight gains of our patients exceeded >4.5% of EDW. Despite advances in the understanding of the pathogenesis of IDH and technologic improvements in reducing the frequency of IDH, other factors influencing excessive intradialytic weight gains cannot always be overcome. As such, additional attention is required to improve patient compliance with dietary sodium restriction. Thus, the focus on these negative results was that our IDH-prone patients were intolerable to sodium and fluid restriction in spite of the strict diet education. We first intended to recruit 30 or more patients into the study, but only 20 patients were included. This small number of enrolled patients could be another limitation of our study.

5. Conclusion

We hypothesized that because of the superior hemodynamic stability of ol-HDF over low-flux HD, ol-HDF allows for easier control of the dry body weight of IDH-prone dialysis patients. However, our study did not show a better benefit of ol-HDF to reach the dry weight compared with low-flux HD in IDH-prone patients. A large-scale study would be necessary to prove its benefit in managing the volume status of IDH-prone dialysis patients.

Acknowledgements

This work was supported by a grant from the Inje University in 2010.

Declaration of Interest

The authors report no conflict of interest. The authors alone are responsible for the content and writing of the paper.

References

[1] Chamney, P.W., Krämer, M., Rode, C., Kleinekofort, W. and Wizemann, V. (2002) A New Technique for Establishing Dry Weight in Hemodialysis Patients via Whole Body Bioimpedance. *Kidney International*, **61**, 2250-2258. http://dx.doi.org/10.1046/j.1523-1755.2002.00377.x

[2] Ozkahya, M., Ok, E., Toz, H., *et al.* (2006) Long-Term Survival Rates in Haemodialysis Patients Treated with Strict Volume Control. *Nephrology Dialysis Transplantation*, **21**, 3506-3513. http://dx.doi.org/10.1093/ndt/gfl487

[3] Reddan, D.N., Szczech, L.A., Hasselblad, V., *et al.* (2005) Intradialytic Blood Volume Monitoring in Ambulatory Hemodialysis Patients: A Randomized Trial. *Journal of the American Society of Nephrology*, **16**, 2162-2169. http://dx.doi.org/10.1681/ASN.2004121053

[4] Agarwal, R., Alborzi, P., Satyan, S. and Light, R.P. (2009) Dry-Weight Reduction in Hypertensive Hemodialysis Patients (DRIP) A Randomized, Controlled Trial. *Hypertension*, **53**, 500-507. http://dx.doi.org/10.1161/HYPERTENSIONAHA.108.125674

[5] Jirka, T., Cesare, S., Di Benedetto, A., *et al.* (2006) Mortality Risk for Patients Receiving Hemodiafiltration versus Hemodialysis. *Kidney International*, **70**, 1524-1524. http://dx.doi.org/10.1038/sj.ki.5001759

[6] Canaud, B., Bragg-Gresham, J., Marshall, M., *et al.* (2006) Mortality Risk for Patients Receiving Hemodiafiltration versus Hemodialysis: European Results from the DOPPS. *Kidney International*, **69**, 2087-2093. http://dx.doi.org/10.1038/sj.ki.5000447

[7] Panichi, V., Rizza, G.M., Paoletti, S., *et al.* (2008) Chronic Inflammation and Mortality in Haemodialysis: Effect of Different Renal Replacement Therapies. Results from the RISCAVID Study. *Nephrology Dialysis Transplantation*, **23**, 2337-2343. http://dx.doi.org/10.1093/ndt/gfm951

[8] Vilar, E., Fry, A.C., Wellsted, D., Tattersall, J.E., Greenwood, R.N. and Farrington, K. (2009) Long-Term Outcomes in Online Hemodiafiltration and High-Flux Hemodialysis: A Comparative Analysis. *Clinical Journal of the American Society of Nephrology*, **4**, 1944-1953. http://dx.doi.org/10.2215/CJN.05560809

[9] Locatelli, F., Altieri, P., Andrulli, S., *et al.* (2010) Hemofiltration and Hemodiafiltration Reduce Intradialytic Hypotension in ESRD. *Journal of the American Society of Nephrology*, **21**, 1798-1807. http://dx.doi.org/10.1681/ASN.2010030280

[10] Moissl, U.M., Wabel, P., Chamney, P.W., *et al.* (2006) Body Fluid Volume Determination via Body Composition Spectroscopy in Health and Disease. *Physiological Measurement*, **27**, 921. http://dx.doi.org/10.1088/0967-3334/27/9/012

[11] Wabel, P., Moissl, U., Chamney, P., *et al.* (2008) Towards Improved Cardiovascular Management: The Necessity of Combining Blood Pressure and Fluid Overload. *Nephrology Dialysis Transplantation*, **23**, 2965-2971. http://dx.doi.org/10.1093/ndt/gfn228

[12] Van Biesen, W., Williams, J.D., Covic, A.C., *et al.* (2011) Fluid Status in Peritoneal Dialysis Patients: The European Body Composition Monitoring (EuroBCM) Study Cohort. *PLoS One*, **6**, Article ID: e17148. http://dx.doi.org/10.1371/journal.pone.0017148

[13] Machek, P., Jirka, T., Moissl, U., Chamney, P. and Wabel, P. (2010) Guided Optimization of Fluid Status in Haemodialysis Patients. *Nephrology Dialysis Transplantation*, **25**, 538-544. http://dx.doi.org/10.1093/ndt/gfp487

[14] Onofriescu, M., Mardare, N.G., Segall, L., *et al.* (2012) Randomized Trial of Bioelectrical Impedance Analysis versus Clinical Criteria for Guiding Ultrafiltration in Hemodialysis Patients: Effects on Blood Pressure, Hydration Status, and Arterial Stiffness. *International Urology and Nephrology*, **44**, 583-591. http://dx.doi.org/10.1007/s11255-011-0022-y

[15] Santoro, A., Mancini, E., Basile, C., *et al.* (2002) Blood Volume Controlled Hemodialysis in Hypotension-Prone Patients: A Randomized, Multicenter Controlled Trial. *Kidney International*, **62**, 1034-1045. http://dx.doi.org/10.1046/j.1523-1755.2002.00511.x

5

Prevalence of the Functional Dyspepsia and Associated Factors in the Chronic Hemodialysis Patients of the National Teaching Hospital "HKM" of Cotonou

Jean Jacques Sehonou[1], Jacques Vigan[2*], Bruno Léopold Agboton[2], Gbètondji Michel Massi[2]

[1]University Clinic of Internal Medicine of the National Teaching Hospital "Hubert K Maga" (CNHU-HKM), Cotonou, Benin
[2]University Clinic of Nephrology and Hemodialysis of the National Teaching Hospital "HKM" of Cotonou, Cotonou, Benin
Email: *vigues2@yahoo.fr

Abstract

Aim: To study the functional dyspepsia in chronic hemodialysis patients of CNHU-HKM of Cotonou. Methods: This descriptive, analytical and cross-sectional study ran from 1 September 2013 to 28 February 2014 in the University Clinic of Nephrology Dialysis of CNHU-HKM of Cotonou. It included all chronic renal failure patients on hemodialysis for at least 9 months prior to the survey. After identifying the patients with upper gastrointestinal disorders, we had submitted to clinical Rome III criteria for functional dyspepsia. Upper endoscopy was performed in patients with clinical criteria of functional dyspepsia. Clinical factors associated, paraclinical and therapeutic were sought by logistic regression in univariate analysis. Data were analyzed using EPI DATA version 3.1. Results: 1) One hundred and thirty-one haemodialysis patients had participated in the study (sex ratio: 1.5, average age 49.6 ± 12.4 years). 2) The prevalence was 71.8% for upper gastrointestinal disorders, 64.9% for dyspeptic syndrome and 1.5% for functional dyspepsia. 3) They were associated to clinical criteria of functional dyspepsia of Roma III, the presence of high blood pressure, hypocalcaemia, treatment with calcic inhibitors and iron supplementation. Conclusion: Functional dyspepsia is uncommon in hemodialysis. The search of an organic cause is imperative for every dyspepsia.

Keywords

Benin, Chronic Haemodialysis, Functional Dyspepsia, Dyspepsia, Upper Gastrointestinal Disorders

---

*Corresponding author.

1. Introduction

The dyspeptic complaint is a difficult syndrome to rigorously characterize every day. It encompasses indeed most of upper gastrointestinal symptoms such as pain or discomfort sitting in the epigastric region [1]. These symptoms contribute and maintain in patients, malnutrition and therapeutic non-compliance that are potent causes of morbidity and mortality in hemodialysis patients [2].

In the general population, dyspepsia is a reason of increasingly frequent consultation and iterative exploration. Its prevalence in the general population varies according to studies, probably in relation with the definition [3]. As a result, it is 29% in Canada [4], 44.1% in the US [5], 38% in the United Kindom [6], 25% in France [7]. In Africa, particularly in Uganda and in Benin, it represents respectively 72% and 77.9% of upper gastrointestinal endoscopy indications in the general population [8] [9].

Two types of dyspepsia are distinguished as it is indicative of a disease (organic dyspepsia), or as it is an isolated symptom (functional dyspepsia) [1]. Functional dyspepsia affects about two thirds of patients with dyspepsia and is one of the difficult and frustrating situations for therapeutic hepato-gastroenterologist [1]. Its prevalence is approximately 23.5%, 64.5% and 67.9% respectively in China, the US and Senegal in the general population [5] [10] [11].

In chronic haemodialysis patients, the prevalence of upper gastrointestinal complications is high. So it is 70.7% in Brunei (South east Asia) [12] and 92% in Morocco [13]. The prevalence of dyspepsia in hemodialysis was 38% in Switzerland [14], 44.7% in Brunei [15] and 58% in Morocco [16]. The prevalence of functional dyspepsia in this particular population of hemodialysis patients is poorly documented.

In Benin, functional dyspepsia represents 33.3% of patients referred for upper endoscopy [9]. The dyspeptic complaints exist in hemodialysis despite the almost systematic prescription of proton pump inhibitors. However, the prevalence of functional dyspepsia is not known. Associated factors have not been studied. Since the installation of the hemodialysis unit of the National Teaching Hospital of Cotonou, no study has been led before on dyspeptic disorders. The scale of these disorders is not known. It is to fill this gap that this study has been initiated.

2. General Purpose

To study functional dyspepsia in chronic hemodialysis of the National Teaching Hospital HKM of Cotonou.

3. Specific Objectives

1) To determine the prevalence of upper gastrointestinal disorders in chronic hemodialysis.
2) To determine the prevalence of dyspepsia in chronic hemodialysis.
3) To determine the prevalence of functional dyspepsia in chronic hemodialysis patients.
4) To identify factors associated with functional dyspepsia among chronic hemodialysis.

4. Framework and Study Methods

4.1. Framework

This study was conducted at National Teaching Hospital "Hubert K. MAGA" (CNHU-HKM) of Cotonou particularly in the University Clinic of Nephrology and Haemodialysis (UCNH). Upper gastrointestinal endoscopies were performed in the endoscopy unit at the Military Hospital of Cotonou (HIA/Cotonou).

4.2. Study Methods

This is a cross-sectional, descriptive and analytical study, which covered 6 months, from 1 September 2013 to 28 February 2014.

Were included, all patients with chronic renal failure undergoing hemodialysis for at least nine (9) months prior to the survey. All patients unable to cooperate due to poor general condition (performance index of World Health Organisation greater than or equal to 2), and all patients who refused to participate in the study were excluded.

In this study, dyspepsia was defined by the presence of one or more upper gastrointestinal (GI) symptoms such as epigastric pain, digestive discomfort, and early satiety in the early meal, gastric fullness after a normal meal, nausea, vomiting, belching, anorexia [17]. Each patient was investigated prior to the start of hemodialysis in search of each of these symptoms. The complaints of nausea and vomiting during dialysis weren't included to the diagnostic of dyspepsia in the study.

The diagnosis of functional dyspepsia was based on Roma III criteria [17]. It was defined when dyspeptic symptom exist for the last 3 months onset, continue at least 6 months prior to diagnosis without no evidence of structural disease (including at upper endoscopy) that is likely to explain the symptom. The associated factors like socio-demographic characteristics (age, gender, occupation, marital status) history and lifestyle, cause of kidney disease, dialysis parameters (hemodialysis age, frequency of sessions, duration of a session, incision, urea reduction rate), biological data and on-going treatments (analgesics, anti-inflammatory drugs, antihypertensive, martial and calcium supplementation) were sought by logistic regression in univariate analysis.

The urea reduction ratio (URR) is computed as follows:

$$URR = \left[1 - \left(\text{post-BUN}/\text{pre-BUN}\right)\right] \times 100\%$$

where BUN is the blood urea nitrogen concentration (BUN) and post-BUN refers to the end of dialysis treatment and pre-BUN to the start of the same dialysis treatment [18].

An upper gastrointestinal endoscopy was performed from dental arches to the second duodenum in all patients with clinical criteria of Roma III to eliminate an organic cause.

Patients were received individually on the day of hemodialysis. A verbal consent of all patients included in this study was obtained before. Blood samples were taken at the beginning of the hemodialysis session. This study was submitted for ethical approval before beginning. Data collected using a survey form was entered in the DATA EPI software version 3.1 and analyzed using STATA/IC11.0 software. The significance level was set at 5% confidence intervals were calculated to 95%.

5. Results

During the study period, 132 hemodialysis patients had responded to our inclusion criteria. One (1) patient had refused to participate in the study for personal reasons. Thus, our study population was reduced to 131 patients.

The limitations of data collection related to the fact that upper gastrointestinal disorders or the diagnosis of dyspepsia is based on subjective symptoms reported by patients. But the majority of patients had more than 2 symptoms. This could reduce the bias. More, according to Rome III criteria, symptoms must last at least six months.

5.1. General Characteristics of the Population

5.1.1. Socio-Demographic Characteristics
The average age of the study population was 49.6 ± 12.4 years, with extremes of 19 and 80 years. The sex ratio was 1.5. Merchants and handicrafts were the most represented. All socio-demographic characteristics are presented in **Table 1**.

5.1.2. History and Lifestyle
The history of hypertension was predominantly found in 70.2% patients. Coffee consumption was observed in 33.6%. The distribution of patients according to history and lifestyle is found in **Table 2**.

5.1.3. Drug Processing
Iron consumption (123; 93.9%) was the most represented, and then came the calcium channel blockers (104; 79.4%) and the inhibitor of enzyme converting (75; 57.2%) (**Table 3**).

5.1.4. Etiology of Chronic Renal Failure
Hypertension and diabetes mellitus predominate as showed in the **Figure 1**.

5.1.5. Parameters of Hemodialysis
The length of times on dialysis of these 131 haemodialysis patients was less than 4 years in 32.8% of cases; and more than 10 years in 26.7% of cases. The distribution of the dialysis parameters is in **Table 4**.

Table 1. Socio-demographic characteristic of the population.

	Number N = 131	Percentage
Age (years)		
<40	29	22.1
40 - 50	34	26.0
50 - 60	37	28.2
≥60	31	23.7
Sex		
Male	78	59.5
Female	53	40.5
Profession		
Merchant, handicraft	54	41.2
Teacher, engineer	28	21.4
FSP, office agent	18	13.7
Unemployed	15	11.4
Other	16	12.2
Marital status		
Live in couple	104	79.4
Live alone	27	20.6

Table 2. Distribution of patients according to the history and lifestyle.

	Frequency	**Percentage**
Antecedents		
Hypertension	92	70.2
Hepatitis C	23	17.6
Diabetes	15	11.5
UGD[*] confirmed	10	7.6
Chronic Glomerular-Nephritis	8	6.1
Hepatitis B	8	6.1
HIV[**]	5	3.8
Digestive tract cancer	0	0.0
Lifestyle		
Coffee consumption	44	33.6
NSAI[***] taking	25	19.1
Alcohol consumption	21	16.0
Cigarette smoking	8	6.1

[*]Ulcer gastroduodenal; [**]Human immunodeficiency virus; [***]Nonsteroidal anti-in-flammatory.

Table 3. Distribution of patients according to drug treatment.

	Frequency	**Percentage**
Inhibitor of enzyme converting	75	57.2
Calcium channel blockers	104	79.4
Iron supplementation	123	93.9

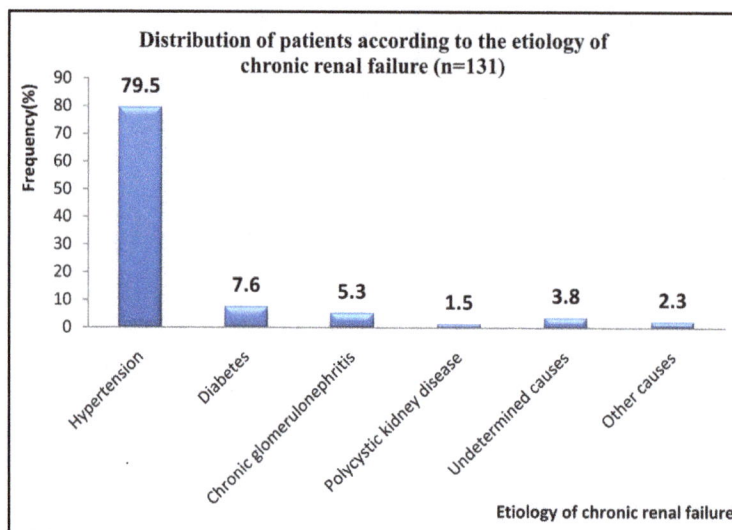

Figure 1. Distribution of patients according to the etiology of chronic renal failure.

Table 4. Distribution of patients according to drug treatment.

	Frequency	Percentage
Length of time on dialysis (year)		
Less than 4	43	32.8
4 - 6	35	26.7
6 - 10	18	13.8
10 et plus	35	26.7
Number of weekly sessions		
Two sessions	122	85.5
Three sessions	19	14.5
Duration of each session		
Four hours	29	22.1
Five hours	102	77.9
Type vascular access		
Arteriovenous fistula	121	92.4
Catheter	10	7.6
Urea reduction rate		
<60%	10	7.6
≥60%	121	92.4

5.2. Prevalence of the Upper Gastrointestinal Disorders in Chronic Hemodialysis Patients

Of the 131 hemodialysis patients, 94% or 71.8% had at least one upper gastrointestinal symptom. The most common were belching (55 patients; 42.0%), dry mouth syndrome (33 patients; 25.2%), dysgeusia (27 patients; 20.6%) and epigastric pain (26 patients; 19.8%) (**Table 5**).

5.3. Prevalence of Dyspepsia in Chronic Hemodialysis Patients

Eighty-five (85) patients had dyspepsia during the investigation, the prevalence of dyspepsia is 64.9% (**Figure 2**).

Table 5. Distribution of patients according to the upper GI symptoms present.

	Frequency	Percentage
Belching	55	42.0
Dry mouth syndrome	33	25.2
Dysgeusia	27	20.6
Epigastric pain	26	19.8
Abdominal discomfort	21	16.0
Anorexia	21	16.0
Heartburn	20	15.3
Nausea	19	14.5
Stomach fullness	13	9.9
Early satiety	11	8.4
Vomiting	11	8.4
Gastric distension sensation	10	7.6
Hematemesis	4	3.1
Metallic taste sensation	1	0.8

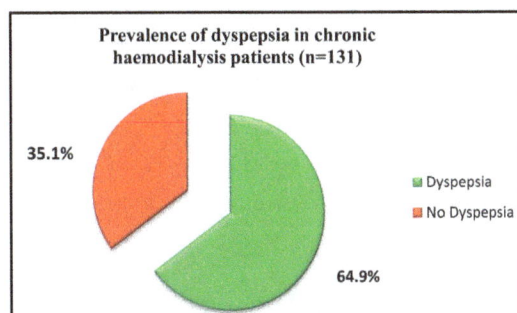

Figure 2. Prevalence of dyspepsia in chronic hemodialysis patients.

5.4. Prevalence of Functional Dyspepsia in Hemodialysis

Twenty (20) patients met the clinical criteria of Roma III where the achievement of upper gastrointestinal endoscopy was required. Two patients had refused to do this endoscopy. Of the remaining 18, two (2) patients had no lesion objectified in upper gastrointestinal endoscopy at the time of the survey, a prevalence of functional dyspepsia is 1.5% (2/131) as showed the **Table 6**.

5.5. Analysis of Associated Factors with Clinical Criteria of Functional Dyspepsia in Chronic Hemodialysis

Associated factors were sought in the twenty (20) patients meeting the clinical criteria for functional dyspepsia Roma III.

5.5.1. Factors Associated with Clinical Criteria of Functional Dyspepsia
Among the history, only hypertension was associated with clinical functional dyspepsia. Patients treated with calcium channel blockers had about six (6) times the risk of having clinical criteria of functional dyspepsia than those not taking. On the contrary iron consumption is a protective factor against the occurrence of clinical criteria of functional dyspepsia (OR = 0.83 < 1). Normal calcemia had an protective action (OR = 0.32). Associated factors are presented in **Table 7**.

Table 6. Results after upper endoscopy.

	Frequency (n = 20)	Percentage
Functional dyspepsia (UGE* normal)	2	1.5
Antral erosive gastropathy or congestive	9	6.9
Bulbar ulcer	3	2.3
Antral ulcer	2	1.5
Gastropathy and squamous fundic	1	0.8
Ulcerative and antral burgeoning Neoformation	1	0.8
UGE* refusal	2	1.5

*Upper gastrointestinal endoscopy.

Table 7. Associated factors with clinical criteria of functional dyspepsia.

	Functional dyspepsia n (%)	no functional Dyspepsia n (%)	RC [IC$_{95\%}$]	p
ATCD* of hypertension				**0.02**
NO	2(5.1)	37(94.9)	1	
YES	18(19.6)	74(80.4)	4.50 [0.99 - 20.43]	
CCB**				**0.03**
NO	1(3.7)	26(96.3)	1	
YES	19(18.3)	85(81.7)	5.81 [0.09 - 45.52]	
Iron supplementation				**<0.01**
NO	5(62.5)	3(37.5)	1	
YES	15(12.2)	108(87.8)	0.83 [0.01 - 0.38]	
Serum of calcium				**0.02**
Hypocalcemia	13(23.6)	42(76.4)	1	
Normal (95 - 105 mg/L)	7(9.2)	69(90.8)	0.32 [0.12 - 0.88]	

*History of hypertension; **Calcium channel blockers.

5.5.2. Non-Associated Factors

No factor of socio-demographic, lifestyle, etiology of chronic renal failure and hemodialysis parameters was associated with clinical functional dyspepsia. Non-associated factors are presented in **Table 8**.

6. Discussion

6.1. Prevalence of Upper Gastrointestinal Disorders in Chronic Hemodialysis Patients

Ninety-four (94) patients had at least one of the digestive symptoms above, a prevalence of 71.8%. This result is similar to that found in hemodialysis at Brunei. Indeed in a population of 123 hemodialysis Chong had found that 65.0% had at least one upper gastrointestinal symptoms [15]. Our results are below those found by ELHOUSSNI in hemodialysis patients of Rabat (Morocco) [16]. Definitely, they had found a prevalence of 92.0% of upper gastrointestinal disorder. This is probably related to the very small size of the study population, 24 patients undergoing hemodialysis.

6.2. Prevalence of Dyspepsia in Chronic Hemodialysis Patients

Eighty-five (85) hemodialysis patients had dyspepsia ether a prevalence of 64.9%. These results are below those found in the population of patients referred for upper endoscopy realization of Cotonou. In effect SOSSA and collaborators in 2007 had found a prevalence of 77.9% among patients came for endoscopy [9].

Table 8. Non associated factors with clinical criteria of functional dyspepsia in chronic hemodialysis.

	Functional dyspepsia n (%)	No functional Dyspepsia n (%)	RC [IC$_{95\%}$]	p
Age (year)				0.07
Less than 40	4(13.8)	25(86.2)	1	
40 - 50	8(23.5)	26(76.5)	1.92 [0.51 - 7.20]	
50 - 60	7(18.9)	30(81.1)	1.45 [0.38 - 5.56]	
60 et plus	1(3.2)	30(96.8)	0.20 [0.02 - 1.98]	
Sex				0.05
Male	8(10.3)	70(89.7)	1	
Female	12(22.6)	41(77.4)	2.56 [0.96 - 6.78]	
Profession				0.10
Merchant	8(25.0)	24(75.0)	1	
Other	7(19.4)	29(80.6)	0.72 [0.23 - 2.28]	
Housewife	4(33.3)	8(66.7)	1.50 [0.35 - 6.34]	
Handicraft	1(4.6)	21(95.4)	0.14 [0.01 - 1.23]	
Teacher	0(0.0)	20(100)	-	
PSF*	0(0.0)	9(100)	-	
Marital status				0.10
Live alone	7(25.9)	20(74.1)	1	
Live in couple	13(12.5)	91(87.5)	0.40 [0.14 - 1.15]	
AINS taking				0.19
NON	14(13.2)	92(86.8)	1	
OUI	6(24.0)	19(76.0)	2.07 [0.70 - 6.08]	
Alcohol taking				0.60
NO	16(14.6)	94(85.4)	1	
YES	4(19.0)	17(80.9)	1.38 [0.41 - 4.64]	
Coffee taking				0.24
NO	11(12.6)	76(87.4)	1	
Yes	9(20.5)	35(20.5)	1.77 [0.67 - 4.67]	
URR**				0.19
Less than 60	1(10.0)	9(90.0)	1	
60 and more	19(15.7)	102(84.3)	0.51 [0.19 - 1.37]	

*Public security forces; **Urea reduction rate.

This prevalence found in our study is relatively above that found by some authors. In Morocco, Elhoussni *et al.* in 2011, found a prevalence of 58.0% of dyspepsia in chronic hemodialysis Rabat [16]. This could be related to the definition used dyspepsia. Indeed, epigastric pain and vomiting were not from their definition of dyspepsia. STRID and collaborators at Switzerland in 2008, had in the same way, found a prevalence of 38.0% of dyspepsia in hemodialysis [14].

6.3. The Prevalence of Functional Dyspepsia in Hemodialysis

The prevalence of functional dyspepsia in our study population was 1.5%. This prevalence is well below that found in 2007 in general population who came for endoscopy in Cotonou (Benin) 33.3% [9]. So there is more organic lesion in hemodialysis. This is explained by the fact that chronic renal failure in itself is a cause of organic dyspepsia. In Brazil, Bacci et al. had found a prevalence of 30.0% of functional dyspepsia in hemodialysis patients [19]. This prevalence is far above that found in this study. This could be explained by the fact that they had worked on a very heterogeneous sample consists of hemodialysis patients, chronic renal failure non-hemodialysis and non-renal failure patients.

6.4. Factors Associated with Clinical Criteria of Functional Dyspepsia in Hemodialysis

6.4.1. Factors Associated

Hypertensive hemodialysis patients were 4.5 times more likely to present the clinical criteria of functional dyspepsia than non-hypertensive hemodialysis (OR [95% CI]: 4.50 [0.99 to 20.43]; $p = 0.02$). In opposite BACCI and collaborators in their series had not established a statistically significant relationship between hypertension and functional dyspepsia [19]. These results could be explained by the heterogeneity of their study population. Other history such as diabetes, chronic glomerulonephritis, hepatitis B and C, infection with HIV and peptic ulcer disease were not associated with functional dyspepsia. These factors are often not taken into account in the different studies.

Consumption of calcium channel blockers was associated with clinical criteria of functional dyspepsia (5.81 [0.09 to 45.52]; $p = 0.03$). Patients who consumed calcium channel blockers had about six (6) times the risk of developing clinical criteria of functional dyspepsia than those who did not consume. Indeed calcium channel blockers have the mode of action to prevent the intracellular penetration of calcium in skeletal muscle but also in smooth muscle fibers. Or intracellular calcium is the activator of muscle contraction [20]. The intracellular calcium deficiency entails the consumption of calcium channel blockers would explain disorders of gastric motility responsible for the clinical criteria of functional dyspepsia observed.

Iron consumption mean while, was also associated with clinical criteria of functional dyspepsia as a protective factor (0.83 [0.01 to 0.38]; $p < 0.01$). Indeed, according to the literature, iron consumption is the cause of irritation of the digestive tract and thus represent an organic cause of dyspepsia [1].

Consumption converting enzyme inhibitor is not associated with the occurrence of clinical criteria of functional dyspepsia (1.14 [0.43 to 3.01]; $p = 0.78$).

Normal calcemia had a protective action against clinical criteria of functional dyspepsia (0.32 [0.12 - 10.99]; $p = 0.02$). This could be explained by the fact that calcium is involved in neuromuscular excitability. Hypocalcaemia could therefore be obvious clinically by neuromuscular and sensory signs such paraesthesia, hypoesthesia, muscle spasms disrupting gastric motility [21]. Salles Junior et al. and Altay et al. had also found no statistically significant relationship between serum calcium and the occurrence of dyspepsia [22] [23].

6.4.2. Non-Associated Factors

Clinical criteria of functional dyspepsia were showed in all age groups in our study, there was no significant association between age and clinical functional dyspepsia. Bacci et al. in opposite found a significant association between the occurrence of functional dyspepsia and age of their patients. Indeed they had observed that more patients are young, more the risk of occurrence of functional dyspepsia seems present [19].

Sex is not associated with the occurrence of clinical functional dyspepsia in our study ($p = 0.05$). The same observations were made by SOSSA and collaborators ($p = 0.05$) [9]. It is the same for Bacci et al. ($p = 0.21$) [19].

The profession of our patients was not associated with clinical functional dyspepsia ($p = 0.10$). This is a variable that is rarely taken into account in the different studies.

The anti-inflammatory intake was not associated with clinical functional dyspepsia (2.07 [0.70 to 6.08]; $p = 0.19$). Bradette reveals that certain medications such as anti-inflammatory play an important role in the development of dyspepsia [24].

Alcohol consumption was not associated with clinical functional dyspepsia (1.08 [0.41 - 4.64]; $p = 0.60$). The same observations were made by Bacci et al. ($p = 0.40$) [19].

Coffee consumption was not associated with the occurrence of clinical functional dyspepsia (1.77 [0.67 to 4.67]; $p = 0.24$). Coffee consumption is rarely taken into account as variable in studies.

No statistically significant association was found between the etiology of chronic kidney disease and clinical functional dyspepsia signs. In the literature, no correlation was observed between the etiology of renal disease and the occurrence of functional dyspepsia [19]. Salles Junior et al. had also found no link between the etiology of renal disease including: hypertension ($p = 0.72$), diabetes ($p = 0.16$), chronic glomerulonephritis ($p = 0.20$) and dyspepsia [22].

A statistically significant association was not found between the length of time on dialysis and clinical functional dyspepsia ($p = 0.50$). Salles Junior *et al.* had also found no link between seniority dialysis and dyspepsia ($p = 0.87$) [22]. The type of vascular access used for hemodialysis was not associated with clinical functional dyspepsia ($p = 0.21$). The literature does not provide information on the influence of vascular kind on the occurrence of functional dyspepsia.

The urea reduction rate was not significantly associated with the occurred of clinical functional dyspepsia. The literature provides more data of the Kt/V parameter. Indeed Salles Junior *et al.* and Altay *et al.* have found that the Kt/V was not significantly associated with the onset of dyspepsia [22] [23].

7. Conclusions

The prevalence of dyspepsia is 64.9% in hemodialysis patients of the National Teaching Hospital "HKM" of Cotonou and of functional dyspepsia according to Rome III diagnostic criteria which is 1.5%. Factors associated with clinical criteria of functional dyspepsia are: history of hypertension, treatment with calcium channel blockers, iron supplementation and calcemia.

This low prevalence of functional dyspepsia suggests an active search for an organic cause by the realization of aoeso-gastro-duodenal endoscopy in these patients.

Declaration of Conflict of Interest

None.

References

[1]   Peyrin-Biroulet, L. and Bigard, M.A. (2005) Dyspepsie. *EMC-Hépato-Gastroentérologie*, **2**, 105-123. http://dx.doi.org/10.1016/j.emchg.2005.01.003

[2]   Avram, M.M., Fein, P.A., Rafiq, M.A., Scholth, T., Chattopad-Hyay, J. and Mittman, N. (2006) Malnutrition and Inflammation as Predictors of Mortality in Peritoneal DIALYSIS Patients. *Kidney International Supplements*, **104**, 4-7.

[3]   Olomos, J.A., Pogorelsky, V., Tobal, F., Marcolongo, M., Salis, G., Higa, R., *et al.* (2006) Uninvestigated Dyspepsia in Latin America: A Population-Based Study. *Digestive Diseases and Sciences*, **51**, 1922-1929. http://dx.doi.org/10.1007/s10620-006-9241-y

[4]   Tougas, G., Hwang, P. and Paterson, W.G. (1998) Dyspeptic Symptoms in the General Canadian Population: Prevalence and Impact on Quality of Life. *Gastro-Enterology*, **114**, A312. http://dx.doi.org/10.1016/S0016-5085(98)81265-1

[5]   Shaib, Y. and El-Serag, H.B. (2004) The Prevalence and Risk Factors of Functional Dyspepsia in Multiethnic Population in the United States. *The American Journal of Gastroenterology*, **99**, 2210-2216. http://dx.doi.org/10.1111/j.1572-0241.2004.40052.x

[6]   Moayyedi, P. and Masson, J. (2002) Clinical and Economic Consequences of Dyspepsia in the Community. *Gut*, **50**, 10-12. http://dx.doi.org/10.1136/gut.50.suppl_4.iv10

[7]   Humair, J.P., Stalder, H. and Armenian, B. (2002) Dyspepsie. *Primary Care*, **2**, 459-467.

[8]   Ogwang, D.M. (2003) Dyspepsia: Endoscopy Findings in Uganda. *Tropical Doctor*, **33**, 175-177.

[9]   Sossa, B.R. (2007) Aspects cliniqueset socio-économiques de la dyspepsie à Cotonou. Thèse de Médecine FSS, Cotonou, No. 1380, 104.

[10]   Li, Y., Nie, Y., Sha, W. and Su, H. (2002) The Link between Psychosocial Factors and Functional Dyspepsia: An Epidemiological Study. *CMJ*, **115**, 1082-1084.

[11]   Mbengue, M., Diouf, M., Ka, M., Dangou, J.M., Ba-Seck, A., Ndiaye, M.F., *et al.* (1998) Dyspepsie fonctionnelle et *Hélicobacter pylori* à Dakar. *Médecine d'Afrique Noire*, **45**, 386-388.

[12]   Chong, V.H. and Tan, J. (2013) Prevalence of Gastrointestinal and Psychosomatic Symptoms among Asian Patients Undergoing Regular Hemodialysis. *Nephrology*, **18**, 97-103. http://dx.doi.org/10.1111/nep.12000

[13]   El-Filali, E.H., Layine, A., Aimad, I., Zamd, M., Medkouri, G., Hachim, K., *et al.* (2009) Manifestations digestives hautes chez les patients hémodialysés chroniques. *Nephrologie et thérapeutique*, **5**, 436-471.

[14]   Strid, H., Fjell, A., Simren, M. and Björnsson, E.S. (2009) Impact of Dialysis on Gastroesophageal Reflux, Dyspepsia, and Proton Pump Inhibitor Treatment in Patients with Chronic Renal Failure. *European Journal of Gastroenterology &*

Hepatology, **21**, 137-142. http://dx.doi.org/10.1097/MEG.0b013e3283200047

[15] Chong, V.H. (2010) Impact of Duration of Hemodialysis on Gastrointestinal Symptoms in Patients with End Stage Renal Failure. *Journal of Gastrointestinal and Liver Diseases*, **19**, 462-463.

[16] Elhoussni, S., Sabri, S., Mouram, H., Loko, S., Daoudi, F.Z., Errebih, H., *et al.* (2011) Apport de la fibroscopie oeso-gastroduodénale chez l'hémodialysé chronique. *Néphrologie & Thérapeutique*, **7**, 411-447. http://dx.doi.org/10.1016/j.nephro.2011.07.357

[17] Bruley des Varannes, S. (2011) Prise en charge de la Dyspepsie fonctionnelle. *Post'U FMC-HGE*, 65-74.

[18] Held, P.J., Port, F.K., Wolfe, R.A., Stannard, D.C., Carroll, C.E., Daugirdas, J.T., Bloembergen, W.E., Greer, J.W. and Hakim, R.M. (1996) The Dose of Hemodialysis and Patient Mortality. *Kidney International*, **50**, 550-556. http://dx.doi.org/10.1038/ki.1996.348

[19] Bacci, M.R. and Chehter, E.Z. (2013) Dyspepsia among Patients with Chronic Kidney Disease: A Cross Sectional Study. *International Archives of Medicine*, **6**, 43. http://dx.doi.org/10.1186/1755-7682-6-43

[20] Combes, A. (2005) Inhibiteurs calciques et dérives nitrés La Collection Hippocrate ECN CARDIO PHARMACO: 2-3.

[21] Soubai, R.B., Abourazzak, F.E. and Harzy, T. (2012) Hypocalcemie: Mise au point pratique. *Revue Marocaine de Rhumatologie*, **21**, 4-9.

[22] Salles Junior, L.D., Santos, P.R., dos Santos, A.A. and de Souza, M.H.L. (2013) Dyspepsia and Gastric Emptying in End-Stage Renal Disease Patients on Haemodialysis. *BMC Nephrology*, **14**, 275. http://dx.doi.org/10.1186/1471-2369-14-275

[23] Altay, M., Turgut, F., Akay, H., Kanbay, M., Babali, A., Akcay, A., *et al.* (2008) Dyspepsia in Turkish Patients on Continuous Ambulatory Peritoneal Dialysis. *International Urology and Nephrology*, **40**, 211-217. http://dx.doi.org/10.1007/s11255-007-9324-5

[24] Bradette, M. (2002) L'approche de la dyspepsie. *Le Médecin du Québec*, **37**, 43-52.

6

Levetiracetam-Associated Acute Kidney Injury and Drug Reaction with Eosinophilia and Systemic Symptoms (DRESS) Syndrome

Mathieu Leblanc[1], Martin Plaisance[2]*

[1]Internal Medecine Residency Program, Faculté de Médecine et des Sciences de la santé, Université de Sherbrooke, Sherbrooke, Canada
[2]Nephrology Division, Department of Medicine, Centre Hospitalier Universitaire de Sherbrooke, Sherbrooke, Canada
Email: *Martin.Plaisance@Sherbrooke.ca

Abstract

DRESS syndrome is a severe drug induced reaction. Acute kidney injury (AKI) is sometimes present in the form of an acute interstitial nephritis. We present the case of a 75-year-old man with glioblastoma who developed a DRESS two months after starting levetiracetam and a few days after stopping dexamethasone. His skin and kidneys improved after removing levetiracetam and introducing again corticosteroids. DRESS has been reported more frequently with other antiepileptics, rarely with levetiracetam. Clinicians should add this drug to the list of potential causes of AKI.

Keywords

Acute Kidney Injury, DRESS Syndrome, HSV-1, Levetiracetam

1. Background

Drug reaction with eosinophilia and systemic symptoms (DRESS) syndrome is a rare and potential fatal disease that usually follows introduction of a drug. Antiepileptics are the predominant agents reported [1]. The reaction produces nonspecific constitutional symptoms including fever, lymphadenopathy and malaise, as well as symptoms related to organ involvement, the liver being the organ most commonly affected. 10 to 30 percent of DRESS syndromes include an acute interstitial nephritis [2]. Allopurinol is the drug most often associated with renal involvement, but cases linked to phenytoin, dapsone, penicillin, nonsteroidal anti-inflammatory drug (NSAID)

---

*Corresponding author.

and other drugs have been reported [2]. Cases of DRESS syndrome secondary to levetiracetam have been described in the literature [3] [4] but, to our knowledge, none with renal involvement. Two cases of acute interstitial nephritis not in the setting of DRESS have been reported [5]. Herein, we report a new case of DRESS syndrome with acute kidney injury, most probably an acute interstitial nephritis secondary to levetiracetam.

2. Case Report

A 75-year-old man was started on levetiracetam 500 mg twice a day October 3rd, 2013 for partial seizures following a neurosurgical procedure to remove a glioblastoma, done August 28th, 2013. Dexamethasone 4 mg twice a day had also been prescribed three days before the operation. Ezetimibe was the only other medication taken by the patient. He had no history of heart disease. He had been taking it for several years for dyslipidemia. It was stopped on admission January 9th, 2014. No NSAID had been taken in the months prior to the events. He had not received chemotherapy, only radiotherapy.

Dexamethasone was slowly tapered and discontinued on December 15th, 2013. In the following days, the patient developed malaise, fatigue and a generalize pruritic maculopapular rash on his trunk, proximal limbs and his face. He never accused chest pain or shortness of breath. Levetiracetam was switched to phenytoin December 31st. At that time, his temperature was 38.2°C, his serum creatinine level had increased from 75 µmol/L (day of the surgery) to 108 µmol/L. Four days later, his symptoms worsened and his creatinine level raised to 139 µmol/L. Vancomycin and clindamycin were tried for a few days. On January 9th, his creatinine level was 465 µmol/L. He never had low blood pressure which on average was 125/75. He did not have invasive arterial procedure or contrast. It was his first acute kidney injury. Cervical lymphadenopathy and numerous buccal aphthous ulcers were new findings at the physical exam. The most notable laboratory abnormality was a leucocytosis at 11,000 white blood cells/mm³ with an important eosinophilia at 4700 mm³. His urinary analysis was normal. Urinary protein/creatinine ratio was minimal at 0.26 g/g. A renal echography showed hyperechogenic cortex without obstruction. AST and ALT were normal. Viral culture of the buccal ulcers was positive for HHV-1. EBV serology showed past infection. HBV and HCV serologies were negative.

Because DRESS syndrome with severe renal involvement was suspected, a dose of prednisone 50 mg was given without proceeding to a skin or kidney biopsy. The following day, creatinine level was 512 µmol/L. Intravenous pulses of methylprednisolone 500 mg IV were given even though the rash already showed some improvement. Two days later, the creatinine level decreased to 457 µmol/L. Prednisone 100 mg daily was given for seven days, followed by prednisone 50 mg daily for one week with a 5 mg decrease each week until complete discontinuation. At discharge, on January 16th, the creatinine level was down to 171 µmol/L, the eosinophils count was 600 mm³ and the rash showed complete resolution.

Unfortunately, the patient had a relapse of his diffuse rash at the end of January while the prednisone was at 40 mg daily (**Figure 1**). Serum creatinine level was then 130 µmol/L. Since DRESS syndrome is known to last longer than other drug related skin reaction, it was probably still the reaction from levetiracetam but phenytoin being one of the more typical drug associated with DRESS, it was changed to valproate. The skin rash slowly

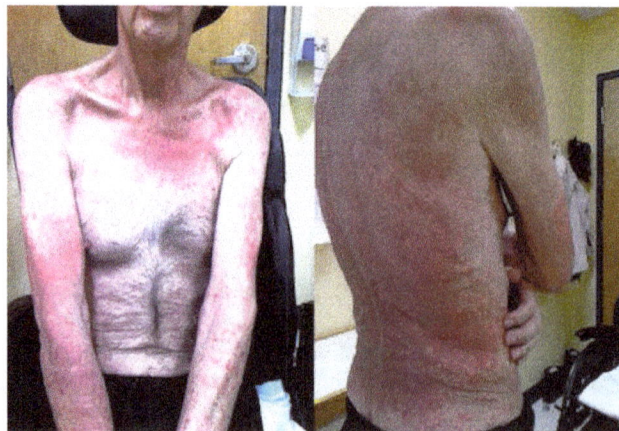

Figure 1. Rash on patient's thorax and arms (left panel) and back (right panel).

resolved and the last creatinine level was 88 μmol/L in July 2014. No further episode of skin rash or acute kidney injury was noted. Sadly, the patient suffered a relapsed from his brain cancer and is now in palliative care.

3. Discussion

A diagnosis of DRESS syndrome should be suspected in a patient with a new drug exposure who develops a skin eruption, eosinophilia or atypical lymphocytosis and systemic involvement like interstitial nephritis, but also hepatitis, pneumonitis or myocarditis.

Presentation typically occurs two to eight weeks after initiation of the offending agent. The presence of dexamethasone could explain the longer delay (10 weeks) in our case. A definite proof of drug reaction requires rechallenge after resolution of the disease. In severe reactions such as this one, it would be unethical to do so, we must thus work with probability linked to chronology.

Aromatic antiepileptic drugs and allopurinol are the most frequently reported culprits [1]. Non-aromatic antiepileptic drugs such as levetiracetam were initially thought to be safe, but at least three cases of DRESS syndrome in patients taking this substance were reported [3] [4], none included renal involvement. Renal involvement is rare in the literature, except for allopurinol that causes renal dysfunction in 84% of the cases in the literature and 43% of the cases reported in the French Pharmacovigilance Database [6]. We herein describe, to the best of our knowledge, the first case of a DRESS with renal involvement caused by levetiracetam. We presume this kidney impairment to be an acute interstitial nephritis but no kidney biopsy was deemed necessary to start treatment with corticosteroids.

The pathophysiology of DRESS syndrome is not well described. Part of it seems to include herpes virus reactivation [7] and expansion of activated T lymphocytes, but there is no clear evidence if the drug reaction is the primary trigger or an amplificater of a subclinical viral infection [8] [9]. Links have been found mainly with HHV-6, but also in HHV-7 and EBV reactivation [9]. To our knowledge, HSV-1 reactivation has not been reported in DRESS syndrome. In this case, serology for HHV-6 was not performed.

The European Registry of Severe Cutaneous Adverse Reactions (RegiSCAR) proposed a score in 2007 to help clinicians in confirming or excluding the diagnosis of DRESS [10]. The criteria of this system are: fever greater than 38.5°C; enlarged lymph nodes; eosinophilia; atypical lymphocytosis; skin involvement; organ involvement; resolution greater than 15 days; and evaluation of other potential causes (ANA, blood cultures, serology for hepatitis A virus, hepatitis B virus, hepatitis C virus, chlamydia and/or mycoplasma or other appropriate serology). With this score, more than five points indicates a definite case. Our patient had a calculated score of six points indicating a definite diagnostic: 2 for the eosinophilia, 2 for the skin involvement, 1 for enlarged lymph nodes, 1 for kidney involvement, 1 for other potential cause, −1 for fever not ≥38.5°C (it was 38.2°C).

Prompt identification and discontinuation of the offending drug is the mainstay of the management. Once done, the rash and the organ involvement usually resolve gradually between six or nine weeks, but about 20 percent of the patients experience persistence of symptoms with remissions and relapses of the syndrome [11]. No treatment has been evaluated in randomized trials but it is generally accepted that patients with severe organ involvement should be treated with systemic corticosteroids on the basis of case reports and retrospective studies. The French Society of Dermatology published in 2010 a consensus on therapeutic management of the syndrome [12]. The recommendation was to treat patients with any signs of severity, including renal involvement, with systemic steroid equivalent to one mg/kg/day of prednisolone. Use of intravenous immunoglobulin (IVIG) at two g/kg over five days for life-threatening situation including kidney failure was also part of the recommendation, but benefits of IVIG remain controversial with the publication of newest articles showing contradictory results [13] [14]. The last recommendation of that consensus is to combine ganciclovir to steroid in severe cases with confirmation of a major viral reactivation of HHV-6.

4. Conclusion

This first case of acute kidney injury in a DRESS syndrome following introduction of levetiracetam confirms this antiepileptic drug as a rare cause of potentially severe acute renal insufficiency.

Acknowledgements

We thank Tanya Fayad for her thorough review of the manuscript and helpful advices.

Conflict of Interest Statement

None to declare.

References

[1]   Kardaun, S.H., Sekula, P., Valeyrie-Allanore, L., *et al.* (2013) Drug Reaction with Eosinophilia and Systemic Symptoms (DRESS): An Original Multisystem Adverse Drug Reaction. Results from the Prospective RegiSCAR Study. *British Journal of Dermatology*, **169**, 1071-1080. http://dx.doi.org/10.1111/bjd.12501

[2]   Chen, Y.C., Chui, H.C. and Chu, C.Y. (2010) Drug Reaction with Eosinophilia and Systemic Symptoms: A Retrospective Study of 60 Cases. *Archives of Dermatology*, **146**, 1373-1379. http://dx.doi.org/10.1001/archdermatol.2010.198

[3]   Hall, D.J. and Fromm, J.S. (2013) Drug Reaction with Eosinophilia and Systemic Symptoms Syndrome in a Patient Taking Phenytoin and Levetiracetam: A Case Report. *Journal of Medical Case Reports*, **7**, 2. http://dx.doi.org/10.1186/1752-1947-7-2

[4]   Gomez-Zorrilla, S., Ferraz, A.V., Pedros, C., Lemus, M. and Pena, C. (2012) Levetiracetam-Induced Drug Reaction with Eosinophilia and Systemic Symptoms Syndrome. *Annals of Pharmacotherapy*, **46**, e20. http://dx.doi.org/10.1345/aph.1R084

[5]   Mahta, A., Kim, R. and Kesari, S. (2012) Levetiracetam-Induced Interstitial Nephritis in a Patient with Glioma. *Journal of Clinical Neuroscience*, **19**, 177-178. http://dx.doi.org/10.1016/j.jocn.2011.08.007

[6]   Peyrière, H., Dereure, O., Breton, H., *et al.* (2006) Variability in the Clinical Pattern of Cutaneous Side-Effects of Drugs with Systemic Symptoms: Does a DRESS Syndrome Really Exist? *British Journal of Dermatology*, **155**, 422-428. http://dx.doi.org/10.1111/j.1365-2133.2006.07284.x

[7]   Descamps, V., Valance, A., Edlinger, C., *et al.* (2001) Association of Human Herpesvirus 6 Infection with Drug Reaction with Eosinophilia and Systemic Symptoms. *Archives of Dermatology*, **137**, 301-304.

[8]   Takahashi, R., Kano, Y., Yamazaki, Y., Mizukawa, Y. and Shiohara, T. (2009) Defective Regulatory T Cells in Patients with Severe Drug Eruptions: Timing of the Dysfunction Is Associated with the Pathological Phenotype and Outcome. *Journal of Immunology*, **182**, 8071-8079. http://dx.doi.org/10.4049/jimmunol.0804002

[9]   Picard, D., Janela, B., Descamps, V., *et al.* (2010) Drug Reaction with Eosinophilia and Systemic Symptoms (DRESS): A Multiorgan Antiviral T Cell Response. *Science Translational Medicine*, **2**, 46-62. http://dx.doi.org/10.1126/scitranslmed.3001116

[10]   Kardaun, S.H., Sidoroff, A., Valeyrie-Allanore, L., *et al.* (2007) Variability in the Clinical Pattern of Cutaneous Side-Effects of Drugs with Systemic Symptoms: Does a DRESS Syndrome Really Exist? *British Journal of Dermatology*, **156**, 609-611. http://dx.doi.org/10.1111/j.1365-2133.2006.07704.x

[11]   Cacoub, P., Musette, P., Descamps, V., *et al.* (2011) The DRESS Syndrome: A Literature Review. *The American Journal of Medicine*, **124**, 588-597. http://dx.doi.org/10.1016/j.amjmed.2011.01.017

[12]   Descamps, V., Ben-Saïd, B., Sassolas, B., *et al.* (2010) Management of Drug Reaction with Eosinophilia and Systemic Symptoms (DRESS). *Annales de Dermatologie et de Vénéréologie*, **137**, 703-708. http://dx.doi.org/10.1016/j.annder.2010.04.024

[13]   Joly, P., Janela, B., Tetart, F., *et al.* (2012) Poor Benefit/Risk Balance of Intravenous Immunoglobulins in DRESS. *Archives of Dermatology*, **148**, 543-544.

[14]   Singer, E.M., Wanat, K.A. and Rosenbach, M.A. (2013) A Case of Recalcitrant DRESS Syndrome with Multiple Autoimmune Sequelae Treated with Intravenous Immunoglobulins. *JAMA Dermatology*, **149**, 494-495. http://dx.doi.org/10.1001/jamadermatol.2013.1949

7

Mechanical Complications of Peritoneal Dialysis

Marwa Miftah[1], Mohammed Asseban[2], Aicha Bezzaz[1], Adil Kallat[2], Ali Iken[2], Yassine Nouini[2], Loubna Benamar[1]

[1]Department of Nephrology-Dialysis-Kidney Transplants, Rabat Ibn Sina University Hospital, Rabat, Morocco
[2]Urology A Department, Rabat Ibn Sina University Hospital, Rabat, Morocco
Email: assebanmh@hotmail.com

Abstract

Introduction: The key to a successful chronic peritoneal dialysis is a permanent and safe access to the peritoneal cavity. The mechanical complications of peritoneal dialysis (MCPD) are a major cause of the failure of the technique. The aim of the study was to define the prevalence of peritoneal dialysis (PD) mechanical catheter complications, to determine the time and the factors associated with their occurring. Materials and Methods: A retrospective study was conducted between January 2009 and January 2014 at the nephrology, dialysis and renal transplants department of Ibn Sina university hospital in Rabat. We included all patients who were on peritoneal dialysis and presented mechanical complications. These mechanical catheter complications are represented by catheter migration or obstruction, inguinal or umbilical hernias, early and late peritoneal dialysate leakage, subcutaneous cuff extrusion and hemoperitoneum. Results: MCPD were noted in 23 of the 62 patients (37% of cases). Onset time of complications was 24.8 ± 18.9 months [3 - 60 months]. Among these complications, we noted a catheter migration (65.2%), postoperative hematoma (21.7%), cracking or perforation of catheter (17.4%), epiploic aspiration (17.4%), sleeve externalization (17.4%), catheter obstruction (13%), hemoperitoneum (13%), hernia (22%; 13% umbilical and 8.7% inguinal), early dialysate leakage (13%), and pleuroperitoneal leakage (8.7%). The average age of our patients was 54.9 ± 15.5 years [21 - 81 years old], with a male predominance and a sex ratio of 2.28. The average body mass index (BMI) was 25.4 kg/m^2. Diabetic patients represent 48.7% of our series. In our study, MCPD represent 13% of causes of transfer to hemodialysis (HD). Conclusion: Prevention of MCPD remains crucial. It is based on good patient education on hygiene and handling errors but also periodic retraining of patients and caregivers.

Keywords

Chronic Renal Failure, Peritoneal Dialysis, Tenckhoff Catheter (TK), Insertion, Mechanical Complications

1. Introduction

Peritoneal dialysis (PD) is a renal replacement technique that occupies an important place in the management of end-stage renal failure. It can be considered as a first-line treatment, temporary or permanent depending on the patient. The results of the PD in terms of morbidity and mortality are equivalent than those of hemodialysis (HD), and better in terms of quality of life [1].

The PD is introduced in Morocco for the first time in 1980, and then quickly abandoned. Through a pilot experiment at the Ibn Sina University Hospital of Rabat, started in 2006 to respond to medical and social needs, the PD was developed as a technique for renal replacement therapy [2].

The key to a successful chronic PD is a permanent and safe access to the peritoneal cavity. Indeed, the occurrence of mechanical catheter complications is a common cause of transfer to HD (8% - 20% of patients treated with PD); a good management of the catheter insertion and knowledge of various complications and their resolutions are paramount [3].

MCPD constitute 24% of PD complications and are represented by catheter migration or obstruction, inguinal or umbilical hernias, early and late peritoneal dialysate leakage, subcutaneous cuff extrusion, and rarely by hemoperitoneum [4].

Contributing factors depend on each type of complication and the most contributing factor implicated in the migration of catheter is constipation. The factor implicated in hernia and fluid leakage is hyperpressure intraperitoneal.

The aim of our study was to determine the prevalence of MCPD, define their nature and identify the time and the factors associated with their occurrence.

2. Materials and Methods

In January 2014, we conducted at the PD unit of Ibn Sina university hospital in Rabat, a retrospective study of 5 years: from January 2009 to January 2014 we identified all patients undergoing peritoneal dialysis who presented during their follow a MCPD. Patients with infectious complications were excluded.

These complications are diagnosed by malfunction of catheter, defined by three situations:
- An impossible drainage after normal infusion;
- An impossible or incomplete drainage with slow speed after slow infusion;
- Impossible drainage and infusion.

MCPD are represented by:
- Displacement or obstruction of catheter;
- Epiploic aspiration;
- Inguinal or umbilical hernias;
- Early and late peritoneal dialysate leakage;
- Cracking or perforation of catheter and
- Hemperitoneum.

We collected from patient medical records the following variables: age, sex, initial nephropathy, duration of PD follow, number of days between insertion of PD catheter and start of exchange, onset time of complications in relation to catheter insertion.

We investigated the contributing factors of MCPD and risk factors of their occurring by comparing patients who had complications and those who did not have.

Statistically, the data were entered and analyzed using SPSS 13.0 software. Quantitative variables were expressed as mean, and standard deviation, and we used the Student t test to compare these variables. Qualitative variables were expressed as numbers and percentages and comparison was made using the Chi2 test.

Implantation Technique of Peritoneal Dialysis Catheter

The PD catheter insertion is performed in the operating room under the most stringent aseptic conditions. We use PD catheter with dacron double sleeve.

Before surgery, the patient performs a bowel preparation by a cleansing enema followed by a general toilet antiseptic (iodised polyvidone) an extensive shaving (from nipples to mid-thigh) and a thorough cleaning of the umbilicus. The site of the emergence of TK is identified preoperatively and marked on the skin taking into account the length and type of the catheter.

Several types of anesthesia can be proposed to patients:

- The local anesthetic, frequently used, can be proposed in premedicated patients and patients's lean body weight. However, it does not control the peritoneal sensitivity and is not conducive to a good hemostasis. It often requires a stronger analgesia;
- General anesthesia which allows correct curarisation and provides comfort to the patient and the operator.

Catheter was inserted by a mini-laparotomy. The peritoneal surgical approach was lateral or paramedian to promote good attachment of deep sleeve and minimize the risk of hernias and leakage. The deep sleeve is placed in the muscles of the anterior abdominal wall or within the pre-peritoneal space. The second subcutaneous sleeve is placed near the skin and a distance of two inches from the orifice of emergence which must always be directed downward. Immediately after insertion in the operating room, the function of the catheter is verified in infusion and drainage, making sure of catheter's permeability and leaks's absence. This is done by injecting 50 ml of 0.9% saline. Care should be taken to never aspire injected liquid to avoid epiploic aspiration. Abdominal plain film is made two hours after waking patient to ensure the correct positioning of catheter in the pouch of Douglas.

3. Results

During five years, we found mechanical complications in 23 from 62 patients followed in peritoneal dialysis unit. The prevalence was 37% after a mean period of 24.8 ± 18.9 months [3 - 60 months]. The initial nephropathy is shown in **Table 1**. In our patients, the average age was 54.9 ± 15.5 years [21 - 81 years old], and the sex ratio (M/F) was 2.28 with a male predominance. The body mass index (BMI) was 25.4 kg/m^2. Diabetic patients accounted for 48.7%. Only 4.5% of patients had undergone cesarean abdominal surgery prior to PD.

Among the mechanical complications of the RFP, we noted: catheter's migration in 65.2%, postoperative hematoma in 21.7%, cracking or perforation of catheter in 17.4%, epiploic aspiration in 17.4%, sleeve externalization in 17.4%, catheter obstruction in 13%, hemoperitoneum in 13%, hernia in 22% (13% umbilical and 8.7% inguinal), early dialysate leakage in 13%, and pleuroperitoneal leakage in 8.7% of cases (**Table 2**).

Table 1. Initial nephropathy in patients followed in PD unit.

Initial Nephropathy	Percentage (%)
Diabetic Nephropathy	33.9%
Chronic Interstitial Nephritis	16.1%
Chronic Glomerular Nephritis	14.5%
Polycystic Kidney Disease	9.7%
Undetermined Nephropathy	25.8%

Table 2. Distribution of different mechanical complications.

Mechanical Complications	Number = 23	%
Catheter Migration	15	65.2%
Postoperative Hematoma	5	21.7%
Cracking or Perforation	4	17.4%
Epiploic Aspiration	4	17.4%
Sleeve Externalization	4	17.4%
Obstruction	3	13%
Hemoperitoneum	3	13%
Umbilical Hernia	3	13%
Inguinal Hernia	2	8.7%
Early Dialysate Leaks	3	13%
Pleuro-Peritoneal Leaks	2	8.7%

The time of occurrence to complications in relation to insertion of catheter was variable and depended on several factors. Thus, the average time to catheter's migration was 4.4 months [0 - 20 months], to epiploic aspiration was 21 days [0 - 2 months], to inguinal hernia was 8 months [4 - 12 months], to umbilical hernia was 20 months [12 - 36 months], to early leakage was 3 days [0 - 6 days], to pleuroperitoneal leakage was 30 months [12 - 48 months], to cracking or perforation was 25.6 months [1 to 48] and to hemoperitoneum was 7.1 months [2 - 16 months] (**Table 3**).

The main contributing factor in the migration of catheter was constipation in 13 cases (86.6%). The contributing factor to catheter obstruction was fibrin deposition in 2 cases (60%) and blood clot in 1 case (30%). The catheter perforation was accidental by use of sharp equipment (**Table 4**).

The treatment of these complications depends on mechanical contributing factors; it is either medical or surgical. Thus, treatment of the catheter migration was by transit accelerators in 80% of cases. In the remaining cases, it was surgical, either by repositioning the catheter in 13% or removal of catheter in 7% of cases.

In case of early dialysate leakage, the treatment consisted of a temporary cessation of exchanges for an average duration of 5 days. In case of pleuroperitoneal leaks, patients had a reduction in the volume of exchanges. In one patient a temporary cessation of exchanges was necessary.

Catheter cracking was treated by shortening of catheter in 2 cases and extension replacement in 2 cases.

The treatment of obstruction by a blood clot or fibrin deposition was by heparin dose of 1 ml/liter of dialysate, while the treatment of epiploic aspiration was surgical.

Three of five patients who had a hernia (two umbilical and inguinal) underwent surgical treatment.

To evaluate risk factors of mechanical complications in PD, we compared two groups of patients, the first with mechanical complications (n = 23) and the second without complications (n = 38).

Univariate analysis showed that age was a protective factor of mechanical complications (**Table 5**).

Mechanical complications of PD KT are implicated as a cause of transfer to HD in 13% of cases after a mean period of 13 months.

Table 3. Time to onset of mechanical complications PD.

Type of Complication	Average Time
Catheter Migration	4.4 months (0 - 20)
Inguinal	8 months (4 - 12)
Umbilical Hernia	20 months (12 - 36)
Pleuro-Peritoneal Leak	30 months (12 - 48)
Early Leak	3 days (0 - 6 days)
Cracking or Perforation	25.6 months (1 - 48)
Epiploic Aspiration	21 days (0 - 60)
Hemoperitoneum	7.1 months (2 - 16)
Obstruction	2.2 months (0.5 - 4)
Sleeve Externalization	24 months (12 - 36)

Table 4. Contributing factors for mechanical complications PD.

Complications	Contributing Factor
Migration	Constipation: 13 cases
Obstruction	Fibrin Deposition: 2 cases Blood Clot: 1 case
Perforation of Catheter	Accidentel (Sharp Equipment): 3 cases (Patient)
Hernia	Hyperpressure Intraperitoneal: 4 cases
Externalization	Catheter Traction: 2 cases
Hemoperitoneum	Menstruation: 1 case Anticoagulant Treatment: 1 case Abdominal Trauma:1 case

Table 5. Risk factor for mechanical complications.

Parameters	No Mechanicals Complications (N = 38)	Mechanicals Complications (N = 23)	p
Age	45.4 ± 16	55 ± 15	0.033
Delay (Median)	12j	7j	0.717
Surgical Operation	21.1%	4.3%	0.087
BMI kg/m^2	24.1 ± 4	25.4 ± 3	0.37
Diabetes	23.7%	41%	0.116

4. Discussion

According to Stefano *et al.* [5] the prevalence of mechanical complications in PD is 32.7%, it is 30% according to the French PD register. In our series we found a prevalence of 37%, which is slightly higher.

The prevalence of catheter dysfunction varies between 0% - 22% depending on the area, the type of catheter and insertion technique [6] [7]. Recent studies have shown that epiploic aspiration was the major cause of malfunction of catheter [8]. In our series the catheter migration was the most common cause; it represents 65% of MCPD followed by epiploic aspiration in 17.4% and catheter obstruction in 13%.

Early complications included leakage, catheter dysfunction, hemoperitoneum, while late complications are defined by hernias, pleuroperitoneal leaks and sleeve externalization [9]-[11].

In our series the median time to onset of leakage was 3 days, of epiploic aspiration was 21 days, of catheter obstruction was 2.2 months, and of catheter migration was 4.4 months which joined the literature as early complications.

In 86% of catheter displacement, the promoting factor was constipation that we treated by transit accelerators with a success rate of 90%.

Hernias of the abdominal wall are commonly observed in both the general population and in PD patients. Their number increases with age, obesity or emaciation and dehiscence of the abdominal wall. The increase of intra-abdominal pressure may be secondary to chronic constipation, bronchitis or mass syndrome (polycystic hepato-renal) [12]. The infusion of dialysate remains the main predisposing factor to hernia, the threshold for intra-abdominal pressure that must not exceed is 18 inches of water [13]. The PD population had at least two of these contributing factors.

The incidence of dialysate leaks is from 5% to 20% [14]. In our study we found dialysate leaks in five patients; three early dialysate leaks (13% of MCPD) and two pleuroperitoneal leakages (8.7% of MCPD). Early dialysate leaks appear in less than 30 days after catheter insertion and are often at the site of emergence [15]. In our series the time to onset of early leaks was three days after catheter insertion. Catheter leaks have two major problems: the first is temporary cessation of PD (use of hemodialysis) and the second is the risk of infection, peritonitis or infection in site of emergence [7]. In our series treatment of early dialysate leaks was temporary cessation of exchanges with an average duration of five days.

The hemoperitoneum occurs in 3% - 4% of the MCPD. It is considered as a benign complication and not a risk factor for peritonitis or failure of technique [16]. In our series hemoperitoneum present 13% of MCPD after an average period of 7 months [2 to 16 months], whereas in the literature it occurs after an average period of 10.5 months [1 to 37 months].

To determine factors associated to MCPD, we have not been able to determine a significant relationship between these factors and MCPD as in the literature [17].

The externalization of the sleeve is either due to melting of edema, progressive cachexia or traction on the KT, treated by peeling the dacron. In our series we found 4 cases of externalization of the sleeve (17.4% of CMDP), which are due in half of the cases to the traction on the KT. All patients underwent a coat.

In our series we studied the group with and the group without CMDP. We compared the age, diabetes, prior surgery and BMI of these two groups of patients so we can determine factors associated with CMDP. And as the data from the literature we were not able to determine a significant relationship between these factors and the CMDP [17].

The CMDP is the second major cause of output from the PD technique after peritonitis, it prevalence varies between 8% - 20% of all outputs [18]. In our series the CMDP are a cause of failure of the technique in 13% of cases.

5. Conclusions

The success of PD depends on a functional and sustainable peritoneal access. Successful access based primarily on the operator expertise. The catheter insertion must be done by a trained operator. The main cause of MCPD was due to displacement of catheter which is stressful for the patient and the PD team.

Many insertion techniques can be adopted, but it is recommended to entrust this practice to experienced operators who will use the technique they control the best.

The PD technique suffers from a lack of interest in Morocco in comparison with hemodialysis and renal transplantation. Its various infectious complications as well as mechanical complications do not explain its low implementation in the treatment of end-stage renal disease (ESRD). Prevention of MCPD is key; it is based on good patient education on hygiene and handling errors but also periodic retraining of patients and caregivers.

References

[1]   Chanliau, J. and Kessler, M. (2011) Peritoneal Dialysis for ESRD Patients: Financial Aspects. *Néphrologie & Thérapeutique*, **7**, 32-37. http://dx.doi.org/10.1016/j.nephro.2010.10.004

[2]   Haddiya, I., Skalli, Z., Lioussfi, Z., Radoui, A., Ouzeddoun, N., Ezaitouni, F., *et al.* (2010) Peritoneal Dialysis: A Satisfying Experience of a Misknown Technique in Rabatat the University Hospital. *Néphrologie & Thérapeutique*, **6**, 569-575. http://dx.doi.org/10.1016/j.nephro.2010.07.017

[3]   Flanigan, M. and Gokal, R. (2005) Peritoneal Catheters and Exit-Site Practices toward Optimum Peritoneal Access: A Review of Current Developments. *Peritoneal Dialysis International*, **25**, 132-139.

[4]   Singh, N., Davidson, I., Minhajuddin, A., Gieser, S., Nurenberg, M., Saxena, R. (2010) Risk Factors Associated with Peritoneal Dialysis Catheter Survival: A 9-Year Single-Center Study in 315 Patients. *The Journal of Vascular Access*, **11**, 316-322.

[5]   Santarelli, S., Zeiler, M., Marinelli, R., Monteburini, T., Federico, A. and Ceraudo, E. (2006) Videolaparoscopy as Rescue Therapy and Placement of Peritoneal Dialysis Catheters: A Thirty-Two Case Single Centre Experience. *Nephrology Dialysis Transplantation*, **21**, 1348-1354. http://dx.doi.org/10.1093/ndt/gfk041

[6]   Schaubel, D.E., Blake, P.G. and Fenton, S.S. (2001) Trends in CAPD Technique Failure: Canada, 1981-1997. *Peritoneal Dialysis International*, **21**, 365-371.

[7]   Scarpioni, R. (2003) Acute Hydrothorax in a Peritoneal Dialysis Patient: Long-Term Efficacy of Autologous Blood Cell Pleurodesis Associated with Small-Volume Peritoneal Exchanges. *Nephrology Dialysis Transplantation*, **18**, 2200-2201. http://dx.doi.org/10.1093/ndt/gfg335

[8]   Zakaria, H.M. (2011) Laparoscopic Management of Malfunctioning Peritoneal Dialysis Catheters. *Oman Medical Journal*, **26**, 171-174. http://dx.doi.org/10.5001/omj.2011.41

[9]   Fleisher, A.G., Kimmelstiel, F.M., Lattes, C.G. and Miller, R.E. (1985) Surgical Complications of Peritoneal Dialysis Catheters. *The American Journal of Surgery*, **149**, 726-729. http://dx.doi.org/10.1016/S0002-9610(85)80174-4

[10]   Farooq, M.M. and Freischlag, J.A. (1997) Peritoneal Dialysis: An Increasingly Popular Option. *Seminars in Vascular Surgery*, **10**, 144-150.

[11]   Peppelenbosch, A., van Kuijk, W.H., Bouvy, N.D., van der Sande, F.M. and Tordoir, J.H. (2008) Peritoneal Dialysis Catheter Placement Technique and Complications. *Nephrology Dialysis Transplantation*, **1**, 23-28.

[12]   Morris-Stiff, G., Coles, G., Moore, R., Jurewicz, A. and Lord, R. (1997) Abdominal Wall Hernia in Autosomal Dominant Polycystic Kidney Disease. *British Journal of Surgery*, **84**, 615-617. http://dx.doi.org/10.1002/bjs.1800840509

[13]   Del Peso, G., Bajo, M.A., Costero, O., Castro, M.J., Gil, F. and Selgas, R. (2001) Mechanical Complications of Abdominal Wall in Patients Treated with Peritoneal Dialysis. *Peritoneal Dialysis International*, **21**, 24S.

[14]   García-Ureña, M.A., Rodríguez, C.R., Vega Ruiz, V., Carnero Hernández, F.J., Fernández-Ruiz, E., Vazquez Gallego, J.M. and Velasco García, M. (2006) Prevalence and Management of Hernias in Peritoneal Dialysis Patients. *Peritoneal Dialysis International*, **26**, 198-202.

[15]   Szeto, C.C. and Chow, K.M. (2004) Pathogenesis and Management of Hydrothorax Complicating Peritoneal Dialysis. *Current Opinion in Pulmonary Medicine*, **10**, 315-319. http://dx.doi.org/10.1097/01.mcp.0000127901.60693.d0

[16]   Tse, K.C., Yip, P.S., Lam, M.F., Li, F.K., Choy, B.Y., Chan, T.M. and Lai, K.N. (2002) Recurrent Hemoperitoneum Complicating Continuous Ambulatory Peritoneal Dialysis. *Peritoneal Dialysis International*, **22**, 488-491.

[17]   Singh, N., Davidson, I., Minhajuddin, A., Gieser, S., Nurenberg, M. and Saxena, R. (2010) Risk Factors Associated with Peritoneal Dialysis Catheter Survival: A 9-Year Single-Center Study in 315 Patients. *Journal of Vascular Access*, **11**, 316-322.

[18] Kolesnyk, I., Dekker, F.W., Boeschoten, E.W. and Krediet, R.T. (2010) Time-Dependent Reasons for Peritoneal Dialysis Technique Failure and Mortality. *Peritoneal Dialysis International*, **30**, 170-177. http://dx.doi.org/10.3747/pdi.2008.00277

8

The Efficacy of Ferumoxytol in Peritoneal Dialysis Patients: A Short Scientific Report

Sayed Husain[1], Hani Judeh[2], Manaf Alroumoh[3], Farhana Yousaf[4], Prince Mohan[5], Ahla Husain[4], Chaim Charytan[4], Bruce Spinowitz[4]

[1]Cape Fear Valley Hospital NC, Fayetteville, USA
[2]St. Luks/Roosevelet Hospital, New York, USA
[3]South Texas Regional Medical Center, San Antonio, USA
[4]New York Hospital Queens, New York, USA
[5]Columbia Medical University, New York, USA
Email: hus9007@hotmail.com

Abstract

One of the major elements contributing to anemia in Chronic Kidney Disease (CKD) patients is iron deficiency. Iron supplementation in oral form is often not tolerated and ineffectively absorbed. Intravenous (IV) infusion is time consuming and is inconvenient in Peritoneal Dialysis (PD) patients self-treating at home. A new preparation of iron, ferumoxytol, is a carbohydrate-coated, paramagnetic iron oxide nanoparticle, which can be administered as a bolus intravenous injection, allowing the PD patient to more easily comply with current IV iron dosing regimens. Few studies have been done to evaluate the efficacy of ferumoxytol in PD population. We retrospectively reviewed the medical records of peritoneal dialysis patients who received at least one dose of ferumoxytol between January 2010 and August 2010 and observed that 17 patients showed an improvement in hemoglobin (Hb) to 1 gm/dl within a month of treatment along with a decrease in epoetin dosage in subsequent weeks.

Keywords

Anemia, Ferumoxytol, Peritoneal Dialysis

1. Introduction

Anemia is a common finding in chronic kidney disease patients and is attributed to lack of iron deficiency along with decreased production of erythropoietin by the kidneys. Erythropoiesis-stimulating agents (e.g., epoetin alfa, darbepoetin alfa), lead to iron deficiency from hemoglobin synthesis [1].

In peritoneal dialysis patients there is impaired release of iron from its stores such as macrophages of the reticuloendothelial system in the liver, spleen, and bone marrow. Commonly referred to as reticuloendothelial blockade, it causes a functional iron deficiency in which iron is present but not usable for hemoglobin synthesis. As a result to overcome this blockade and iron deficit from erythropoiesis stimulating agents and blood loss, use of intravenous iron has been successful in treating anemia [2]. United States Food and Drug Administration on June 30, 2009 approved ferumoxytol for the treatment of iron deficiency anemia in adults with chronic kidney disease. The approved dosage regimen is an intravenous dose of 510 mg, followed by a second dose 3 - 8 days later. The drug is given undiluted at a rate of up to 1 ml/second (30 mg/sec). If response in monitoring parameters is not seen (hemoglobin level, ferritin level, transferrin saturation, blood pressure) then regimen can be repeated again [3].

Ferumoxytol is a super-paramagnetic iron oxide nanoparticle that has a polyglucose carboxy-methylether coating. It has a molecular weight of 731 kD. *In vitro* studies have demonstrated that ferumoxytol contains or releases less free (labile) iron than its counterparts. As a result, ferumoxytol can be safely and rapidly administered intravenously in relatively high doses without acute adverse reactions [4].

To our knowledge, very few studies have been done to assess the efficacy of furomxytol on peritoneal dialysis patients. Retrospectively, we reviewed the medical records of peritoneal dialysis patients aged 18 years, who received at least one dose of ferumoxytol and analyzed the hematologic changes over a period of 4 months. The primary objective of this study was to analyze improvement in hemoglobin after the administration of ferumoxytol.

2. Method

Study design: A retrospective analysis was conducted on 9 males and 8 females aged 53.5 ± 16.6 years with average weight of 83.94 ± 22.8 kg peritoneal dialysis patients being treated with ferumoxytol for anemia at New Hospital Queens/Cornell University clinic between January 2010 and August 2010. Approval for retrospective analysis was approved by our local research review committee.

The primary objective was to evaluate the effect of ferumoxytol on hemoglobin, hematocrit, ferritin and iron saturation and compare the results of the iron profile pre and post Feraheme dosing.

The study population consisted of end stage renal disease patients on peritoneal dialysis with lab data meeting the iron deficient criteria per our institute, iron transferrin saturation of <20% or serum ferritin of <500 ug/dl. With the exception of 2 patients all others received two doses of the drug. Time elapsed between two consecutive ferumoxytol doses were on an average 10 days. Epoetin dosing interval was not altered and changes in the amount of the erythropoietin stimulating agent was made according to hematologic parameters as per institute guidelines. After initial ferumoxytol dosage, subsequent administration was done based on the response of the iron profile. Data on hemoglobin, ferrtin and TSAT were collected at baseline and then on a monthly basis for 4 months. We did not exclude iron depleted patients or with co-morbidities that would effect furomoxytol and ESA response.

3. Result

The analysis of Hb (**Table 1**) revealed an overall effect (p = 0.05), and an increase in Hb value from baseline and 12 weeks post furomoxytol Hb levels increased from 10.4 gm/dl to 11.3 gm/dl, p < 0.05. A similar decline in was observed in the use of epoeitin to less than 10,000 Units/week and remain constant till the end of the 4 month period. Comparison of Hb between baseline and week 16 were not significant.

The primary objective of the study was to determine an improvement in Hb range following ferumoxytol administration. At the end point all of the patients showed increase in Hb by 1 gm/dl. Changes in TSAT and ferritin were significant from baseline and increased by three fold.

4. Discussion

Ferumoxytol has the expected efficacy of an intravenous iron compound, with improvements in anemia and iron being evident as early as 4 weeks post ferumoxytol. Additionally, significant decrease in monthly epoetin dose

Table 1. Trends of hemoglobin and iron parameters during ferumoxytol therapy.

Lab	Baseline	4 Wk Post Feraheme	8 Wk Post Feraheme	12 Wk Post Feraheme	16 Wk Post Feraheme
Hemoglobin (g/dL)	10.4 ± 1.0	11.0 ± 0.9*	11.3 ± 0.9*	11.3 ± 1.0*	10.9 ± 1.2
Hematocrit (%)	32.3 ± 3.9	33.8 ± 3.5*	34.6 ± 3.2*	34.6 ± 3.4*	33.6 ± 3.
Ferritin (µg/dL)	279 ± 152	625 ± 248*	743 ± 259*	N/A	640 ± 367*
TSAT (%)	18.1 ± 6.3	37.4 ± 14.7*	36.9 ± 23.7	N/A	32.9 ± 12.9*
Epoetin (U)/week	39,573	29,764	27,058	27,329*	26,585

was noted at 12 weeks post ferumoxytol dosing. Ferumoxytol is a desirable therapeutic option in peritoneal dialysis patients, who typically visit the clinic at monthly intervals.

Alternative iron therapies would require lengthy infusions, or frequent visits to achieve comparable iron delivery. No direct comparisons of ferumoxytol with other parenteral iron preparations have been done in PD to the best of our knowledge; Ferumoxytol may be safely administered intravenously at a much more rapid rate (30 mg/sec) than currently available iron products. Our study has the limitation because of its observation nature and sample size. Ferumoxytol was not directly compared with other formulations (sodium ferric gluconate, iron sucrose, iron dextran)

5. Conclusion

In this short-term study (4 months), ferumoxytol therapy was demonstrated to be effective and safe in patients with PD and anemia. It is equally effective when compared to other intravenous iron formulations (iron sucrose) in increasing hemoglobin levels [5]. With a greater proportion of patients achieving increases of 1 g/dl, the ability to administer intravenous ferumoxytol 510 mg in less than 30 seconds makes it a convenient treatment option for outpatient treatment.

References

[1] Eschbach, J.W., Egrie, J.C., Downing, M.R., Browne, J.K. and Adamson, J.W. (1987) Correction of the Anemia of End-Stage Renal Disease with Crecombinant Human Erythropoietin: Results of a Combined Phase I and II Clinical Trial. *New England Journal of Medicine*, **316**, 73-78. http://dx.doi.org/10.1056/NEJM198701083160203

[2] Gotloib, L., Silverberg, D., Fudin, R. and Shostak, A. (2006) Iron Deficiency Is a Common Cause of Anemia in Chronic Kidney Disease and Can Often Be Corrected with Intravenous Iron. *Journal of Nephrology*, **19**, 161.

[3] AMAG Pharmaceuticals, Inc. (2009) Feraheme (Ferumoxytol) Package Insert. Lexington.

[4] Balakrishnan, V.S., Rao, M., Kausz, A.T., *et al.* (2009) Physicochemical Properties of Ferumoxytol, a New Intravenous Iron Preparation. *European Journal of Clinical Investment*, **39**, 489-496. http://dx.doi.org/10.1111/j.1365-2362.2009.02130.x

[5] Iain, C.M., *et al.* (2014) A Randomized Comparison of Ferumoxytol and Iron Sucrose for Treating Iron Deficiency Anemia in Patients with CKD *CJASN ePress*. http://dx.doi.org/10.2215/CJN.05320513

9

Mortality in Kidney Transplantation

Karima Boubaker, Madiha Mahfoudhi*, Amel Gaieb Battikh, Hayet Kaaroud, Ezzeddine Abderrahim, Taieb Ben Abdallah, Adel Kheder

Department of Internal Medicine A, Charles Nicolle Hospital, Tunis, Tunisia
Email: *madiha_mahfoudhi@yahoo.fr

Abstract

It's a retrospective study whose aim was to evaluate the incidence and the mortality in a population including 329 patients who received first kidney transplants from a living donor in 269 cases and cadaveric donor in 60 cases at Internal Medicine A department between June 1986 and December 2003. Aetiologies of mortality in our kidney transplant recipients were determined. There were 157 males and 75 females having an average age of 30.8 years. After a period of follow-up of 5.64 years, 51 patients (21.98%) died. Aetiologies of mortality were multiple and were known in approximately 98% of cases. Infections were observed in 25 cases. Cancer was observed in 7 cases (13.72%). Patient survival was not affected by gender, donor age or cause of donor death. Infections represent the major cause of mortality in our patients even many years after kidney transplantation. The maximum of death occurred in the 8th year after kidney transplantation.

Keywords

Kidney Transplantation, Aetiology, Mortality

1. Introduction

Kidney transplantation is the treatment of choice for patients with end-stage renal failure. However such patients are increasingly older and have additional co-morbid conditions leading to high mortality rates after transplantation. This poor prognosis of allograft recipients is due to an interaction between high prevalence of classic risk factors and inherent conditions to kidney transplantation [1]. Hence, cardiovascular death rate is higher than in the general population, even after stratifying for age, sex, and race. The aim of this review is to evaluate retrospectively the incidence and aetiologies of mortality in our kidney transplant recipients.

2. Material and Methods

The study population included 329 patients who received first kidney transplants from a living donor in 269

---

*Corresponding author.

cases and cadaveric donor in 60 cases at Internal Medicine A department between June 1986 and December 2003. Exclusion criteria were death occurred during kidney transplantation.

We collected all causes of mortality occurred in these patients. We studied age, sex, aetiologies of death and patient survival rates.

All patients received induction immunosuppression during the first few days after receiving the allograft. The induction agent has evolved over the years from Minnesota ALG, to monoclonal antilymphocyte antibodies OKT3 and thymoglobulin. None of the patients had received monoclonal anti-CD25 anti-bodies.

Initiation of cyclosporine treatment post-transplant was delayed until the serum creatinine was ≤2.5 mg/dl. All patients were started on cyclosporine microemulsion (Neoral). Prior to 1995, most patients received azathioprine (Imuran) in addition to cyclosporine. However since 1995, all patients received mycophenolate mofetil (Cellcept) instead of azathioprine as part of triple immunosuppression protocol that also included Neoral and prednisone. None of the patients were treated by sirolimus (Rapamycin).

Clinical data were obtained mainly from an electronic database that contains all the clinical and laboratory information in our patients. Age, sex, cause of end-stage renal disease (glomerulonephritis, diabetes, or other causes), pretransplant cardiovascular disease, vascular calcifications, time from first treatment for end-stage renal disease to kidney transplantation and acute tubular necrosis were recorded.

Delayed graft function is defined as the need for dialysis within 1 week after kidney transplantation.

Data in the manuscript are expressed as means ± standard deviation of the mean unless indicated otherwise. Statistical analysis used STATVIEW logician.

3. Results

There were 157 males and 75 females aged mainly of 30.8 years (16 - 61 years).

After a period of follow-up of 5.64 years (0 - 17.2 years), 51 patients (21.98%) died.

The maximum of death occurred in the 8th year after kidney transplantation.

Aetiologies of mortality were multiple and were known in approximately 98% of cases (**Table 1**).

Infection were observed in 25 cases (49.01%): no specific infection in 19 cases, pulmonary aspergillosis in 1case, tuberculosis in 2 cases, listeriosis in 1case, varicelle in 1 case and perforation of CMV intestinal lesions in 1 case. Cancer was observed in 7 cases (13.72%) with cerebral localisation in 2 cases, hepatic in 1case, gastric in 1case, maxillary in 1case, cutaneous in 1 case and renal lymphoma in 1case. Cirrhosis was observed in 6 cases (11.76%), pulmonary emboli in 2 cases (3.92%). Other causes were observed in 11 cases (21.56 %).

The 1-, 5-, 10- and 20-year patient survival rates were 99.60%, 91.20%, 80.60% and 62.70% respectively (**Figure 1**). Patient survival was not affected by gender, donor age or cause of donor death.

4. Discussion

Since the initial successful kidney transplantation in humans, the field of kidney transplantation has made significant progress.

Patient survival and graft survival have improved tremendously. High comorbidity is associated with an increased risk for patient death but not for graft failure or acute cellular rejection, both in the perioperative period and after first 3 months of kidney transplantation [2].

Indeed, based on age and number of co morbid conditions, kidney transplant recipients have been successfully classified to have low, medium, or high risk of death [3] [4].

The most common comorbid conditions found in literature were posttransplant diabetes mellitus diabetes (30%) and heart failure (12%) [2] [5]. The occurrence of fatal and nonfatal cardiovascular events after successful kidney transplantation not only relates to baseline cardiovascular risk factors present at transplantation, but also to immunosuppressive drugs and post transplantation traditional and non-traditional risk factors. Posttransplantation anemia is an independent risk factor for cardiovascular morbidity and mortality in kidney transplant recipients. There are multiple causes of Posttransplantation anemia such as impaired kidney function, iron deficiency, medications, infections, acute rejection, inflammation, and erythropoietin deficiency.

Current guidelines recommend evaluation for hemoglobin level of less than 12 g/dL and treatment when the value falls less than 11 g/dL and a target of 11 to 12 g/dL. Additional treatments may entail removing the cause of the anemia, nutritional supplementation, and/or an erythrocyte stimulating agent [6]. In our study, we found 2

Survival Rate

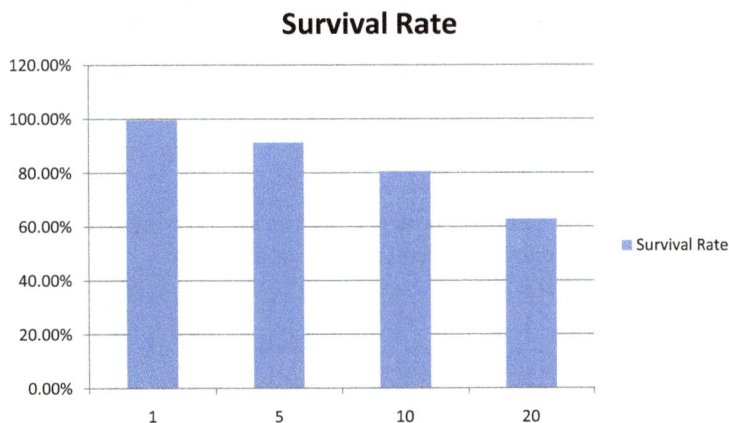

Figure 1. Survival rate histogram.

Table 1. Aetiologies of mortality in our series.

Aetiologies of mortality	Number of patients
Infections	25
Cancers	7
Cirrhosis	6
Pulmonary emboli	2
Other causes	11

cases of pulmonary emboli.

Other important risk factors of co morbidity are immunosuppressive regimen, metabolic disorders and infections [2]. Infection-related mortality was observed in 49.01% of cases in our study. They were specific infection in almost the half of the cases. Indeed, in the last decade, infection-related mortality among kidney transplant recipients has not decreased. Although better control of invasive viral infections has been achieved, bacterial and fungal invasive infections remain important causes of mortality in this population. Cytomegalovirus infection in kidney transplant recipients causes decreased patient survival. It was a case of death in one of our patients.

Early targeted treatment interventions groups at high risk for poor outcomes may be indicated and, consequently, help minimize mortality [2].

In our series, the maximum of death occurred in the 8th year after kidney transplantation. This may be due to either elevated frequency of infections caused by prolonged immunosuppression or high carcinogenic risk of the prescribed treatment.

Twelve variables independently predicted death: age, race, cause of kidney failure, body mass index, comorbid disease, smoking, employment status, serum albumin level, year of first renal replacement therapy, kidney transplantation, time to transplant wait-listing and time on the wait list [7].

Increasing donor age (but not recipient age), recipient diabetes, and grafts from adult offspring were independently associated with poorer patient survival in the first 3 years after transplantation [8]. Poorer graft survival was independently associated with donor age older than 59 years, and female recipients [8].

Cancer related mortality is observed in 13.72% of cases in our study. In fact, immunosuppression in solid organ transplant recipients is associated with increased risk of a broad range of cancers. Increased cancer risk mainly for Kaposi's sarcoma, non-Hodgkin's lymphoma, melanoma, and lip cancer, is rapidly reversible on reduction or cessation of immunosuppression regimen [9].

Our 1-, 5-, 10- and 20-year patient survival rates were 99.60%, 91.20%, 80.60% and 62.70% respectively, were better than those recently published with non-extended criteria donors [10] [11].

In the quoted study, however, a decidedly inferior graft survival was seen among extended criteria donor organs, 87.4% and 66.4% at 1 and 5 years, respectively [10]. In fact expanded criteria deceased kidneys render a survival benefit, but should be given principally to patients over the age of 40 years and when the waiting list is long.

Patient survival is reduced among recipients aged >50 years compared with those <50 years of age and in female-to male donations [10].

5. Conclusion

Infections represent the major cause of mortality even many years after kidney transplantation. Cancer origin should also be considered in kidney transplantation mortality.

Conflict of Interests

The authors declare no conflict of interests.

References

[1]   Sarnak, M.J., Levey, A.S., Schoolwerth, A.C., Coresh, J., Culleton, B., Hamm, L.L., *et al.* (2003) Kidney Disease as a Risk Factor for Development of Cardiovascular Disease: A Statement from the American Heart Association Councils on Kidney in Cardiovascular Disease, High Blood Pressure Research, Clinical Cardiology, and Epidemiology and Prevention. *Circulation*, **108**, 2154-2169. http://dx.doi.org/10.1161/01.CIR.0000095676.90936.80

[2]   Hernández, D., Rufinoa, M., González-Posadaa, J.M., Estupiñán, S., Pérez, G., Marrero-Miranda, D., *et al.* (2008) Predicting Delayed Graft Function and Mortality in Kidney Transplantation. *Transplantation Reviews*, **22**, 21-26. http://dx.doi.org/10.1016/j.trre.2007.09.007

[3]   Wright, L.F. (1991) Survival in Patients with End-Stage Renal Disease. *American Journal of Kidney Diseases*, **17**, 25-28. http://dx.doi.org/10.1016/S0272-6386(12)80245-9

[4]   Miskulin, D.C., Meyer, K.B., Martin, A.A., Fink, N.E., Coresh, J., Powe, N.R., *et al.* (2003) Comorbidity and Its Change Predict Survival in Incident Dialysis Patients. *American Journal of Kidney Diseases*, **41**, 149-161. http://dx.doi.org/10.1053/ajkd.2003.50034

[5]   Gnatta, D., Keitel, E., Heineck, I., Cardoso, B.D., Rodrigues, A.P., Michel, K., *et al.* (2010) Use of Tacrolimus and the Development of Posttransplant Diabetes Mellitus: A Brazilian Single-Center, Observational Study. *Transplantation Proceedings*, **42**, 475-478. http://dx.doi.org/10.1016/j.transproceed.2010.02.021

[6]   Blosser, C.D. and Bloom, R.D. (2010) Post Transplant Anemia in Solid Organ Recipients. *Transplantation Reviews*, **24**, 89-98. http://dx.doi.org/10.1016/j.trre.2010.01.006

[7]   Van Walraven, C., Austin, P.C. and Knoll, G. (2010) Predicting Potential Survival Benefit of Renal Transplantation in Patients with Chronic Kidney Disease. *CMAJ*, **182**, 666-672. http://dx.doi.org/10.1503/cmaj.091661

[8]   Fuggle, S.V., Allen, J.E., Johnson, R.J., Collett, D., Mason, P.D., Dudley, C., *et al.* (2010) Factors Affecting Graft and Patient Survival after Live Donor Kidney Transplantation in the UK. *Transplantation*, **89**, 694-701. http://dx.doi.org/10.1097/TP.0b013e3181c7dc99

[9]   van Leeuwen, M.T., Webster, A.C., McCredie, M.R., Stewart, J.H., McDonald, S.P., Amin, J., *et al.* (2010) Effect of Reduced Immunosuppression after Kidney Transplant Failure on Risk of Cancer: Population Based Retrospective Cohort Study. *BMJ*, **340**, c570. http://dx.doi.org/10.1136/bmj.c570

[10]   Shaheen, M.F., Shaheen, F.A., Attar, B., Elamin, K., Al Hayyan, H. and Al Sayyari, A. (2010) Impact of Recipient and Donor Nonimmunologic Factors on the Outcome of Deceased Donor Kidney Transplantation. *Transplantation Proceedings*, **42**, 273-276. http://dx.doi.org/10.1016/j.transproceed.2009.12.052

[11]   Merion, R.M., Ashby, V.P., Robert, M.A., *et al.* (2005) Deceased-Donor Characteristics and the Survival Benefit of Kidney Transplantation. *JAMA*, **294**, 2726. http://dx.doi.org/10.1001/jama.294.21.2726

10

Recent Advances in Treatment for Uremic Pruritus

Hiromichi Suzuki[1*], Hiroshi Omata[2], Hiroo Kumagai[3]

[1]Department of Nephrology, Saitama Medical University, Moroyama, Japan
[2]Center for Oriental and Integrated Medicine, Saitama Medical University, Moroyama, Japan
[3]Department of Nephrology and Endocrinology, National Defense Medical College, Tokorozawa, Japan
Email: [*]iromichi@saitama-med.ac.jp

Abstract

This review highlights recent advances in pathophysiology and treatment for uremic pruritus, especially focusing on various interventions. Pruritus in patients on hemodialysis (HD) and peritoneal dialysis (PD) still remains an unresolved issue. Recently, the efficacy and safety of nalfurafine hydrochloride have been reported in Japan, and at present, more than thirty thousand patients receive this new drug. In comparison with the efficacy of this new drug, acupuncture, a form of traditional Japanese therapy, has been validated for relief of symptoms of pruritus. In this review, various interventions for relief of symptoms of pruritus as well as recent studies on its pathophysiology will be introduced. This review will be helpful for treatment of pruritus in patients on dialyzed therapy in clinical practice.

Keywords

Itch, Dialysis, Ultraviolet, Topical Ointment, Acupuncture, Opioid Antagonists, Nalfurafine

1. Introduction

Uremic pruritus remains a frequent concern for hemodialysis patients with the most frustrating and disabling symptoms. Nearly 90% of patients on dialysis suffer from pruritus. Until present, there have been a lot of reviews discussing the pathophysiology and treatment of pruritus [1]-[14]. Previously, the word "uremic pruritus" has been used for symptoms of itching because it is a common skin derangement in patients with advanced renal failure. However, the usage of "uremic" may cause confusion because pruritus is not found in patients with acute kidney injury. In this regard, Paitel *et al.* [9] recently proposed the term, "chronic kidney disease (CKD)-asso-

---

[*]Corresponding author.

ciated pruritus" instead of "uremic pruritus" as a more precise nomenclature. In this review, the words "uremic pruritus", "CKD-associated pruritus" and "pruritus" are used interchangeably because the authors would like to respect each author's contribution. The prevalence of CKD-associated pruritus was found to range from 15% - 90% of patients [15] [16]. Recent data from the Dialysis Outcomes and Practice Patterns Study (DOPPS) reported that the prevalence of CKD-associated pruritus was 42% [17].

2. Clinical Characteristics of CKD-Associated Pruritus

In patients with CKD, skin lesions are usually not found. Generally, skin lesions are secondary changes such as excoriations with or without impetigo, linear crusts, papules, and ulcerations. Half of patients have generalized itching, and in the other half, pruritus is localized to the back, limbs, chest or head. Pruritus is intermittent or prolonged over hours and days, and becomes worse at night [18] [19]. Mettang & Krener [14] stated in their review that the diagnosis of uremic pruritus may be challenging because many patients with end-stage renal disease (ESRD) are suffering from other diseases, such as cardiovascular diseases, diabetes mellitus, chronic liver or hematological diseases, which may provoke itching either by itself or by medication given to treat these entities.

3. Why Is Pruritus Problematic?

A recent longitudinal study of CKD-associated pruritus in HD patients have clearly demonstrated that significant associations were found among itching intensity, severity, and health-related quality of life (HR-QOL) measures in domains such as mood, social relations, and sleep. In Japan, Narita et al. [16] recruited a total of 1773 patients on HD and evaluated the severity of pruritus with a visual analogue scale (VAS). Four hundred and fifty-three patients had severe pruritus with a VAS score of more than or equal to 7.0. Further, 70% of these patients complained of sleep disturbances. From these data, it is clear that patients who suffer from pruritus also have a lower HR-QOL including sleep disturbances which may lead to poor prognosis.

4. Pathogenesis of Itch

The exact pathophysiological mechanisms of CKD-associated pruritus still remain unexplained. Recently, the role of opioid μ-receptors in the central nervous system and skin has been focused on as a promising candidate in the pathophysiological mechanism of itch [20]. Further, a more recent report showed an imbalance between the antagonistic activities of μ- and κ-opioid receptors in favor of μ-receptor activation in CKD-associated pruritus [21].

In conjunction with other advances in the pathophysiology of itch, some central imaging studies on itch using positron emission tomography (PET) and functional magnetic resonance image (fMRI) have provided further information on itch processing in the brain [22]. In these studies, the premotor areas, prefrontal cortex, anterior cingulate cortex, and cerebellum were found to be activated. When comparing the brain areas involved in itch and pain processing, a large overlap between the two sensations was identified. However, this comparison is based on only a few studies and is largely regarded as preliminary.

The itch-selective spinal neurons from a distinct pathway project from lamina I of the spinal cord to the ventrocaudal part of the nucleus medialis, which projects to the anterior cingulate and dorsal insular cortices. The supraspinal processing of itch and its corresponding scratch response in humans have recently been investigated by PET and fMRI. Induction of itch by histamine application coactivates the anterior cingulate and insular cortices, premotor and supplementary motor areas, cerebellum, primary somatosensory cortex, and thalamus. As done earlier for pain sensation, particular aspects of the itch sensation are correlated with the activation of certain brain areas; spatial and temporal aspects may be processed in the primary somatosensory cortex, planning of the scratch response in the premotor and supplementary motor cortices, and affective and motivational aspects in the anterior cingulate and insular cortices.

In addition, slow-conducting c-fibers that transduce itch spinal have recently been discovered [23], and these new findings will develop further our understanding of the neurobiology of itch.

5. Treatment for CKD-Associated Pruritus

5.1. Modification of Dialysis Techniques

Introduction of the use of biocompatible dialysis membranes has reduced the prevalence of pruritus in HD patients [7]. However, it still remains uncertain whether alterations in dialysis therapy including changes in dialysis membrane can reduce pruritus [24] [25] or not [26]. Hiroshige *et al.* [27] analyzed data on 59 HD patients, who did not have disorders in calcium and phosphate metabolism, and found that more than 60% of them suffered from disabling pruritus possibly related to chronic uremia. Blood urea nitrogen (BUN) and plasma β_2-microglobulin, both of which are biochemical factors that are associated with the prevalence of pruritus and dialysis efficacy, were investigated and calculated by urea kinetics. Significantly higher values of BUN and plasma β_2-microglobulin were observed just before the dialysis session in pruritic patients with lower dialysis efficacy as estimated by Kt/V urea and normalized protein catabolic rate (nPCR), respectively. After 3 months without changing the dialysis prescriptions, 16 patients with a mean Kt/V urea and an nPCR of 1.28 and 1.22 g/kg/day, respectively, experienced significant reductions in the degree of pruritus as estimated by the pruritic score, from 12.6 ± 5.1 to 6.3 ± 3.2 ($P < 0.001$). Twenty-two patients with a mean Kt/V urea and an nPCR of 1.09 and 1.01, respectively, continued to suffer severe pruritus (score: 12.3 ± 4.7 to 12.7 ± 6.4, $P =$ NS). In 9 of 22 patients with prolonged severe pruritus, dialysis efficacy was heightened with an increase in dialyzer membrane area of more than 0.3 m^2. Seven of 9 patients with increased dialysis prescription had significant reductions in the mean pruritic score, from 12.6 ± 4.8 to 6.3 ± 2.4, which was inversely related to the significant increase of Kt/V urea from 1.05 ± 0.25 to 1.24 ± 0.33 ($P < 0.05$); among patients whose dialysis prescription did not change, only one had a significant reduction in pruritic score. The authors concluded that higher dialysis efficacy with good nutritional state reduces the prevalence and degree of pruritus in HD patients.

Previously, Graf *et al.* [28] reported that lowering the dialysate magnesium concentration can restore nerve conduction velocity towards normal in patients receiving HD, and this could be the reason for the complete disappearance of pruritus in the study by Hiroshige *et al.* [24]. In contrast, Carmichael *et al.* [29] failed to demonstrate a beneficial effect of reduction in magnesium on pruritus. In their trial, although they showed that a magnesium-free dialysis fluid corrected hypermagnesaemia, it failed to improve renal itch. In addition, the fall in serum magnesium concentration was associated with an increased concentration of parathyroid hormone, as previously noted, with the potential of producing renal osteodystrophy in the long term. It is therefore difficult to generalize the findings from the study by Hiroshige and colleagues.

The role of calcium in the dialysate was discussed by Kyriazi *et al.* [30], who showed that reduction in dialysis calcium concentrations from 1.75 to 1.0 mmol/L was associated with a $41.421\% \pm 8.47\%$ ($P < 0.05$) relief from itching in 4 HD patients, indicating that at least in some uremic individuals, ionized calcium (iCa) has a pivotal role in the neuropathophysiology of CKD-associated pruritus. It has been postulated that calcium contributes to itching by influencing the degranulation of cutaneous mast cells, thus appearing to be a modifier rather than an initiator of CKD-associated pruritus.

Polymethylmethacrylate (PMMA) artificial kidney (AK) has been reported to adsorb more serum cytokines than other high-flux AK. In 30 patients with severe uremic pruritus out of 300 chronic patients in a single center who entered this prospective study, the dialyzers were changed to PMMA AK for 4 weeks. There were no significant differences in the laboratory assay results including predialysis serum BUN, creatinine (Cr), β_2 microglobulin, calcium, phosphate, calcium-phosphate product, intact parathyroid hormone (iPTH), ferritin, hematocrit, high-sensitivity C-reactive protein (hsCRP), interleukin (IL)-1β, IL-2, IL-6, IL-18, tumor necrosis factor (TNF)-α, and Kt/V. PMMA AK was effective in reducing the pruritus score from 23.46 ± 11.94 to 7.38 ± 6.42 ($P < 0.001$). The effect of uremic pruritus relief appeared after 1 week of PMMA AK use. In spite of this study, the mechanism for the beneficial effect of PMMA AK on uremic pruritus remains to be determined. However, it is proposed that PMMA AK may be a useful adjuvant therapy in chronic HD patients with severe uremic pruritus.

In line with this study, Kato *et al.* [31] conducted a 6-month prospective and crossover trial to investigate the effect of PMMA membrane for renal itching. They examined the role of the TNF-α system in pruritus in hemodialysis patients through assessment of the degree of skin itching and measurement of circulating levels of TNF-α and soluble TNF receptors (sTNFR-I, sTNFR-II) in 19 HD patients, who were complicated with prolonged severe pruritus for 6 months. However, no association was found between the degree of pruritus and circulating sTNFR-I and II values. Skin itching scale was significantly decreased from 2.7 ± 0.2 to 2.1 ± 0.3 following the use of PMMA membrane for 3 months ($P < 0.05$). In contrast, there was no change in itching scale during 3 months of conventional therapy (2.2 ± 0.3 versus 2.2 ± 0.3, $P =$ NS). PMMA itself did not affect serum TNF-α and sTNFR values as compared to conventional dialyzer membranes. These findings suggested that the PMMA dialyzer can improve renal itching, but not through modification of the TNF-α system.

5.2. Topical Treatments

Emollients have been shown to be beneficial in patients with CKD-associated pruritus [32]-[34]. In general, emollients are proposed for use as first-line treatment. Among emollients, aqueous gels have been shown to reduce pruritus; previously, Okada and Matsumoto [35] demonstrated that emollients with high water content effectively reduced itch. In their report, 20 HD patients were divided into two groups; one group was treated with an aqueous gel containing 80% water (ADJUPEX Ensemble gel, ADJUPEX Co. Ltd., Tokyo, Japan) and another group did not receive any emollient treatment. The aqueous gel consisted of 80 g of water and 20 g of aloe vera extract, silk powder, naturally-derived vitamin E, squalane, and other naturally-derived ingredients. The gel contained no synthetic surfactants, artificial fragrance, color mineral oil, synthetic antioxidants, or alcohol. The emollient was applied twice daily for 2 weeks. VAS scores for itching at 2 weeks were significantly decreased compared with that at week 0. In addition, skin dryness was significantly improved. The results showed that an aqueous gel containing high water content effectively improves itching in HD patients with mild uremic pruritus. Besides, psychological discomfort also improved.

These findings corroborated those that were already reported by Itai et al. [36], who examined the effects of aromatherapy (odorless condition, lavender, and hiba oil) on mood and anxiety in 14 female patients who were being treated with chronic HD. A control period consisting of natural hospital smells was established before each test session, and then aromatic test conditions including lavender and hiba oil aromas were systematically compared with odorless conditions. The effects of aromatherapy were measured using the Hamilton rating scale for depression (HAMD) and the Hamilton rating scale for anxiety (HAMA). Hiba oil aroma significantly decreased the mean scores of HAMD and HAMA, and lavender aroma significantly decreased the mean scores of HAMA. The mean scores of HAMD and HAMA in odorless conditions were not significantly different from those of the control conditions. These results indicate that in chronic HD patients, hiba oil is an effective, non-invasive treatment for depression and anxiety.

In another study, a cream with structured physiological lipids (DMS, Derma Membrane Structure) and endogenous cannabinoids was tested for 3 weeks in 21 subjects with pruritus [34]. A significant reduction in pruritus was noted during the test product application using both scales for itching intensity assessment ($P < 0.0001$). Pruritus was significantly decreased at the end of the 3-week treatment ($P = 0.02$) as compared to before treatment, and was completely eliminated in eight patients (38.1%). However, the symptoms worsened slightly 2 weeks after test discontinuation, although it was still significantly less intensive than before treatment ($P < 0.001$). During the follow-up period, pruritus appeared again in 2 of these 8 subjects, but disappeared in an additional 2 patients. Therefore, at follow-up, 14 days after the end of the treatment, 8 patients (38.1%) were still free from itch. Further, xerosis was also observed in all test subjects. A 3-week treatment period resulted in complete reduction of xerosis in 17 patients (81%). During follow-up 14 days after the end of the therapy, symptoms of dry skin appeared again in 4 patients, while 13 patients (61.9%) still had smooth skin. Xerosis scores were significantly reduced during the whole study period. After discontinuation of the trial, the scores for dry skin increased, although the difference between day 21 (end of the therapy) and follow-up visit did not reach statistical significance. At follow-up visit, xerosis remained significantly less intensive as compared to the beginning of the study. The test product was very well-tolerated by all patients (100%). At the end of the treatment period, 11 patients (52.4%) found the final result of the treatment satisfactory, 8 patients (38.1%) considered it as very satisfactory, and only 2 patients (9.5%) stated that the result of the therapy was unsatisfactory. This is considered the first study to evaluate topical application of a preparation containing endocannabinoids in the treatment of uremic pruritus. In this preliminary open study, they demonstrated that the preparation with structured natural lipids and endocannabinoids could be of help in controlling itching and xerosis in patients on maintenance HD. Based on the present knowledge, the exact mechanism of antipruritic action of the tested cream could only be hypothesized. Although the antipruritic action of the evaluated preparation could be related to the its moisturizing effect, it is very probable that the observed decrease in pruritus with this therapy was not only the result of the improvement in dry skin. Based on these findings, these effects could be influenced by additional active ingredients of endocannabinoids. Dvorak et al. [37] showed that cannabinoid receptor agonists significantly reduced histamine-induced itch and vasodilatation by topical application of them before administration of histamine. In addition, N-palmitoylethanolamine was demonstrated to down-modulate mast cell degranulation induced either by neurogenic- or immune-mediated stimuli [38].

Another naturally-derived agent that may be helpful in reducing pruritus is capsaicin, which is an alkaloid extracted from the common pepper plant and marketed as a topical analgesic. Capsaicin owes its potential antipruritic properties to desensitization of nociceptive nerve endings depleting the peripheral neurons of substance P and perhaps blocking the conductor of pain or pruritus. Moreover, it is highly likely that capsaicin preferentially activates nociceptive fibers and probably, by acting as an analgesic, indirectly affects itch inhibition. However, the painful burning sensation associated with capsaicin use frequently leads to treatment withdrawal.

Breneman et al. [39] carried out an open-label, uncontrolled trial and a double-blind, vehicle-controlled trial to evaluate the efficacy and safety of capsaicin 0.025% cream in the treatment of localized areas of pruritus in patients undergoing long term HD. Eight of nine evaluable patients in the open-label trial reported marked relief or complete resolution of itching during the study period, and 2 of 5 evaluable patients in the double-blind trial reported complete resolution of itching in the capsaicin-treated arm with no or minimal improvement in the vehicle-treated arm. Twelve patients in the open-label trial and two in the double-blind trial were unevaluable. No serious treatment-related adverse reactions occurred.

Further, Tarng et al. [40] reported that 19 HD patients with idiopathic, moderate (n = 5) to severe (n = 14) pruritus were examined in a double-blind, placebo-controlled, crossover study, and 17 of them completed the study. Topical capsaicin or placebo base cream was applied to localized areas of pruritus 4 times a day. The severity of pruritus and treatment-related side effects (cutaneous burning/stinging sensations, dryness, or erythema) were evaluated weekly. The results showed that 1) 14 of 17 patients reported marked relief, and 5 of these 14 patients had complete remission of pruritus during capsaicin treatment ($P < 0.001$); 2) capsaicin was significantly more effective than placebo ($P < 0.001$), and a prolonged antipruritic effect was observed 8 weeks posttreatment; 3) no serious side effects were noted during the study; and 4) there were no significant changes in serum concentrations of albumin, calcium, phosphorus, alkaline phosphatase, or iPTH during the treatment with either capsaicin or placebo. According to their results, this study provides indirect evidence that in idiopathic pruritus in some patients on maintenance HD, substance P may be transmitted from the peripheral sensory neurons to the central nervous system because local application of capsaicin depletes the peripheral neurons of substance P and may block the conduction of pruritus. Moreover, the unique pharmacological effect of topical capsaicin may be able to markedly improve the pruritus of certain patients.

In another study, Weisshaar et al. [41] reported that 11 pruritic patients on HD and 10 controls were treated with capsaicin 0.05% liniment on the upper back three times daily for 5 days. Study parameters investigated were wheal and flare reactions, itch, and alloknesis (perifocal itch sensation induced by usually non-itching stimuli) after serotonin and histamine iontophoresis in treated and untreated skin. There were no significant differences in any parameter before and after HD. In both groups, itching was not significantly reduced by capsaicin as compared to untreated skin. Itching, however, was significantly lower in capsaicin-pretreated patients when comparing to controls. They summarized that topical capsaicin showed some antipruritic potency in HD patients in this experimental model and may therefore be considered as a co-medication in HD patients.

In addition to the components described above, essential fatty acids and their derivatives are necessary for normal cutaneous function and are thus proposed as potential treatments of pruritus. Tamimi et al. [42] found that primrose oil rich in the essential fatty acid gamma-linolenic acid (GLA) may be beneficial in alleviating pruritus, although findings did not reach statistical significance. Chen et al. [43] hypothesized that transepidermal absorption of GLA or its metabolites mediate a local anti-inflammatory and immunoregulatory effect, providing relief from pruritus. They found that GLA-rich cream was better than placebo-based cream for alleviating uremic pruritus, thus it is a useful adjuvant in the management of refractory uremic pruritus.

A new topically active antipruritic medication has been derived from the Amazonian Medicine Sangre de Grado [44]. The reported antipruritic effect on itch induced by insect bite was convincing, based on its role as a potent inhibitor of sensory afferent nerves. Moreover, Sangre de Grado is an effective analgesic and anti-inflammatory agent when applied topically.

In addition to naturally-derived agents, chemical formulations, such as Tacrolimus, have also been studied. Tacrolimus is a calcineurin inhibitor that reduces the synthesis of IL-2 by lymphocytes. Pauli-Magnus et al. [45] reported that 3 patients on PD, severely suffering from CKD-associated pruritus and previously treated, to no avail, with other potentially effective modalities, were recruited. The patients evaluated pruritus using VAS, ranging from 0 to 10, and a detailed pruritus score 3 days prior to and during the treatment phase. Patients were instructed to apply a tacrolimus ointment 0.03% twice daily, for a period of 7 days, to areas most affected by CKD-associated pruritus. In all 3 patients, CKD-associated pruritus was reduced dramatically right from the start of treatment. Two days after treatment was stopped, pruritus slowly recurred. No side effects were noted during or after the treatment period.

Duque *et al.* [46] reported that in an attempt to confirm these findings, they conducted a randomized, double-blind, vehicle-controlled study to assess the efficacy of tacrolimus ointment 0.1% for the treatment of HD-related pruritus. The results of this study did not demonstrate that tacrolimus ointment 0.1% was more effective than vehicle in relieving uremic pruritus. Topical steroids were also prescribed to these patients, probably based on the assumption that drugs used for itch in other conditions may also work on uremic pruritus, however, the absence of controlled studies and potential serious side effects of these agents dampen the routine prescription of such drugs to HD patients.

5.3. Ultraviolet Irradiation

Ultraviolet, especially narrowband UVB, has been proposed as a potential therapeutic agent for pruritus. Although exact mechanisms of UVB therapy in CKD-associated pruritus is unknown, some possible explanations have been proposed such as inactivation of circulating pruritogenic substances [47] [48], suppression of histamine release from cutaneous mast cells [49], and reduction of cutaneous nerve fibers [50] [51]. Blachley *et al.* [52] reported that 17 patients presenting with severe pruritus were treated thrice weekly with total body exposure to either UVA or UVB light. UVB light resulted in resolution of pruritus in all cases. UVA light was without any significant effect. Skin biopsies obtained before and after UV phototherapy revealed elevated contents of calcium, magnesium, and phosphorus in all pruritic patients. The resolution of pruritus following UVB treatment was associated with a reduction in skin phosphorus to values comparable with nonpruritic uremics or healthy volunteers. Uremic pruritus may be due to increased skin divalent ion content resulting in microprecipitation of calcium or magnesium phosphate. The mechanism by which UVB improves pruritus is not clear, but it has been suggested that it may in part be due to its ability to reduce cytokine production by lymphocytes.

5.4. Acupuncture

Acupuncture can be defined as the stimulation of anatomical points on the body using a variety of techniques for therapeutic purposes. The acupuncture technique that has been most often studied scientifically involves penetrating the skin with thin, solid, metallic needles that are manipulated by the hands or by electrical stimulation. Acupuncture has been practiced in China and other Asian countries for thousands of years, and is one of the key components of traditional medicine in the East Asia area, although it has developed differently in each region.

Recently, Kim *et al.* [53] reported a systemic review of acupuncture for treating uremic pruritus in patients with ESRD. According to their analysis, all of the included subjects reported beneficial effects of acupuncture. Che-yi *et al.* [54] randomized 40 patients with refractory uremic pruritus into two groups; in group 1 (n = 20), acupuncture was applied unilaterally at the Quchi (LI11) acupoint thrice weekly for 1 month, and in group 2 (controls, n = 20), acupuncture was applied at a non-acupoint 2 cm lateral to Quchi (LI11) thrice weekly for 1 month. Subjects responded to a pruritus score questionnaire given before and at the end of the 1 month treatment and at a 3-month follow-up. The results of the pruritus scores were analyzed with the repeated measures general linear model to examine the effect of acupuncture on pruritus scores. In their findings, pruritus scores before and after acupuncture, and at the 3-month follow-up were 38.3 ± 4.3, 17.3 ± 5.5, and 16.5 ± 4.9 in group 1, and 38.3 ± 4.3, 37.5 ± 3.2, and 37.1 ± 5 in group 2 (controls), respectively. Laboratory tests showed no significant differences between the two groups. Pruritus scores were significantly lower after acupuncture and at the 3-month follow-up with a significance of $P < 0.001$. From these findings, the authors concluded that acupuncture at the Quchi (LI11) acupoint is an easy, safe, and effective method of relieving uremic pruritus.

In another study by Gao *et al.* [55], 68 cases were randomly divided by half into two groups, acupuncture or drug administration with chlor-trimenton and topical ointment for 2 weeks. While receiving HD treatment, the acupuncture group received treatment at Quchi (LI11) with lifting-thrusting reducing method, and Zusanli (ST36) with lifting-thrusting reinforcing method for 30 min. In patients who received acupuncture therapy, after one course of treatment, 24 of 34 cases (70.6%) had complete alleviation of pruritus, 9 cases (26.5%) had obvious alleviation of pruritus, and 1 case had no improvement.

Sakurada *et al.* [56] reported that almost one-third of HD patients had undergone acupuncture or had a desire to try acupuncture treatment to manage common complications. Similar findings were also reported by Shapiro *et al.* [57] in an observational study. Further, electro-acupuncture was performed on 7 HD patients with pruritus. It was noted that all the patients experienced partial or complete symptom relief during or after the electro-acupuncture treatment. Complete relief after one session of acupuncture treatment was reported in 6 patients and effects lasted up to one year.

There were very few undesirable side effects reported during and after acupuncture treatment. The mechanisms of action of acupuncture are of utmost interest. As described in the section on the pathophysiology of pruritus, it is likely that acupuncture may modulate pruritus through the endogenous opioids system. As pain and pruritus have similar pattern of activation, acupuncture analgesia is initiated by stimulation, in the muscles, of high-threshold small-diameter neurons. These nerves are able to send messages to the spinal cord and then activate the spinal cord, brain stem, and hypothalamic neurons, which, in turn, trigger endogenous opioid mechanisms.

Our group recently demonstrated a marked improvement of symptoms related with pruritus. Acupuncture was administered in 12 HD patients 1 to 3 times a week for one year. With improvement of these symptoms, QOL as evaluated by short form 36 (SF-36) health survey showed a marked increase in physical activity and sleep quality (personal communication). Interestingly, the BUN levels were significantly decreased, and those of hemoglobin increased although it did not reach statistical significance (**Figures 1-3**).

5.5. Rubdown with Japanese Dry Towels

Our group examined the effects of "rubdown with Japanese dry towels" on CKD-associated pruritus. This method is a traditional Japanese alternative medical treatment to strengthen the barrier function of the skin. Briefly, subjects were naked or wore minimal clothing to maximally expose the skin of their body. Then, the subjects prepared three sets of Japanese dry towels made with cotton. These towels were cleansed with water and then dried under sunlight. After drying, the subjects gently rubbed their whole body with these towels, and if possible, this procedure was carried out in direct sunlight. The results are shown in **Figure 4**. The mechanism by which this traditional Japanese alternative medical procedure aids in symptom relief may be because skin-rubbing produces secretion of corticosteroid hormone through stimulation of the thalamus [58]. Further, skin-rubbing eliminates the bacterial flora on the surface of the skin [59]. In combination with ultraviolet rays, skin-rubbing may prevent intrusion of c-fiber from the dermis into the epidermis which is one of the causes of itch [20] [60].

5.6. Opioid Antagonists

The use of opioid antagonists in uremic pruritus was first brought to our attention by Andersen *et al.* [61] when they published a case report about a terminally ill uremic patient successfully treated by naloxone for persistent

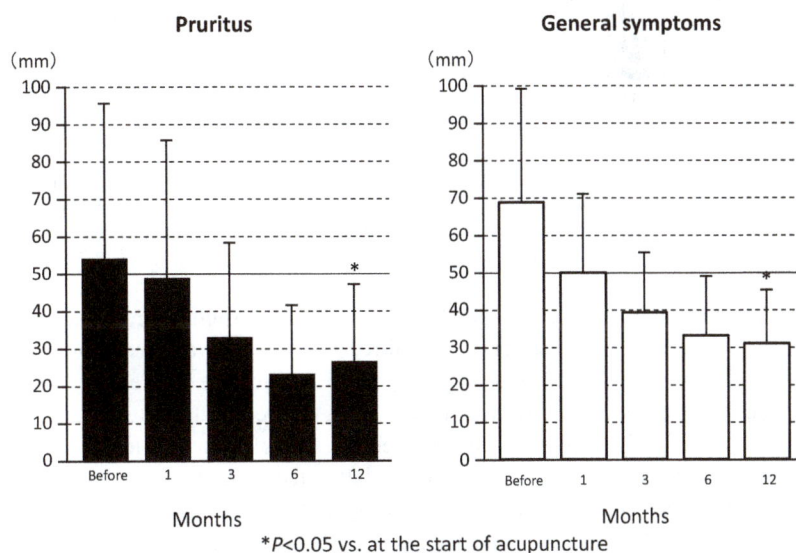

*P<0.05 vs. at the start of acupuncture

Figure 1. Changes in pruritus and general symptoms related with hemodialysis therapy by acupuncture 1 to 3 times a week for one year. Acupuncutre 1 to 3 times a week for one year produced a marked improvement in pruritus and general symptoms in patients with hemodialysis. * indicates $P < 0.05$.

Energy

Sleep

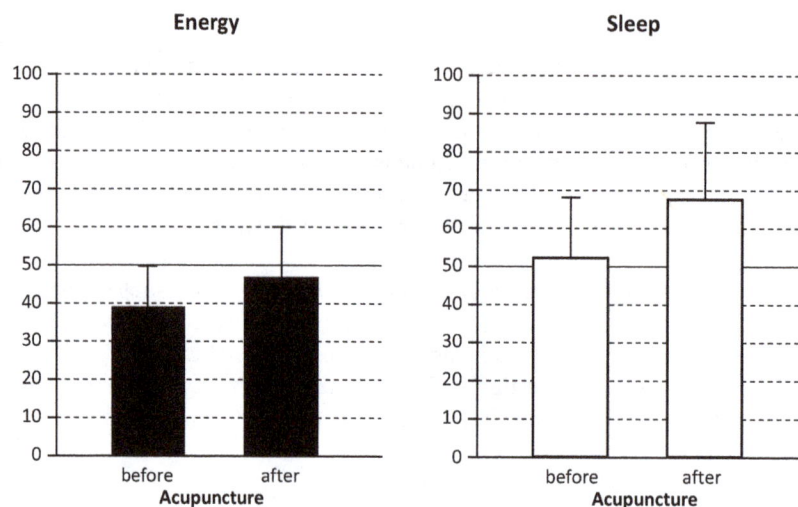

Figure 2. Changes in energy level and sleep of patients with hemodialysis by acupuncture 1 to 3 times a week for one year as evaluated by SF-36. Acupuncutre 1 to 3 times a week for one year produced a marked improvement in energy level and sleep in patients with hemodialysis.

Blood urea nitrogen

Hemoglobin

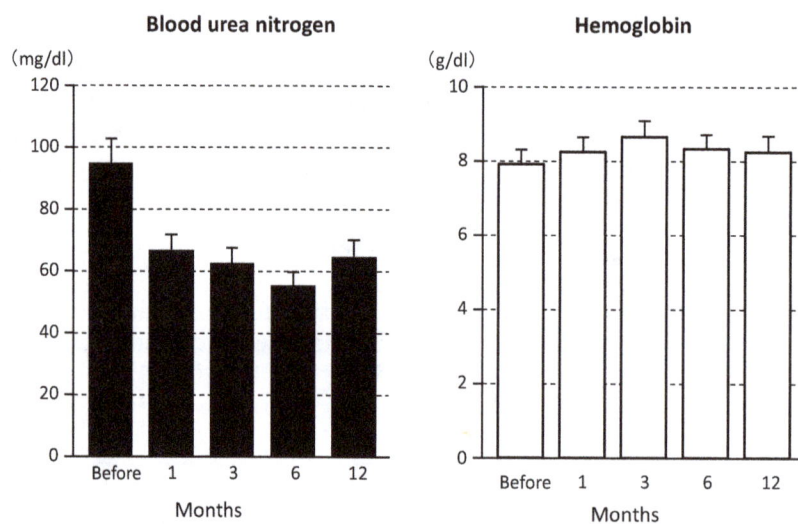

Figure 3. Changes in blood urea nitrogen and hemoglobin levels by acupuncture 1 to 3 times a week for one year. Acupuncutre 1 to 3 times a week for one year produced a marked improvement in blood urea nitrogen and hemoglobin levels in patients with hemodialysis.

itching. However, few studies were published, and these had conflicting findings. While Peer *et al.* [62] showed in a small placebo-controlled clinical trial that naltrexone, which is a μ-receptor antagonist, is effective, Pauli-Magnus *et al.* [45] failed to demonstrate any efficacy of naltrexone in the treatment of uremic pruritus. Later, Legroux-Crespel *et al.* [63] conducted a comparative study between naltrexone and loratadine, and concluded that naltrexone is not effective and not well-tolerated because of frequent side effects, except in a small subset of patients. More recently, another perspective was elaborated regarding the use of a κ-agonist, for κ-receptor stimulation inhibits μ-receptor effects both peripherally and centrally, and hence might inhibit itching induced by substance P. In line with this concept, Wikstrom *et al.* [64] conducted two multicenter, randomized, double-blind, placebo-controlled studies that enrolled 144 patients with uremic pruritus to receive post-dialysis intravenous treatment with either nalfurafine, a novel κ-receptor agonist, or placebo for 2 to 4 weeks. Statistically significant reductions in itching, itching intensity, excoriations, and sleep disturbances were noted in the nalfurafine group as compared to the placebo group.

In light of all these findings, Toray Industries, Inc., Japan, recently developed nalfurafine, with refined opioid receptor affinity and selectivity, as an agent for relief of pruritus [65] [66]. In studies using animal models, nalfurafine exerted antipruritic activity not only for antihistamine-sensitive itch, but also for antihistamine-resistant itch [67] [68].

Kumagai *et al.* [69] carried out a prospective, randomized, double-blind comparative study for 2 weeks to compare the antipruritic effect of oral nalfurafine (2.5 and 5.0 µg) with a placebo in 337 patients. The mean pruritus value as assessed by VAS was 75.2 mm during the pre-observation period, which decreased significantly to 50.9 in weeks 2. The mean decrease in VAS from baseline was significantly larger in the 2 µg (n = 112, P = 0.0001) and 5 µg (n = 114, P = 0.0002) nalfurafine groups than in the placebo group (n = 111). However, adverse drug reactions (ADRs) occurred in 103 patients, and the incidence was 25.0% in the 2.5 µg group, 35.1% in the 5 µg group, and 16.2% in the placebo group. The most common ADR was insomnia, observed in 24 of the 226 nalfurafine patients (22.3%). It is interesting to note that the group that received placebo also had a similar decrease in itching. It is well known that placebo-induced expectancies have been shown to decrease pain in a manner reversible by opioid antagonists. This phenomenon is corroborated by the findings of Wager *et al.* [70], who demonstrated using fMRI that placebo analgesia was related to decreased brain activity in pain-sensitive brain regions, including the thalamus, insula, and anterior cingulate cortex.

Further, Kumagai *et al.* [71] carried out an open-label study examining the effects and ADRs of 52-week oral administration of nalfurafine hydrochloride in 211 HD patients with treatment-resistant itch. They found that the mean pruritus values as assessed by the VAS was 75.2 mm during the pre-observation period, which decreased significantly to 50.9 and 30.9 mm in weeks 52, indicating a long-lasting efficacy. ADRs occurred in 103 patients. Frequent ADRs were insomnia (19.4%), constipation (7.1%), and increased blood prolactin (3.3%).

6. Advantages and Disadvantages in Modalities for Treatment for Hemodialyzed Patients with Pruritus

The modalities discussed in this review are summarized in the **Table 1**.

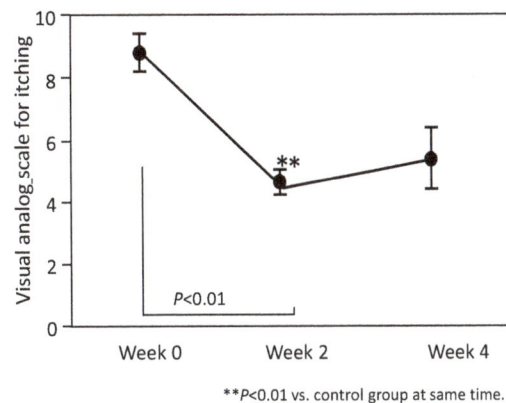

**P<0.01 vs. control group at same time.

Figure 4. Effect of rubdown with Japanese dry towels on change in visual analog scale for itching. Manipulation by rubdown with Japanese dry towels produced a marked reduction in pruritus using the visual analog scale. ** indicates $P < 0.01$.

Table 1. Comparison of various modalities for treatment for hemodialyzed patients with pruritus.

Modality	Advantages	Disadvantages
Modification of dialysis techniques	Easy	Not always effective
Emollients	Use for first-line treatment	Needs a large amount
Ultraviolet irradiation	Effective	Unclear for mechanisms
Acupuncture	Safe and effective	Needs technique
Rubdown with Japanese dry towels	Easy and safe	Not always effective
Opioid antagonists	Effective	Expensive

7. Future Perspectives

As stated in this review, recent advances in pathophysiology of itch and treatment for CKD-associated pruritus have improved this condition remarkably, however, there are still a lot of obstacles to overcome in order to achieve satisfactory comfort and relief from unpleasant symptoms stemming from pruritus. It is therefore of the utmost importance for investigators and physicians to study and research in this area.

References

[1] Stahle-Backdahl, M. (1989) Uremic Pruritus. Clinical and Experimental Studies. *Acta Dermato-Venereologica. Supplementum*, **145**, 1-38.

[2] Stahle-Backdahl, M. (1992) Pruritus in Hemodialysis Patients. *Skin Pharmacology and Physiology*, **5**, 14-20. http://dx.doi.org/10.1159/000211011

[3] Stahle-Backdahl, M. (1995) Uremic Pruritus. *Seminars in Dermatology*, **14**, 297-301. http://dx.doi.org/10.1016/S1085-5629(05)80051-3

[4] Manenti, L., Tansinda, P. and Vaglio, A. (2009) Uraemic Pruritus: Clinical Characteristics, Pathophysiology and Treatment. *Drugs*, **69**, 251-263. http://dx.doi.org/10.2165/00003495-200969030-00002

[5] Yosipovitch, G., Greaves, M.W. and Schmelz, M. (2003) Itch. *The Lancet*, **361**, 690-694. http://dx.doi.org/10.1016/S0140-6736(03)12570-6

[6] Lugon, J.R. (2005) Uremic Pruritus: A Review. *Hemodialysis International*, **9**, 180-188. http://dx.doi.org/10.1111/j.1492-7535.2005.01130.x

[7] Kosmadakis, G.C. and Zerefos, N. (2006) Uremic Pruritus. *The International Journal of Artificial Organs*, **29**, 938-943.

[8] Greaves, M.W. (2007) Recent Advances in Pathophysiology and Current Management of Itch. *Annals Academy of Medicine Singapore*, **36**, 788-792.

[9] Patel, T.S., Freedman, B.I. and Yosipovitch, G. (2007) An Update on Pruritus Associated with CKD. *American Journal of Kidney Diseases*, **50**, 11-20. http://dx.doi.org/10.1053/j.ajkd.2007.03.010

[10] Narita, I., Iguchi, S., Omori, K. and Gejyo, F. (2008) Uremic Pruritus in Chronic Hemodialysis Patients. *Journal of Nephrology*, **21**, 161-165.

[11] Berger, T.G. and Steinhoff, M. (2011) Pruritus and Renal Failure. *Seminars in Cutaneous Medicine and Surgery*, **30**, 99-100. http://dx.doi.org/10.1016/j.sder.2011.04.005

[12] Greaves, M.W. (2010) Pathogenesis and Treatment of Pruritus. *Current Allergy and Asthma Reports*, **10**, 236-242. http://dx.doi.org/10.1007/s11882-010-0117-z

[13] Kfoury, L.W. and Jurdi, M.A. (2012) Uremic Pruritus. *Journal of Nephrology*, **25**, 644-652. http://dx.doi.org/10.5301/jn.5000039

[14] Mettang, T. and Kremer, A.E. (2014) Uremic Pruritus. *Kidney International*. [Equib ahead of print] http://dx.doi.org/10.1038/ki.2013.454

[15] Pontremoli, R., Sofia, A., Ravera, M., Nicolella, C., Viazzi, F., Tirotta, A., *et al.* (1997) Prevalence and Clinical Correlates of Microalbuminuria in Essential Hypertension: The MAGIC Study. *Hypertension*, **30**, 1135-1143. http://dx.doi.org/10.1161/01.HYP.30.5.1135

[16] Narita, I., Alchi, B., Omori, K., Sato, F., Ajiro, J., Saga, D., *et al.* (2006) Etiology and Prognostic Significance of Severe Uremic Pruritus in Chronic Hemodialysis Patients. *Kidney International*, **69**, 1626-1632. http://dx.doi.org/10.1038/sj.ki.5000251

[17] Pisoni, R.L., Wikstrom, B., Elder, S.J., Akizawa, T., Asano, Y., Keen, M.L., *et al.* (2006) Pruritus in Haemodialysis Patients: International Results from the Dialysis Outcomes and Practice Patterns Study (DOPPS). *Nephrology Dialysis Transplantation*, **21**, 3495-3505. http://dx.doi.org/10.1093/ndt/gfl461

[18] Gilchrest, B.A., Stern, R.S., Steinman, T.I., Brown, R.S., Arndt, K.A. and Anderson, W.W. (1982) Clinical Features of Pruritus among Patients Undergoing Maintenance Hemodialysis. *JAMA Dermatology*, **118**, 154-156. http://dx.doi.org/10.1001/archderm.1982.01650150016012

[19] Dar, N.R. and Akhter, A. (2006) Clinical Characteristics of Uremic Pruritus in Patients Undergoing Haemodialysis. *Journal of the College of Physicians and Surgeons-Pakistan*, **16**, 94-96.

[20] Tominaga, M. and Takamori, K. (2014) Sensitization of Itch Signaling: Itch Sensitization—Nerve Growth Factor, Semaphorins.

[21] Kumagai, H., Matsukawa, S., Sasamura, H., Hayashi, M. and Saruta, T. (2004) Prospects for a Novel κ-Opioid Recep-

tor Agonist, TRK-820, in Uremic Pruritus. In: Yoshipovitch, G., Ed., *Itch Basic Mechanisms and Therapy*, Marcel Dekker, New York, 279-286.

[22] Walter, B., Sadlo, M.N., Kupfer, J., Niemeier, V., Brosig, B., Stark, R., Vaitl, D. and Gieler, U. (2005) Brain Activation by Histamine Prick Test-Induced Itch. *Journal of Investigative Dermatology*, **125**, 380-382.

[23] Schmelz, M., Hilliges, M., Schmidt, R., Ørstavik, K., Vahlquist, C., Weidner, C., *et al.* (2003) Active "Itch Fibers" in Chronic Pruritus. *Neurology*, **61**, 564-566. http://dx.doi.org/10.1212/01.WNL.0000078193.64949.08

[24] Liakopoulos, V., Krishnan, M., Stefanidis, I., Savaj, S., Ghareeb, S., Musso, C., *et al.* (2004) Improvement in Uremic Symptoms after Increasing Daily Dialysate Volume in Patients on Chronic Peritoneal Dialysis with Declining Renal Function. *International Urology and Nephrology*, **36**, 437-443. http://dx.doi.org/10.1007/s11255-004-8788-9

[25] Szepietowski, J.C., Reich, A. and Szepietowski, T. (2005) Emollients with Endocannabinoids in the Treatment of Uremic Pruritus: Discussion of the Therapeutic Options. *Therapeutic Apheresis and Dialysis*, **9**, 277-279. http://dx.doi.org/10.1111/j.1774-9987.2005.00271.x

[26] Novak, M.J., Sheth, H., Bender, F.H., Fried, L. and Piraino, B. (2008) Improvement in Pittsburgh Symptom Score Index after Initiation of Peritoneal Dialysis. *Advances in Peritoneal Dialysis*, **24**, 46-50.

[27] Hiroshige, K., Kabashima, N., Takasugi, M. and Kuroiwa, A. (1995) Optimal Dialysis Improves Uremic Pruritus. *American Journal of Kidney Diseases*, **25**, 413-419. http://dx.doi.org/10.1016/0272-6386(95)90102-7

[28] Graf, H., Kovarik, J., Stummvoll, H.K. and Wolf, A. (1979) Disappearance of Uraemic Pruritus after Lowering Dialysate Magnesium Concentration. *British Medical Journal*, **2**, 1478-1479. http://dx.doi.org/10.1136/bmj.2.6203.1478-a

[29] Carmichael, A.J., Dickinson, F., McHugh, M.I., Martin, A.M. and Farrow, M. (1988) Magnesium Free Dialysis for Uraemic Pruritus. *British Medical Journal*, **297**, 1584-1585. http://dx.doi.org/10.1136/bmj.297.6663.1584

[30] Kyriazis, J. and Glotsos, J. (2000) Dialysate Calcium Concentration of ≤1.25 mmol/l: Is It Effective in Suppressing Uremic Pruritus? *Nephron*, **84**, 85-86. http://dx.doi.org/10.1159/000045546

[31] Kato, A., Takita, T., Furuhashi, M., Takahashi, T., Watanabe, T., Maruyama, Y. and Hishida, A. (2001) Polymethyl-methacrylate Efficacy in Reduction of Renal Itching in Hemodialysis Patients: Crossover Study and Role of Tumor Necrosis Factor-Alpha. *Artificial Organs*, **25**, 441-447. http://dx.doi.org/10.1046/j.1525-1594.2001.025006441.x

[32] Morton, C.A., Lafferty, M., Hau, C., Henderson, I., Jones, M. and Lowe, J.G. (1996) Pruritus and Skin Hydration during Dialysis. *Nephrology Dialysis Transplantation*, **11**, 2031-2036. http://dx.doi.org/10.1093/oxfordjournals.ndt.a027092

[33] Twycross, R., Greaves, M.W., Handwerker, H., Jones, E.A., Libretto, S.E., Szepietowski, J.C. and Zylicz, Z. (2003) Itch: Scratching More than the Surface. *QJM: An International Journal of Medicine*, **96**, 7-26. http://dx.doi.org/10.1093/qjmed/hcg002

[34] Szepietowski, J.C., Szepietowski, T. and Reich, A. (2005) Efficacy and Tolerance of the Cream Containing Structured Physiological Lipids with Endocannabinoids in the Treatment of Uremic Pruritus: A Preliminary Study. *Acta Dermatovenerologica Croatica*, **13**, 97-103.

[35] Okada, K. and Matsumoto, K. (2004) Effect of Skin Care with an Emollient Containing a High Water Content on Mild Uremic Pruritus. *Therapeutic Apheresis and Dialysis*, **8**, 419-422. http://dx.doi.org/10.1111/j.1526-0968.2004.00175.x

[36] Itai, T., Amayasu, H., Kuribayashi, M., Kawamura, N., Okada, M., Momose, A., *et al.* (2000) Psychological Effects of Aromatherapy on Chronic Hemodialysis Patients. *Psychiatry and Clinical Neurosciences*, **54**, 393-397. http://dx.doi.org/10.1046/j.1440-1819.2000.00727.x

[37] Dvorak, M., Watkinson, A., McGlone, F. and Rukwied, R. (2003) Histamine Induced Responses Are Attenuated by a Cannabinoid Receptor Agonist in Human Skin. *Inflammation Research*, **52**, 238-245.

[38] Facci, L., Dal Toso, R., Romanello, S., Buriani, A., Skaper, S.D. and Leon, A. (1995) Mast Cells Express a Peripheral Cannabinoid Receptor with Differential Sensitivity to Anandamide and Palmitoylethanolamide. *Proceedings of the National Academy of Sciences of the United States of America*, **92**, 3376-3380. http://dx.doi.org/10.1073/pnas.92.8.3376

[39] Breneman, D.L., Cardone, J.S., Blumsack, R.F., Lather, R.M., Searle, E.A. and Pollack, V.E. (1992) Topical Capsaicin for Treatment of Hemodialysis-Related Pruritus. *Journal of the American Academy of Dermatology*, **26**, 91-94. http://dx.doi.org/10.1016/0190-9622(92)70013-6

[40] Tarng, D.C., Cho, Y.L., Liu, H.N. and Huang, T.P. (1996) Hemodialysis-Related Pruritus: A Double-Blind, Placebo-Controlled, Crossover Study of Capsaicin 0.025% Cream. *Nephron*, **72**, 617-622. http://dx.doi.org/10.1159/000188949

[41] Weisshaar, E., Dunker, N. and Gollnick, H. (2003) Topical Capsaicin Therapy in Humans with Hemodialysis-Related Pruritus. *Neuroscience Letters*, **345**, 192-194. http://dx.doi.org/10.1016/S0304-3940(03)00511-1

[42] Tamimi, N.A., Mikhail, A.I. and Stevens, P.E. (1999) Role of γ-Linolenic Acid in Uraemic Pruritus. *Nephron*, **83**, 170-171. http://dx.doi.org/10.1159/000045498

[43] Chen, Y.C., Chiu, W.T. and Wu, M.S. (2006) Therapeutic Effect of Topical Gamma-Linolenic Acid on Refractory Uremic Pruritus. *American Journal of Kidney Diseases*, **48**, 69-76. http://dx.doi.org/10.1053/j.ajkd.2006.03.082

[44] Miller, M.J.S., Vergnolle, N., McKnight, W., Musah, R.A., Davison, C.A., Trentacosti, A.M., *et al.* (2001) Inhibition of Neurogenic Inflammation by the Amazonian Herbal Medicine Sangre de Grado. *Journal of Investigative Dermatology*, **117**, 725-730.

[45] Pauli-Magnus, C., Mikus, G., Alscher, D.M., Kirschner, T., Nagel, W., Gugeler, N., *et al.* (2000) Naltrexone Does Not Relieve Uremic Pruritus: Results of a Randomized, Double-Blind, Placebo-Controlled Crossover Study. *Journal of the American Society of Nephrology*, **11**, 514-519.

[46] Duque, M.I., Thevarajah, S., Chan, Y.H., Tuttle, A.B., Freedman, B.I. and Yosipovitch, G. (2006) Uremic Pruritus Is Associated with Higher kt/V and Serum Calcium Concentration. *Clinical Nephrology*, **66**, 184-191. http://dx.doi.org/10.5414/CNP66184

[47] Gilchrest, B.A., Rowe, J.W., Brown, R.S., Steinman, T.I. and Arndt, K.A. (1979) Ultraviolet Phototherapy of Uremic Pruritus: Long-Term Results and Possible Mechanism of Action. *Annals of Internal Medicine*, **91**, 17-21. http://dx.doi.org/10.7326/0003-4819-91-1-17

[48] Shultz, B. and Roenigk, H. (1980) Uremic Pruritus Treated with Ultraviolet Light. *Journal of American Medical Association*, **243**, 1836-1837. http://dx.doi.org/10.1001/jama.1980.03300440038023

[49] Imazu, L.E., Tachibana, T., Danno, K., Tanaka, M. and Imamura, S. (1993) Histamine-Releasing Factor(s) in Sera of Uraemic Pruritus Patients in a Possible Mechanism of UVB Therapy. *Archives of Dermatological Research*, **285**, 423-427. http://dx.doi.org/10.1007/BF00372137

[50] Fjellner, B. and Hagermark, O. (1982) Influence of Ultraviolet Light on Itch and Flare Reactions in Human Skin Induced by Histamine and the Histamine Liberator Compound 48/80. *Acta Dermato-Venereologica*, **62**, 137-140.

[51] Wallengren, J. and Sundler, F. (2004) Phototherapy Reduces the Number of Epidermal and CGRP-Positive Dermal Nerve Fibres. *Acta Dermato-Venereologica*, **84**, 111-115. http://dx.doi.org/10.1080/00015550310022899

[52] Blachley, J.D., Blankenship, D.M., Menter, A., Parker III, T.F. and Knochel, J.P. (1985) Uremic Pruritus: Skin Divalent Ion Content and Response to Ultraviolet Phototherapy. *American Journal of Kidney Diseases*, **5**, 237-241. http://dx.doi.org/10.1016/S0272-6386(85)80115-3

[53] Kim, K.H., Lee, M.S., Choi, S.M. and Ernst, E. (2010) Acupuncture for Treating Uremic Pruritus in Patients with End-Stage Renal Disease: A Systematic Review. *Journal of Pain and Symptom Management*, **40**, 117-125. http://dx.doi.org/10.1016/j.jpainsymman.2009.11.325

[54] Che-Yi, C., Wen, C.Y., Min-Tsung, K. and Chiu-Ching, H. (2005) Acupuncture in Haemodialysis Patients at the Quchi (LI11) Acupoint for Refractory Uraemic Pruritus. *Nephrology Dialysis Transplantation*, **20**, 1912-1915. http://dx.doi.org/10.1093/ndt/gfh955

[55] Gao, H., Zhang, W. and Wang, Y. (2002) Acupuncture Treatment for 34 Cases of Uremic Cutaneous Pruritus. *Journal of Traditional Chinese Medicine*, **22**, 29-30.

[56] Sakuraba, H., Takeuchi, H., Takeuchi, M., Syoji, M. and Moriyama, T. (2007) Questionnaire Survey of Complaints and Accupuncutre Treatment in Maintenance Hemodialysis Patients. *Nihon Toseki Igakkai Zasshi*, **40**, 513-516. http://dx.doi.org/10.4009/jsdt.40.513

[57] Shapiro, R., Stockard, H. and Schank, A. (1986) Successful Treatment of Uremic Pruritus with Acupuncutre. *American Journal of Acupuncture*, **14**, 235-242.

[58] Antoni, F. (1986) Hypothalamic Control of Adrenocorticotropin Secretion: Advances Since the Discovery of 41-Redue Corticotropin-Releasing Factor. *Endocrine Reviews*, **7**, 351-378. http://dx.doi.org/10.1210/edrv-7-4-351

[59] Percival, S.L., Emanuel, C., Cutting, K.F. and Williams, D.W. (2012) Microbiology of the Skin and the Role of Biofilms in Infection. *International Wound Journal*, **9**, 14-32. http://dx.doi.org/10.1111/j.1742-481X.2011.00836.x

[60] Tominaga, M. and Takamori, K. (2013) An Update on Peripheral Mechanisms and Treatments of Itch. *Biological and Pharmaceutical Bulletin*, **36**, 1241-1247. http://dx.doi.org/10.1248/bpb.b13-00319

[61] Andersen, L.W., Friedberg, M. and Lokkegaard, N. (1984) Naloxone in the Treatment of Uremic Pruritus: A Case History. *Clinical Nephrology*, **21**, 355-356.

[62] Peer, G., Kivity, S., Agami, O., Fireman, E., Silverberg, D., Blum, M. and Iaina, A. (1996) Randomised Crossover Trial of Naltrexone in Uraemic Pruritus. *Lancet*, **348**, 1552-1554. http://dx.doi.org/10.1016/S0140-6736(96)04176-1

[63] Legroux-Crespel, E., Cledes, J. and Misery, L. (2004) A Comparative Study on the Effects of Naltrexone and Loratadine on Uremic Pruritus. *Dermatology*, **208**, 326-330. http://dx.doi.org/10.1159/000077841

[64] Wikstrom, B., Gellert, R., Ladefoged, S.D., Danda, Y., Akai, M., Ide, K., *et al.* (2005) κ-Opioid System in Uremic Pruritus: Multicenter, Randomized, Double-Blind, Placebo-Controlled Clinical Studies. *Journal of the American Society of Nephrology*, **16**, 3742-3747. http://dx.doi.org/10.1681/ASN.2005020152

[65] Seki, T., Awamura, S., Kimura, C., Ide, S., Sakano, K., Minami, M., *et al.* (1999) Pharmacological Properties of TRK-820 on Cloned μ-, δ- and κ-Opioid Receptors and Nociceptin Receptor. *European Journal of Pharmacology*, **376**, 159-167. http://dx.doi.org/10.1016/S0014-2999(99)00369-6

[66] Nagase, H., Hayakawa, J., Kawamura, K., Kawai, K., Takezawa, Y., Matsuura, H., *et al.* (1998) Discovery of a Structurally Novel Opioid κ-Agonist Derived from 4,5-Epoxymorphinan. *Chemical and Pharmaceutical Bulletin* (*Tokyo*), **46**, 366-369. http://dx.doi.org/10.1248/cpb.46.366

[67] Wakasa, Y., Fujiwara, A., Umeuchi, H., Endoh, T., Okano, K., Tanaka, T. and Nagase, H. (2004) Inhibitory Effects of TRK-820 on Systemic Skin Scratching Induced by Morphine in Rhesus Monkeys. *Life Sciences*, **75**, 2947-2957. http://dx.doi.org/10.1016/j.lfs.2004.05.033

[68] Togashi, Y., Umeuchi, H., Okano, K., Ando, N., Yoshizawa, Y., Honda, T., *et al.* (2002) Antipruritic Activity of the κ-Opioid Receptor Agonist, TRK-820. *European Journal of Pharmacology*, **435**, 259-264. http://dx.doi.org/10.1016/S0014-2999(01)01588-6

[69] Kumagai, H., Ebata, T., Takamori, K., Muramatsu, T., Nakamoto, H. and Suzuki, H. (2010) Effect of a Novel κ-Receptor Agonist, Nalfurafine Hydrochloride, on Severe Itch in 337 Haemodialysis Patients: A Phase III, Randomized, Double-Blind, Placebo-Controlled Study. *Nephrology Dialysis Transplantation*, **25**, 1251-1257. http://dx.doi.org/10.1093/ndt/gfp588

[70] Wager, T.D., Rilling, J.K., Smith, E.E., Sokolik, A., Casey, K.L., Davidson, R.J., *et al.* (2004) Placebo-Induced Changes in FMRI in the Anticipation and Experience of Pain. *Science*, **303**, 1162-1167. http://dx.doi.org/10.1126/science.1093065

[71] Kumagai, H., Ebata, T., Takamori, K., Miyasato, K., Muramatsu, T., Nakamoto, H., *et al.* (2012) Efficacy and Safety of a Novel κ-Agonist for Managing Intractable Pruritus in Dialysis Patients. *American Journal of Nephrology*, **36**, 175-183. http://dx.doi.org/10.1159/000341268

11

Subjective Burden on Family Carers of Hemodialysis Patients

Magda M. Bayoumi

Medical Surgical Nursing, Nursing College, King Khalid University, Abha, Saudi Arabia
Email: mbayeome@kku.edu.sa

Abstract

Background: Hemodialysis (HD) is an important objective burden (task) on patient with end stage renal disease (ESRD) and the caregiver has a subjective burden which contributes to lifestyle changes, which result in depression, anxiety declining physical health, social isolation and financial strain. Aim: To evaluate the subjective burden on family caregiver who cares patient on maintenance hemodialysis therapy. Methods: Fifty main family caregivers for each patient on HD and the instrument were used by Caregiver Burden Interview (CBI) completed by caregiver as a major of subjective response to care giving. Results: The present study findings demonstrated that main age of caregiver was 40 (11.0) years, two thirds of females, and they were mostly married (78.0%) with children. The total family caregiver burden reported was 43.3 (21.7), role strain 50.0 (25.4) and the personal strain 39.5 (19.7). The total caregivers' burden significantly positively correlated with the patients' age (r = 0.461) and negatively correlated with patients' level of education (r = −0.290). Moreover the role strain, personal strain and total caregiver burden scores were statistically and significantly negatively correlated with their age (r = −0.444) and level of education (r = −0.416) and the total burden scores were ranked as moderately to severely burdened all family caregivers. Conclusion: Caregivers' appraisal, coping strategies, interpersonal relationship issues, and social support would need to be considered for caregivers of patients maintained on HD.

Keywords

Dialysis, Burden, Family Caregiver, Saudi Arabia

1. Introduction

Dialysis patients are at increasing risk of physical, cognitive and emotional impairment related to many factors: such as length of dialysis duration, dialysis populations' ages, high prevalence of cardiovascular risk factors and multiple metabolic disturbances [1]. Accordingly, the mainstay of therapy for end stage renal disease (ESRD) hemodialysis (HD) places a burden in terms of the need for ongoing medical intervention and treatment time [2]. It is essential to properly control the symptoms and complications of ESRD and work towards the full rehabilitation of the renal patient [3]. Related to burden of HD described, a number of physical symptoms that they found were stressful, feeling sick, fatigue, insomnia, heart problems, and decreased mobility. The theme of stressors is composing of participants' experiences of physical, psychological, and logistical stressors. However, the stressors were defined by patients' experience, responses and preparatory behaviors to those stressors, regrets and advice [4]. As well, most chronically ill patients are cared for by an informal support system comprised of family members. Moreover caring for patients with chronic and disabling disease is associated with the caregivers' experiencing physical and psychological distress, limitations to their personal and social activities, and financial burden [5]. Especially the experience of a wife caregiver has been described as a mixture of anger, helplessness, guilt and isolation and was deemed to have lost freedom, because they had relinquished recreational and social activities [6].

The patients, who are physically and/or mentally unable to provide the necessary treatment for themselves, require a caregiver to assume major responsibility for their treatment [7], whereas the burden of family caregivers leads to negative consequences not only for themselves but also for patients, other family members, and health care system. Moreover for caregivers, burden negatively affects caregiver's physical, emotional, and economic status [8].

Family caregiver is the most important person who cares for patient. However, when care is provided for a long time, he/she may experience the burden [9]. This in turn may result in a more negative impact on the emotional and social aspects of caregivers' lives [10].

In fact, those families which maintain primary responsibility for the care of hemodialysis patients are not well understood. Although recent studies have shown that some family members find caregiving to be burden and stressful, while others derive self satisfaction for caregiving, there is no study evaluating the subjective burden on family caregiver of hemodialysis patients in the Kingdom of Saudi Arabia. Therefore this study aimed to evaluate the subjective burden on family caregiver who cares patient on maintenance hemodialysis therapy.

2. Materials and Methods

2.1. Design and Study Population

We conducted a cross-sectional survey of 50 caregivers for their patients enrolled in the Security Forces Hospital, Riyadh, Saudi Arabia. To be eligible, a patient should have been on maintenance hemodialysis therapy for more than 3 months, regardless of age or sex. A caregiver is defined in this study as the family member who provides the physical help and support to the patient and takes the responsibility of ensuring patient's compliance with physician's dietary instructions, pharmacological prescriptions, and the dialysis routine.

2.2. Questionnaires and Data Collection

Caregivers' Background: age, sex, work status, marital status, level of education, health problem and other burden on family caregiver such as other patient in family, financial burden related to needs of caregivers' life or health problems.

2.2.1. Caregiver Burden Interview

This consisted of a 22-item self-report instrument; the Caregiver Burden Interview (CBI) was completed by caregivers as a measure of subjective response to caregiving. The instrument was translated into Arabic language. Final form was reached by consensus of experts. It was tested by a pilot study to investigate the feasibility and clarity of the tool and its translation. The dimensions of the subjective burden tool have been determined by Zarit [11]. The scales represent the dimensions of personal strain and role strain.

2.2.2. Scoring

The burden interview is scored by summing the responses of the individual items. Higher scores indicate greater caregiver distress. The level of subjective burden was determined according to the following scoring: (0 - 20) little to no burden, (21 - 40) Mild to Moderate, (41 - 60) Moderate to severe burden and (61 - 88) Sever burden.

2.3. Preparatory Phase

During this phase, the research was developing the research tools. Certain of these were obtained from authors through E-mail. Then started the process of translation, and review by experts for finalization. It has also involved preparation of the settings for the study.

2.4. Field Work

Personal interviews with the caregivers were scheduled at study settings. The researcher started to take an appointment was set with the caregiver at the hospital, at home, or at the workplace. The time for filling the questionnaire sheet from the caregiver took 10 - 15 minutes.

2.5. Limitation of the Study

The tool was lengthy, and sometimes needed more than one meeting with the caregiver. Moreover, an appointment with main caregiver may canceled regarding to caregiver time and re-scheduled again.

2.6. Ethical Consideration

The researcher met with director of the dialysis unit and explained the aim and process of the study. Caregiver's verbal consents were obtained. Complete confidentiality of any obtained information was ensured. The researcher has also assured the administration that the conduction of the study will not affect the work in the study settings.

2.7. Statistical Analysis

The SPSS version 18.0 statistical software packages for statistical analysis. Data were presented using descriptive statistics in the form of frequencies and percentages for qualitative variables, and means and standard deviations for quantitative variables. For multiple group comparisons of quantitative data, one-way analysis of variance test (ANOVA) was used. Pearson correlation analysis was used for assessment of the inter-relationships among quantitative variables. Multiple stepwise backward regression analysis was used, and analysis of variance for the full regression models were done. Statistical significance was considered at p-value < 0.05.

3. Results

The characteristics of caregivers in the sample are displayed in **Table 1**, the most of caregivers were female, Unemployed/housewife, with Basic/intermediate level of education. Moreover mostly married, and have children, with an age 52.0% more the 40 of years on average. Not all caregiver were enjoying a perfect health, since more half of them did report having health problems.

Table 2 demonstrates the scores of caregivers' burden and its components. Significant variation in caregivers burden was evident with a total score ranging from (41 - 60) Moderate to severe burden, When broken down to reflect levels of severity, the mean burden scores (43.3 + 21.7) were ranked as moderate to severe burden on family caregiver.

Table 3: The correlation between caregivers' burden scores and patients' age, duration of illness and level of education. It points to statistically significant positive correlation between total caregivers' burden score and patients' age. Conversely, total caregivers' burden score was negatively and significantly correlated to patients' level of education (r = −0.290), and positively and significantly correlated with patients' age (r = 0.461).

Table 4: Correlations between caregivers' burden scores and their age, education, and patient's duration of illness, it shows statistically significant negative correlation between total caregivers' burden score and it components to and caregivers' age and level of education.

4. Discussion

Dialysis therapy is an important objective burden (task) associated with care of patient with ESRD. Science many patients on HD require a caregiver to take care of them, with their daily living and medical needs, alternatively, objective caregiver burden, on one hand, is comprised of those tasks or burden required to care for the

Table 1. The caregivers' personal characteristics.

	Hemodialysis (n = 50)	
	No.	%
Age (years):		
<30	10	20.0
30 - 40	14	28.0
40+	26	52.0
Range		
Mean (SD)	40.6 (11.0)	
Gender:		
Male	15	30.0
Female	35	70.0
Relation to patient:		
Spouse/children	31	62.0
Others	19	38.0
Education:		
Illiterate	10	20.0
Basic/intermediate	22	44.0
High	18	36.0
Marital status:		
Married	39	78.0
Unmarried	11	22.0
Have children:		
No	8	16.0
Yes	42	84.0
Job:		
Unemployed/housewife	30	60.0
Working	20	40.0
Have health problems:		
No	18	36.0
Yes	32	64.0
Dialysis duration (months): Mean (SD)	75.1 (62.8)	

Table 2. The caregivers' burden scores.

	Hemodialysis (n = 50)	
	Mean	SD
Caregiver burden:		
Role	50.0	25.4
Personal	39.5	19.7
Total	43.3	21.7
Overall	1.6	1.5

Table 3. Correlations between caregivers' burden scores and patients' age, duration of illness, and level of education.

	Pearson correlation coefficients		
	Hemodialysis (n = 50)		
	Age	Duration	Education[#]
Caregiver burden:			
Overall	0.25	0.208	−0.22
Total	0.461[**]	0.206	−0.290[*]

[*]Statistically significant at p < 0.05; [**]Statistically significant at p < 0.01; [#]Spearman rank correlation.

Table 4. Correlations between caregivers' burden scores and their age, education, and patient's duration of illness.

	Pearson correlation coefficients		
	Hemodialysis (n = 50)		
	Age	Duration	Education[#]
Caregiver burden:			
Role	−0.386[**]	0.099	−0.334[*]
Personal	−0.473[**]	0.136	−0.458[**]
Total	−0.444[**]	0.124	−0.416[**]
Overall	−0.322[*]	0.132	−0.390[**]

[*]Statistically significant at p < 0.05; [**]Statistically significant at p < 0.01; [#]Spearman rank correlation.

client. On the other hand, subjective burden indicates the extent to which the caregiver "minds" performing these tasks [12].

Belasco and Sesso, studied the burden on family caregiver and found the majority of caregivers were women (84%), married (66%), with a mean age of 46 years, and of low socioeconomic level. Their main types of relationship with patients were wives (38%) and sons or daughters (27%) [13]. Similarly, in the study conducted by Wicks *et al.*, they have reported that the majority of caregivers were spouses (62%), females (76%), employed (67%), and lived with the patient (79%). The mean length of dialysis was 18.6 ± 18.2 months (range 5 to 82 months) for patients receiving renal replacement therapy. Which are close to that of the studied patients in this study. But as regards the unemployed caregivers in the present study were (60%) caring for hemodialysis patients for mean length of dialysis duration 75.1 ± 62.8 months [14].

Other study done by Beanlands *et al.*, were presented that caregivers role of patients on hemodialysis is very important and described specific caring tasks, including dialysis-related activities, management of diet, medications and symptoms in addition the personal caregivers shared a rich repertoire of caregiving abilities and activities that were often supported by a strong knowledge base [15]. However, the present study findings investigate perceived burden and correlates in family caregivers of hemodialysis patients, we found the caregivers remarked burden as moderate to severe similar to recent research reported that majority of the unpaid caregiver having extremely high perceptions of burden [16].

Moreover, the present study findings showed that is statistically significant positive correlation between total caregivers' burden score and patients' age. Conversely, Rioux et al. has reported that a relatively low global burden perceived by caregivers and patients undergoing nocturnal home hemodialysis [17]. Particularly the burden on family caregivers is important predictor may influenced with their level of education and age as showed in the study results, it shows statistically significant negative correlation between total caregivers' burden score and it components to caregivers' age and level of education. Conversely, Suri et al., reported no significant correlation among perceived caregiver burden and demographic factors including age, sex, race and level of education [16]. Moreover, the literature provides conflicting views regarding the significant predictor for caregiving by older people to lead to poor physical health, depression, and even increased mortality. However, younger caregivers must generally juggle work, their own family responsibilities, and sacrifices involving their social lives. Middle-aged caregivers typically worry about missed workdays, interruptions at work, taking leaves of absence, and reduced productivity [18] [19].

Arechabala *et al.* identified the depressive symptoms and degree of fatigue in caregivers of HD patients and found the primary caregivers were female spouses, with an average age of 50 ± 16.1 years. as well as the primary caregivers (43.82%) had depressive symptoms [20]. A positive association ($r = 0.43$, $p < 0.001$) statistically significant was found between self-perceived burden and the presence of depressive symptoms in patients. Caregiver burden contributes to lifestyle changes, which result in depression, anxiety, declining physical health, social isolation, and financial strain for the caregiver [21]-[23].

We found that caregivers of patient on hemodialysis reported increase burden of role strain more than personal strain. In addition, the two dimensions of personal strain and role strain are considered to reflect two important aspects of caregiving. Also, personal strain refers to how personally stressful the experience is, while overload due to role conflict constitutes role strain [24]. Because the caregiver burden contributes to lifestyle changes, which result in depression, anxiety, declining physical health, social isolation, and financial strain for the caregiver [21]-[23].

Finally, the empirical literature on family burden predictors requires more efforts to investigate how sociodemographic, clinical, and personality variables from patients and their relatives may combine to predict higher levels of burden. Plus the cultural differences, community values may play a role to identify the burden.

5. Conclusion

As the ESRD population in Saudi Arabia grows, the management of HD requires an ongoing commitment not only from the patient but also from the family when ongoing lifestyle adjustments become necessary as the disease complications. And there are minimal data regarding the identification of the aspects of caregiver burden, Caregiver's appraisal, coping strategies, interpersonal relationship issues, and social support would need to be considered for caregivers of patients maintained on HD. Nurses could render appropriate knowledge regarding hemodialysis and complications, how to help patients on hemodialysis to cope decrease burden on family caregiver and improve outcome of the patients' care. For further research, studies may investigate caregiver resources on decreasing burden, such as coping and social support especially in the eastern countries.

Acknowledgements

This research project was supported by Deanship of Scientific Research, King Khalid University. Saudi Arabia.

References

[1]   Kalirao, P., Pederson, S., Foley, R.N., Kolste, A., Tupper, D., Zaun, D., Buot, V. and Murray, A.M. (2011) Cognitive Impairment in Peritoneal Dialysis Patients. *American Journal of Kidney Diseases*, **57**, 612-620. http://dx.doi.org/10.1053/j.ajkd.2010.11.026

[2]   Kimmel, P.L., Peterson, R.A., Weihs, K.L., Simmens, S.J., Boyle, D.H., Cruz, I., Umana, W.O., Alleyne, S. and Veis, J.H. (1995) Aspects of Quality of Life in Hemodialysis Patients. *Journal of the American Society of Nephrology*, **6**, 1418-1426.

[3]   Moreno, F.J.M., Lopez Gomez, M.J., Sanz-Guajardo, D., Jofre, R. and Valderrabano, F. (1996) Quality of Life in Dialysis Patients. A Spanish Multicentre Study. *Nephrology Dialysis Transplantation*, **11**, 125-129. http://dx.doi.org/10.1093/ndt/11.supp2.125

[4]   Harwood, L., Locking-Cusolito, H., Spittal, J., Wilson, B. and White, S. (2005) Preparing for Hemodialysis: Patient Stressors and Responses. *Nephrology Nursing Journal*, **32**, 3.

[5]   Choi, K.S. and Eun, Y. (2000) A Theory Construction on the Care Experience for Spouse of Patients with Chronic Illness. *Journal of Korean Academic Nursing*, **30**, 122-136.

[6]   Kumar, S., Matreja, P.S., Gupta, A.K., Singh, A. and Garg, P. (2012) To Assess the Quality of Life (QOL) of Caregivers and Patients Suffering from Chronic Obstructive Pulmonary Disease (COPD). *Journal of Allergy and Therapy*, 2155-6121.

[7]   Gayomali, C., Sutherland, S. and Finkelstein, F.O. (2008) The Challenge for the Caregiver of the Patient with Chronic Kidney Disease. *Nephrology Dialysis Transplantation*, **23**, 3749-3751. http://dx.doi.org/10.1093/ndt/gfn577

[8]   Caqueo-Urizar, A., Gutierrez-Maldonaldo, J. and Miranda-Castillo, C.(2009) Quality of Life in Caregivers of Patients with Schizophrenia: A Literature Review. *Health and Quality of Life Outcomes*, **7**, 1-5.

[9]   Rafiyah, S.I. (2011) Sutharangsee. Review: Burden on Family Caregivers Caring for Patients with Schizophrenia and Its Related Factors. *Nurse Media Journal of Nursing*, 29-41.

[10]   Belasco, A., Barbosa, D., Bettencourt, A.R., *et al.* (2006) Quality of Life of Family Caregivers of Elderly Patients on Hemodialysis and Peritoneal Dialysis. *American Journal of Kidney Diseases*, **48**, 955-963. http://dx.doi.org/10.1053/j.ajkd.2006.08.017

[11]   Zarit, S.H., Todd, P.A. and Zarit, J.M. (1986) Subjective Burden of Husbands and Wives as Caregivers: A Longitudinal Study. *Gerontologist*, **26**, 260-266. http://dx.doi.org/10.1093/geront/26.3.260

[12]   Jones, S.L. (1996) The Association between Objective and Subjective Caregiver Burden. *ARON Psychiatric Nursing*, **10**, 77-84. http://dx.doi.org/10.1016/S0883-9417(96)80070-7

[13]   Belasco, A.G. and Sesso, R. (2002) Burden and Quality of Life of Caregivers for Hemodialysis Patients. *American Journal of Kidney Diseases*, **39**, 805-812. http://dx.doi.org/10.1053/ajkd.2002.32001

[14]   Wicks, M.N., Milstead, E.J. and Hathaway, D.K. (1997) Subjective Burden and Quality of Life End-Stage Renal Disease. *ANNA Journal*, **24**, 527-540.

[15]   Beanlands, H., Horsburgh, M.E., Fox, S., Howe, A., Locking-Cusolito, H., Pare, K. and Thrasher, C. (2005) Caregiving by Family and Friends of Adults Receiving Dialysis. *Nephrology Nursing Journal*, **32**, 621-631.

[16]   Suri, R.S., Larive, B., Garg, A.X., Hall, Y.N., Pierratos, A., Chertow, G.M., Gorodetskeya, I., Kliger, A.S. and FHN Study Group (2011) Burden on Caregivers as Perceived by Hemodialysis Patients in the Frequent Hemodialysis Network (FHN) Trials. *Nephrology Dialysis Transplantation*, **26**, 2316-2322. http://dx.doi.org/10.1093/ndt/gfr007

[17]   Rioux, J.P., Narayanan, R. and Chan, C.T. (2012) Caregiver Burden among Nocturnal Home Hemodialysis Patients. *Hemodialysis International*, **16**, 214-219. http://dx.doi.org/10.1111/j.1542-4758.2011.00657.x

[18]   Cameron, J.I., Franche, R.L., Cheung, A.M., *et al.* (2002) Lifestyle Interference and Emotional Distress in Family Caregivers of Advanced Cancer Patients. *Cancer*, **94**, 521-527.

[19]   Given, B. and Sherwood, P.R. (2006) Family Care for the Older Person with Cancer. *Seminars in Oncology Nursing*, **22**, 43-50. http://dx.doi.org/10.1016/j.soncn.2005.10.006

[20]   Arechabala, M.C., Catoni, M.I., Palma, E. and Barrios, S. (2011) Depression and Self-Perceived Burden of Care by Hemodialysis Patients and Their Caregivers. *Revista Panamericana de Salud Pública*, **30**, 74-79. http://dx.doi.org/10.1590/S1020-49892011000700011

[21]   Cossette, S. and Levesque, L. (1993) Caregiving Tasks as Predictors of Mental Health of Wife Caregivrs of Men with Chronic Obstructive Pulmonary Disease. *Research in Nursing and Health*, **16**, 251-263. http://dx.doi.org/10.1002/nur.4770160404

[22]   Kell-Card, G., Foxall, M.J. and Barron, C. (1993) Loneliness, Depression, and Social Support of Patients with COPD and Their Spouses. *Public Health Nursing*, **10**, 245-251. http://dx.doi.org/10.1111/j.1525-1446.1993.tb00060.x

[23]   Ferrans, C.E. and Powers, M.J. (1992) Psychometric Assessment of the Quality of Life Index. *Research in Nursing and Health*, **15**, 29-38. http://dx.doi.org/10.1002/nur.4770150106

[24]   Whitlatch, C.J., Zarit, S.H. and Von Eye, A. (1991) Efficacy of Interventions with Caregivers: A Reanalysis. *Gerontology*, **31**, 9-14. http://dx.doi.org/10.1093/geront/31.1.9

12

Acute Kidney Injury with Rhabdomyolysis: 25 Years Experience from a Tertiary Care Center

Rubina Naqvi*, F. Akhtar, E. Ahmed, A. Naqvi, A. Rizvi

Sindh Institute of Urology and Transplantation (SIUT), Karachi, Pakistan
Email: *rubinanaqvi@gmail.com

Abstract

Objective: To describe patients presenting with acute kidney injury after rhabdomyolysis at a tertiary renal care center in Pakistan. Patients and Methods: An observational cohort of patients identified as having acute kidney injury (AKI) with rhabdomyolysis, which was diagnosed by rise in creatinine phosphokinase (CK) and lactate dehydrogenase (LDH) more than 4 times the reference range whereas AKI was defined according to RIFLE criteria. On ultrasonography, all patients had normal size non obstructed kidneys, and no other co morbid. Results: Between January1990 to December 2014, 334 patients with rhabdomyolysis and AKI registered to this hospital. Mean age was 28.22 ± 11.22 years with M:F ratio of 3.33:1. Mean values of CK and LDH were 597,749.790 ± 180,461.360 and 4077.026 ± 5050.704 U/L with reference range of 26 - 174 U/L and 91 - 180 U/L respectively. We divided the study population into 4 groups over timeline. Rhabdomyolysis etiology was divided in 3 groups; 1) traumatic, 2) non-traumatic exertional, and 3) non-traumatic non-exertional. In the last group, which spans from 2010-2014, we treated many cases with toxic rhabdomyolysis and main toxin was paraphenylenediamine (PPD). The other causes showed more or less same prevalence over two and a half decade, except non-traymatic exertional which has decreased during last 5 years without any explainable cause. Renal replacement therapy (RRT) was required on arrival in 94% cases. Complete renal recovery was observed in 70%, while 15.86% died and 10% were lost during recovery phase. A small number 2.69% left against medical advice during acute phase of illness and 0.8% developed chronic kidney disease (CKD). Conclusion: The common clinical conditions found associated with rhabdomyolysis and AKI includes trauma, immobilization, sepsis, overexertion, and drugs and toxins. In recent years, we have seen many young patients with PPD poisoning; we have found good renal recovery in patients who survived initial 2 - 3 weeks.

---
*Corresponding author.

Keywords

Acute Kidney Injury, Rhabdomyolysis, RIFLE Criteria, Torture, Toxins, PPD

1. Introduction

Rhabdomyolysis is a syndrome in which muscle pain and necrosis occurs with release of intracellular muscle constituents into the circulation. A variety of events can lead to rhabdomyolysis and this result in rise of Creatinine phosphokinase (CK) levels. Presence of myoglobinuria may or may not be observed. The Symptomatology ranges from simple moderate elevations in serum muscle enzymes to life-threatening disease associated with extreme enzyme elevations, electrolyte imbalances (especially hyperkalemia), and acute kidney injury [1].

The final common pathway for injury in rhabdomyolysis is an increase in intracellular free ionized cytoplasmic and mitochondrial calcium. This may be caused by depletion of adenosine triphosphate (ATP), the cellular source of energy, and/or by direct injury and rupture of the plasma membrane [2] [3].

ATP depletion causes dysfunction of the Na/K-ATPase and Ca^{2+} ATPase pumps that are essential for maintaining the integrity of the muscle cells, resulting in release of muscle enzymes in the circulation. The exact mechanism of myoglobin causing defective glomerular filtration is not known. Previous experimental and clinical studies suggest that intra renal vasoconstriction, direct tubular injury, indirect (ischemic) tubular injury and intra luminal blockade with myoglobin casts all can play a role [4].

New classification of causes of rhabdomyolysis categorizes broadly into three groups, that is: traumatic, non-traumatic exertional and non-traumatic non-exertional. Traumatic includes crush syndrome or prolonged immobilization. Non-traumatic exertional includes marked exertion in untrained individuals, recurrent convulsions, human stampede, hyperthermia, or metabolic myopathies. While non-traumatic non-exertional mainly drugs, toxins and infections [5]-[9].

Detailed history and clinical examination often provide a clue for the cause in an individual.

Many large series have been published in the past, reporting relative frequencies of different etiologies [4] [5] [10]. In the present study, we report AKI secondary to rhabdomyolysis from single tertiary care center, over a period of 25 years.

2. Methods and Patients

An observational cohort of patients identified as having AKI, which was defined according to RIFLE criteria [11], with normal size, non-obstructed kidneys, after rhabdomyolysis, which was defined as rise in CK and lactate dehydrogenase (LDH) more than 4 times the reference range. Study includes all patients with AKI secondary to rhabdomyolysis registered at this institution from January 1990 to December 2014.

For our laboratory, reference ranges for CK and LDH are 26 - 174 and 91 - 180 U/L respectively. All biochemical tests were done on Unicel DxC 800 Synchron Clinical System, Beckman Coulter auto-analyzer.

Myoglobinuria was checked with $(NH_4)_2 \cdot SO_4$ method and markers for myoglobin were checked on pigment casts of histological samples. Renal biopsy was performed in 12 patients where history was dubious and patients reached late. For immunohistochemistry, tissue sections were immersed in peroxidase quenching solution and rinsed with PBS. Primary antibody (polyclonal rabbit anti human Myoglobin, Dako, Glostrup, Denmark) in dilution of 1:400 was applied for 30 - 60 minutes at room temperature followed by PBS rinsing. Secondary antibody (HRP: horse reddish peroxidase. Dako LSAB +/HRP kit, Dako, Glostrup, Denmark) was applied for 10 minutes at room temperature followed by PBS rinsing. Enzyme conjugate was applied for 10 minutes at room temperature followed by PBS rinsing. Chromogen substance (DAB, Dako, Glostrup, Denmark) was applied for 5 - 10 minutes followed by PBS rinsing and light counter stain with Hematoxylin and mounting of slides. The slides were visualized under the light microscope.

The patients who remained on follow up; which expands from first discharge to maximum of 23 years, and not recovered normal renal functions but remain dialysis free were labeled as CKD.

We divided the population in 4 time periods, for observing any change in trends in different causes of rhabdomyolysis. Whereas, rhabdomyolysis was divided in 3 groups based on etiology: Traumatic, which include crush syndrome and prolonged immobilization, torture causing blunt trauma, burn, and electrocution; non-traumatic exertional include prolonged exercises by untrained personnel and prolonged convulsions, whereas; non-traumatic non-exertional include drugs, toxins, and infections. Quantitative variables reported as means ± STD and Qualitative as percentages.

3. Results

A total of 5623 patients with AKI brought to this hospital between January 1990 to December 2014, of these 334 (5.9%) were secondary to rhabdomyolysis. Average age of patients in this group was 28.22 ± 11.29 years, 258 were male and 76 were females.

Traumatic rhabdomyolysis include 28 patients from road traffic accidents, 24 from crush injury (earthquake, collapsed roof and fire arm injuries), prolonged immobilization, electrocution, blunt trauma, burn and 58 cases of torture. Last group includes person beaten up by batons, fists, leather belts, hanging upside down and sits ups given for torture purpose (**Table 1**).

Non traumatic exertional group includes 30 people with prolonged exercise in untrained people, especially in hot weather and 23 epileptic patients brought after status epilepticus (**Table 1**).

Non traumatic non exertional group include infections and poisonings with drugs, substances or venom (**Table 1**).

During different time periods that is initial 10 years, then 5 years, 5 years and 5 years, prevalence of traumatic rhabdomyolysis remains unchanged, non traumatic exertional shown decline during last 5 years, while the last group of non traumatic non exertional rhabdomyolysis has shown dramatic increase of PPD poisoning during last 5 years (**Table 2**).

The main demographic, clinical and laboratory parameters of the study population are given in **Table 3**. Majority patients were young; males were 3.3 times more than females. Majority was in advanced uremia and muscle enzymes were many folds higher than reference range (**Table 3**).

Renal biopsy was done in 12 cases and revealed acute tubular necrosis in all with presence of pigment casts in tubular lumina in 8 cases. Immunohistochemistry for myoglobin was positive in these patients.

The complete recovery from AKI was seen in 70% of patients, highest observed in non-traumatic exertional rhabdomyolysis (83%). Mortality was high in traumatic rhabdomyolysis (22.22%), among these crush injury

Table 1. Causes of rhabdomyolysis (N = 334).

Traumatic = 126	Non Traumatic exertional = 53	Non traumatic, non-exertional = 155
RTA = 28		Poison PPD = 75
Crush injury = 24 (Including fire arm injury = 11)	Prolonged exercise = 30	Alcohol binge = 10 Marihuana Binge = 9
Prolonged immobilization = 3	Recurrent Convulsions = 23	Infections = 35
Electrocution = 3		Scorpion venom = 5 Snake venom = 5
Burn = 1		Drugs over dosage = 4
Blunt trauma = 9		Others = 12
Torture* = 58		

*Torture cases include beaten up by batons, fists, leather belts, hanging upside down, sit-ups.

Table 2. Pattern over different time periods.

Cause of Rhabdomyolysis	1990-1999 (n = 67)	2000 - 2004 (n=35)	2005-2009 (n = 52)	2010-2014 (n = 180)	Total 25 yrs (n = 334)
Traumatic	42 (62)	20 (57)	32 (62)	32 (18)	126 (37.72)
Non-traumatic exertional	21 (31)	10 (28)	13 (52)	9 (5)	53 (15.86)
Non-traumatic non-exertional	4 (6)	5 (14)	7 (13)	139 (77)	155 (46.40)

*% in parenthesis.

was worst which revealed 45.83% mortality as subgroup. For non-traumatic non-exertional group, overall mortality was 12.9% with infection contributing most (14.28%). The poisoning with PPD, which comprises largest of this last group, showed mortality of 6.6% (**Table 4**). Fifty three patients died during acute phase of illness, 26 of these within 24 hours of reaching to hospital. Multi organ failure, sepsis and recurrent hyperkalemia were main causes of mortality in the study population (**Table 5**).

Table 3. Demography and laboratory values (N = 334).

M:F	3.3:1
Age mean ± SD, years	28.221 ± 11.299
Duration of insult mean ± SD, days	7.346 ± 5.510
Hb mean ± SD, g/dl	11.300 ± 2.496
Blood Urea mean ± SD, mg/l	265.895 ± 109.411
Serum Creatinine mean ± SD, mg/l	12.142 ± 5.550
LDH mean ± SD, U/l	4077.026 ± 5050.704
CK mean ± SD, U/l	59,774.790 ± 180,461.356
AST mean ± SD, U/l	1954.298 ± 2397. 769
ALT mean ± SD, U/l	888.95 ± 1100.987

Table 4. Outcome in different groups (N = 334).

Cause	Complete recovery	Partial recovery[**]	LAMA[*]	ESRF	Died
Traumatic = 126	=84	=10	=04		=28
• RTA = 28	15	3	0		10
• Crush injury = 24	10	2	1		11
• Prolonged immobilization = 3	3	0			0
• Electrocution = 3	1	1			1
• Burn = 1	1	0			0
• Other trauma = 9	6	0			3
• Torture = 58	48	4	3		3
Non traumatic Exertional = 53	=44	=02	=00	=01	=06
• Prolonged exercise = 30	28	1	0	0	1
• Recurrent convulsion = 23	16	1	0	1	5
Non traumatic non exertional = 155	=107	=22	=05	=10	=20
• Poison PPD = 75	65	3	2	0	5
• Alcohol binge = 10	4	5	0	0	1
• Marihuana binge = 9	2	5	0	1	2
• Infections = 35	21	5	3	0	5
• Scorpion bite = 5	5	0	0	0	0
• Snake bite = 5	5	0	0	0	0
• Drug over dose = 4	3	1	0	0	0
• Others = 12	2	3	0		7

[*]LAMA: refused treatment and left against medical advice, [**]Partial recovery: trends were towards improvement but didn't turn up for follow up.

Table 5. Cause of death (N = 53).

Cause	No.	%
MOF[*]	17	32.07
Sepsis	29	54.71
Hyperkalemia	6	11.32
G I bleed	1	1.88

[*]Respiratory, circulatory and coagulation along with AKI. 26/53 deaths occurred within first 24 hours of reaching this hospital.

4. Discussion

Rhabdomyolysis has been described for thousands and thousands of years. Old Testament describes rhabdomyolysis in Israelites who consumed quail fed on hemlock [12]. Hemlock poison, also famous to execute Socrates, can cause rhabdomyolysis and acute tubular necrosis (ATN) along with other neurologic symptoms. During spring season, birds consume large amount of buds from plant and when eaten up by humans, toxins disintegrate and cause harm [13].

Musculoskeletal trauma, in particular crush syndrome, accounts for a large proportion of the cases of rhabdomyolysis. Initial reports are from 1908 during Sicilian earthquake in Messina where rescuers searched through the rubble for weeks, and whole families were still being pulled out alive, and later in timeline from German military literature and during the bombing of London in Second World War. Pigmented casts were found in the renal tubules at autopsy; however, at that time pathogenesis was unclear [14] [15].

Additional cases were described during the Korean War [16]. The decreased incidence of posttraumatic AKI during the Vietnam War could be explained on the basis of the faster evacuation techniques and improved fluid resuscitation of affected people [17].

According to previously published studies about 10% - 50% of patients with rhabdomyolysis develop AKI [18]. Whereas with extensive traumatic injuries figure rises up to 85%. Mortality for such patients, *i.e.* severe trauma, rhabdomyolysis and AKI, has been reported up to 20% [19], more so with multi-organ dysfunction syndrome [20].

Rhabdomyolysis and crush syndrome are common results of natural disasters such as earthquakes. Many reports have been published on survivors of earthquakes who suffered from crush injury and AKI [21] [22]. In the present cohort, 10 patients were from earthquake of 2005 in northern area of country [23].

Rhabdomyolysis may complicate a high-voltage electrical injury and lightning strikes. It has been reported in 10% of subjects that survive an electrical shock. The clinical course following an electrical burn is similar to that of a crush injury. Pathogenesis can be ascribed to the electrical disruption of sarcolemmal membranes, with loss of barrier function and massive calcium influx [24] [25].

Non-traumatic myoglobinuria with AKI is a relatively common disease easy to diagnose and has an excellent prognosis [26]. Risk factors for non-traumatic rhabdomyolysis, include malignant hyperpyrexia, malignant neuroleptic syndrome, extreme exertion, recurrent seizures, bacterial and viral infections, use of certain medications, and exercise by untrained personnel especially in hot and humid weather [27]. In our study, we found 15.86% patients with history of prolonged exercise or recurrent convulsions, while 10.47% had infection, and another 27.24% were affected by different toxins. To our surprise number of patients developing rhabdomyolysis after prolonged exercise has markedly decreased during last five years of study for which we have no proper explanation.

Myoglobinuria can be estimated by chemical methods, spectrophotometry and immunologic (radial immunodiffusion, complement fixation, counter immunoelectrophoresis) methods in laboratory [28]. Most simple, "sideroom" method, is to collect 5 ml of urine, mix well with 2.8 gm of $(NH_4)_2 \cdot SO_4$, allow to stand for 5 minutes and then filter, colored supernatant indicates myoglobinuria while colored precipitate hemoglobinuria [27]. Important to mention is the fact that absence of myoglobinuria does not exclude the diagnosis [5].

Non-traumatic rhabdomyolysis has also been reported with alcohol intake, where the cause is not fully understood. The patho-physiology can be quite different between short- and long-term alcohol abuses [29]. Under short-term alcohol intoxication, immobilization or coma induced by ethanol-related central nervous system sedation plays an important role in developing rhabdomyolysis. It causes muscle compression and ischemia, which will accelerate short-term alcohol myotoxicity [30], resulting in a massive breakdown of skeletal muscle over a short period of time.

In long-term alcohol abuse, electrolyte abnormalities (*i.e.*, hypokalemia, hypophosphatemia, or hypomagnesaemia) may play significant causative roles for developing rhabdomyolysis [29] [31].

There is a long list of medications and recreational drugs that can cause rhabdomyolysis by different mechanisms. Any drug that directly or indirectly impairs the production or use of ATP by skeletal muscle, or increases energy requirements that exceed the rate of ATP production, can cause rhabdomyolysis [32].

Heavy metals, insects venoms and snake venom (especially Sea-Snake and Elapids), have been reported to cause rhabdomyolysis [33]-[36]. Scorpion venom has rarely been reported as direct nephrotoxic agent [37] but extensive muscle necrosis at the site of sting which was observed in our studied population as well as reported previously, can give rise to muscle damage severe enough to cause tubular injury with myoglobin. Hemolytic uremic syndrome (HUS) has been reported after scorpion sting as a single case report in literature. [38] [39]

Another toxin, paraphenylenediamine (PPD) has been described as a hair dye since the end of 19th century. Up till now, it is reported to be used in more than 1000 oxidative hair-dyes in the USA [40] [41]. PPD is also used in the photographic or rubber industries. In addition, in many African countries, PPD in its pure form or in combination with other natural coloring extracts like Henna, is used for coloring of palms and soles for cosmetic reasons [42] [43]. Unfortunately, there are also vast numbers of unintended and intended incidents of severe to life threatening intoxication involving this synthetic compound [43] [44]. PPD intoxication leads to a severe clinical syndrome including laryngeal edema, rhabdomyolysis and subsequent renal failure, neurotoxicity and acute toxic hepatitis which *per se* can lead to dark colored urine [44]. In our experience, we have started registering the rhabdomyolysis after intoxication with PPD mainly over last two years, though reports from India and Africa as case reports or case series are there in literature [44]-[46]. In the present study, majority were young females and ingested it as an attempt for committing suicide, as the substance is easily available widely at a low cost. A case series published from India reported complete renal recovery in 61.35% of patients with PPD intoxication, but patient population was small with total cases of 13 in this particular study [44]. In our observation complete renal recovery was seen in 86.66% of PPD intoxication patients Rhabdomyolysis in association with crush injury has been reported with poor prognosis about seven decades ago [15], but with passage of time as understanding of patho-physiology improved and early methods of resuscitation adopted in large catastrophic situations, mortality rate has declined [22]. In the present study, mortality was 46% in crush injury victims but half of these succumbed to death within 24 hours of arrival to this hospital, indicating extent of insult and delay in reaching to this particular tertiary care service and poor infra structure of health facilities in country.

5. Conclusion

This study was conducted over a span of two and a half decades; we have observed changes in the pattern of causes of rhabdomyolysis. During the first decade, torture and blunt trauma was more common while during last five years largest contributing factor was toxic rhabdomyolysis with PPD ingestion. Patients who survived initial period of insult show good renal recovery. Mortality is mostly contributed by multi organ failure and sepsis. Remarkable number of deaths occurred soon after arrival highlighting the need of good supportive, well equipped infra structure at national level.

Conflict of Interest

None.

References

[1]   Miller, M.L. (2014) Clinical Manifestations and Diagnosis of Rhabdomyolysis. Up Todate, Version 11.0.

[2]   Giannoglou, G.D., Chatzizisis, Y.S. and Misirli, G. (2007) The Syndrome of Rhabdomyolysis: Pathophysiology and Diagnosis. *European Journal of Internal Medicine*, **18**, 90. http://dx.doi.org/10.1016/j.ejim.2006.09.020

[3]   Khan, F.Y. (2009) Rhabdomyolysis: A Review of the Literature. *Netherlands Journal of Medicine*, **67**, 272.

[4]   Bosch, X., Poch, E. and Grau, J.M. (2009) Rhabdomyolysis and Acute Kidney Injury. *New England Journal of Medicine*, **361**, 62-72. http://dx.doi.org/10.1056/NEJMra0801327

[5]   Gabow, P.A., Kaehny, W.D. and Kelleher, S.P. (1982) The Spectrum of Rhabdomyolysis. *Medicine (Baltimore)*, **61**, 141-152. http://dx.doi.org/10.1097/00005792-198205000-00002

[6]   Melli, G., Chaudhry, V. and Cornblath, D.R. (2005) Rhabdomyolysis: An Evaluation of 475 Hospitalized Patients. *Medicine (Baltimore)*, **84**, 377. http://dx.doi.org/10.1097/01.md.0000188565.48918.41

[7]   Huerta-Alardín, A.L., Varon, J. and Marik, P.E. (2005) Bench-to-Bedside Review: Rhabdomyolysis—An Overview for Clinicians. *Critical Care*, **9**, 158. http://dx.doi.org/10.1186/cc2978

[8]   Petejova, N. and Martinek, A. (2014) Acute Kidney Injury Due to Rhabdomyolysis and Renal Replacement Therapy: A Critical Review. *Critical Care*, **18**, 224-231. http://dx.doi.org/10.1186/cc13897

[9]   Sheikh, I.A., Shaheen, F.A.M., El Aqeil, N., Alkhader, A. and Karsuwa, S. (1994) ARF Due to Rhabdomyolysis Following Human Setmpede. *Saudi Journal of Kidney Diseases and Transplantation*, **5**, 17-22.

[10] McMahon, G.M., Zeng, X. and Waikar, S.S. (2013) A Risk Prediction Score for Kidney Failure or Mortality in Rhab-

domyolysis. *JAMA Internal Medicine*, **173**, 1821. http://dx.doi.org/10.1001/jamainternmed.2013.9774

[11] Lameire, N., Van Biesen, W. and Vanholder, R. (2006) Acute Renal Failure. *The Lancet*, **365**, 417-430. http://dx.doi.org/10.1016/S0140-6736(05)70238-5

[12] Book of Numbers: The Bible. The New English Bible (1970) Joint Comitee on the New Translation of the Bible. Cambridge University Press, New York, Vol. 11, 31-35.

[13] Rizzi, D., Basile, C. and Di Maggio, A. (1991) Clinical Spectrum of Accidental Hemlock Poisoning: Neurologic Manifestations, Rhabdomyolysis and Acute Tubular Necrosis. *Nephrology Dialysis Transplantation*, **6**, 939-943. http://dx.doi.org/10.1093/ndt/6.12.939

[14] Vanholder, R., Sever, M.S., Erek, E. and Lameire, N. (2000) Rhabdomyolysis. Disease of the Month. *Journal of the American Society of Nephrology*, **11**, 1553-1561.

[15] Bywaters, E.G.L. and Beall, D. (1941) Crush Injuries with Impairment of Renal Function. *British Medical Journal*, **1**, 427-432. http://dx.doi.org/10.1136/bmj.1.4185.427

[16] Smith, L., Post, R., Teschan, P., Abernathy, R., Davis, J., Gray, D., Howard, J., Johnson, K., Klopp, E., Mundy, R., *et al.* (1955) Postraumatic Renal Insufficiency in Military Casualties. II Management, Use of an Artificial Kidney, Prognosis. *American Journal of Medicine*, **18**, 187-198. http://dx.doi.org/10.1016/0002-9343(55)90234-5

[17] Stone, W. and Knepshield, J. (1974) Post Traumatic Acute Renal Insufficiency in Vietnam. *Clinical Nephrology*, **2**, 189-190.

[18] Ward, M. (1988) Factors Predictive of Acute Renal Failure in Rhabdomyolysis. *Archives of Internal Medicine*, **148**, 1553-1557. http://dx.doi.org/10.1001/archinte.1988.00380070059015

[19] Mohaupt, M. (2003) Rhabdomyolysis. *Therapeutische Umschau*, **60**, 391-397. http://dx.doi.org/10.1024/0040-5930.60.7.391

[20] Splendiani, G., Mazzarella, V., Cipriani, S., Zazzaro, D. and Casciani, C. (2001) Dialytic Treatment of Rhabdomyolysis-Induced Acute Renal Failure: Our Experience. *Renal failure*, **23**, 183-191. http://dx.doi.org/10.1081/JDI-100103490

[21] Sever, M., Erek, E., Vanholder, R., Akoglu, E., Yavaz, M., Ergin, H., Tekce, M., Korular, D., Tulbek, M., Keven, K., *et al.* (2001) The Marmara Earthquake: Epidemiological Analysis of the Victims with Nephrological Problems. *Kidney International*, **60**, 1114-1123. http://dx.doi.org/10.1046/j.1523-1755.2001.0600031114.x

[22] Kantarci, G., Vanholder, R., Tuclular, S., Akin, H., Koc, M., Ozrner, C. and Akoglu, E. (2002) Acute Renal Failure Due to Crush Syndrome during Marmara Earthquake. *American Journal of Kidney Diseases*, **40**, 682-689. http://dx.doi.org/10.1053/ajkd.2002.35673

[23] Van Dam, R. (2006) Earthquake in Pakistan—The Renal Disaster Relief Task Force in Action. *EDTNA-ERCA Journal*, **32**, 104-107. http://dx.doi.org/10.1111/j.1755-6686.2006.tb00461.x

[24] Rosen, C., Adler, J., Rabban, J., Sethi, R., Arkoff, L., Blair, J. and Sheridan, R. (1999) Early Predictors of Myoglobinuria and Acute Renal Failure Following Electrical Injury. *The Journal of Emergency Medicine*, **17**, 783-789. http://dx.doi.org/10.1016/S0736-4679(99)00084-0

[25] Brumback, R., Feeback, D. and Leech, R. (1995) Rhabdomyolysis Following Electrical Injury. *Seminars in Neurology*, **15**, 329-334 http://dx.doi.org/10.1055/s-2008-1041040

[26] Grossman, R.A., Hamilton, R.W., Morse, B.M., Penn, A.S. and Goldberg, M. (1974) Nontraumatic Rhabdomyolysis and Acute Renal Failure. *The New England Journal of Medicine*, **291**, 807-811.

[27] Sweny, P. (1989) Pigment Nephropathy: Rhabdomyolysis and Hemolysis. In: Sweny, P., Farrington, K. and Morehead, J.F. Eds., *The Kidney and Its Disorders*, Chapter 22, Blackwell Scientific Publications, Oxford, 348-358.

[28] Markowitz, H. and Wobing, G.H. (1977) Quantitative Methods for Estimating Myoglobin in Urine. *Clinical Chemistry*, **23**, 1689-1693.

[29] Haller, R.G. and Knochel, J.P. (1984) Skeletal Muscle Disease in Alcoholism. *Medical Clinics of North America*, **68**, 91-103.

[30] Song, S.K. and Rubin, E. (1972) Ethanol Produces Muscle Damage in Human Volunteers. *Science*, **175**, 327-328. http://dx.doi.org/10.1126/science.175.4019.327

[31] Knochel, J.P. (1992) Hypophosphatemia and Rhabdomyolysis. *American Journal of Medicine*, **92**, 455-457. http://dx.doi.org/10.1016/0002-9343(92)90739-X

[32] Kakulas, B. (1981) Experimental Myopathies. In: Walton, S.J., Ed., *Disorders of Voluntary Muscle*, Churchill Livingstone, New York, 393-400.

[33] Sitprija, V., Gopalakrishnakone, P. and Martinez-Maldonado, M. (1998) Snake Bite, Rhabdomyolysis, and Renal Failure. *American Journal of Kidney Diseases*, **31**, l-lii. http://dx.doi.org/10.1016/S0272-6386(14)70010-1

[34] Chugh, K.S. (1989) Snake Bite Induced ARF in India. *Kidney International*, **35**, 891-907.

[35] Gold, B.S., Dart, R.C. and Barish, R.A. (2002) Bites of Venoumous Snakes. *The New England Journal of Medicine*, **347**, 346-56. http://dx.doi.org/10.1056/NEJMra013477

[36] Reid, H.A. (1961) Myoglobinuria and Sea Snake Bite Poisoning. *British Medical Journal*, **1**, 1284-1289.

[37] Naqvi, R., Naqvi, A., Akhtar, F. and Rizvi, A. (1998) ARF Developing after a Scorpion Sting. *British Journal of Urology*, **82**, 295.

[38] Mocan, H., Mocan, M.Z. and Kaynar, K. (1998) HUS Following a Scorpion Sting. *Nephrology Dialysis Transplantation*, **13**, 2639-2640.

[39] Valavi, E., Ansari, M.J.A. and Hoseini, S. (2011) ADAMTS-13 Deficiency Following Scorpion Sting. *Saudi Journal of Kidney Diseases and Transplantation*, **22**, 792-795.

[40] Dressler, W.E. and Appelqvist, T. (2006) Plasma/Blood Pharmacokinetics and Metabolism after Dermal Exposure to Para-Aminophenol or Para-Phenylenediamine. *Food and Chemical Toxicology*, **44**, 371-379. http://dx.doi.org/10.1016/j.fct.2005.08.009

[41] Stanley, L.A., Skare, J.A., Doyle, E., Powrie, R., D'Angelo, D., *et al.* (2005) Lack of Evidence for Metabolism of p-Phenylenediamine by Human Hepatic Cytochrome P450 Enzymes. *Toxicology*, **210**, 147-157. http://dx.doi.org/10.1016/j.tox.2005.01.019

[42] Meyer, A., Blomeke, B. and Fischer, K. (2009) Determination of p-Phenylenediamine and Its Metabolites MAPPD and DAPPD in Biological Samples Using HPLC-DAD and Amperometric Detection. *Journal of Chromatography B*, **877**, 1627-1633. http://dx.doi.org/10.1016/j.jchromb.2009.04.008

[43] Shalaby, S.A., Elmasry, M.K., Abd-Elrahman, A.E., Abd-Elkarim, M.A. and Abd-Elhaleem, Z.A. (2010) Clinical Profile of Acute Paraphenylenediamine Intoxication in Egypt. *Toxicology and Industrial Health*, **26**, 81-87. http://dx.doi.org/10.1177/0748233709360200

[44] Chrispal, A., Begum, A., Ramya, I. and Zachariah, A. (2010) Hair Dye Poisoning—An Emerging Problem in the Tropics: An Experience from a Tertiary Care Hospital in South India. *Tropical Doctor*, **40**, 100-103. http://dx.doi.org/10.1258/td.2010.090367

[45] Nagaraja, B.S., Spoorthy, S.S. and Mubarak, H. (2012) Hair Dye Poisoning: Case Report. *International Journal of Clinical Cases and Investigations*, **4**, 43-48.

[46] Fatihi, E.M., Ramdani, B., Benghanem, M.G., Hachim, K. and Zaid, D. (1997) Rhabdomyolysis and Acute Renal Failure Secondary to Toxic Material Abuse in Morocco. *Saudi Journal of Kidney Diseases and Transplantation*, **8**, 131-133.

13

Prevalence and Risk Factors of Hypertension in Hemodialysis

Imen Gorsane, Madiha Mahfoudhi*, Fathi Younsi, Imed Helal, Taieb Ben Abdallah

Internal Medicine A Department, Charles Nicolle Hospital, Tunis, Tunisia
Email: *madiha_mahfoudhi@yahoo.fr

Abstract

The prevalence of hypertension in iterative hemodialysis (HD) remains high and was associated with a high morbidity and mortality. It was a single-center retrospective study including 124 patients on chronic HD in our unit. The prevalence of hypertension was determined from blood pressure (BP) monitoring in beginning, middle and end of dialysis. We defined hypertension as systolic BP (SBP) greater than or equal to 140 mmHg and/or diastolic BP (DBP) greater than or equal to 90 mmHg on at least two measures. We have established a comparative study between the group of hypertensive dialysis and those not hypertensive. The prevalence of hypertension was 69.35% (86/124). The mean age was 57.15 years with a sex ratio of 1.2. Echocardiograms, performed in 64.5% of patients, showed a high prevalence of cardiac consequences of hypertension with left ventricular hypertrophy in 80% of patients and an average ejection fraction of 62%. Diabetes, dialysis one session per week and the non-compliance with lifestyle and dietary rules were significantly associated with hypertension in HD in our study. The effect of HD on BP is dose-dependent. The reduction of BP allows a lower risk of cardiovascular (CV) events and mortality in hypertensive patients.

Keywords

Hemodialysis, Blood Pressure, Hypertension, Ultrafiltration, Volume Expansion

1. Introduction

Hemodialysis patients are at high risk for CV complications. This persists as their most common cause of death. Hypertension remains the most prevalent treatable risk factor in these patients [1]. Control of hypertension is important for reducing morbidity and mortality.

Hypertension is common in HD patients with a prevalence rate of approximately 90%. Appropriate BP targets

---

*Corresponding author.

for these patients remain uncertain. Studies have shown major gaps between recommended practice and real-world clinical performance in hemodialysis populations, including management and control of BP.

The measurement of BP is a simple and reproducible method. The National Kidney Foundation Kidney Disease Outcomes Quality Initiative (NKF-KDOQI) BP targets are pre-HD < 140/90 mm Hg, post-HD < 130/80 mm Hg [2].

Volume overload is a primary factor contributing to hypertension, and attaining true dry weight remains a priority for nephrologists. More, a wide variety of pathophysiological mechanisms are involved.

2. Material and Methods

This was a retrospective study including 124 patients on chronic hemodialysis in our unit conducted in January 2014.

We excluded from the study, patients with advanced diseases such as cancer and New York Heart Association (NYHA) stage IV heart failure and those with average hemodialysis < 6 months. Patients were on bicarbonate dialysis by synthetic membranes of various surfaces, and the duration of dialysis was 4 hours.

A blood pressure monitoring was performed in beginning, middle and end of dialysis as well as the heart rate. BP was taken in sitting position after 5 - 10 minutes of rest. Post-HD values were taken 5 - 10 minutes following dialysis.

The weight is measured at the entrance and exit of the session.

Demographic, clinical data and laboratory parameters were collected from patient's medical records.

Echocardiograms data not exceeding 6 months is collected.

Comparative study of different clinical and biological parameters between the group of hypertensive dialysis patients and those not hypertensive was conducted.

Baseline characteristics were described as means and standard deviations for continuous variables, and frequencies and proportions for categorical variables.

A study of the correlation was made between the various parameters by the statistical test CHI2. p value $\leq$ 0.05 was regarded as significant.

The ethics committee had no objections against this study since it reflects our clinical work habits and did not include supplementary measures (biological or radiological examinations).

3. Results

The prevalence of hypertension was 69.35% (86/124), and it was both systolic and diastolic in 90% of patients. The mean SBP was 170 mmHg. The mean age was 57.15 years [24 - 79 years] with a sex ratio of 1.21. Twenty patients (23.25%) were smokers.

Forty six patients (53.48%) were chronic HD with 3 sessions per week, 27 (31.39%) had two sessions per week and 13 (15.11%) had one session per week. The average hemodialysis was 48.65 months [6 - 300 months]. The interdialytic weight gain was 2.7 kg. Significant residual renal diuresis persisted in 12 patients (13.95%). Thirty nine patients were diabetics (45.34%). The initial nephropathy was diabetic nephropathy in 33 cases (38.37%), hypertensive nephropathy in 28 cases (32.55%), chronic glomerulonephritis in 13 cases (15.11%), chronic interstitial nephritis in 7 cases (8.13%) and chronic kidney disease of unknown etiology in 5 cases (5.81%).

Table 1 shows patient's epidemiological data.

Fifty-seven (66.27%) of the patients said respect the life style and dietary rules.

Only four patients (4.65%) were on ASE. Echocardiograms, performed in 64.5% of patients, showed left ventricular hypertrophy in 80% of patients and an average ejection fraction of 62%.

Table 2 shows clinical and laboratory patient's features.

Sixty per cent of patients were taking antihypertensive treatment. The third of them (19.76%) took three anti hypertensive drugs. Forty five (52.32%) patients were on RAS-blocking drugs.

A comparative study of different clinical and biological parameters between the group of hypertensive dialysis patients and those not hypertensive (**Table 3**), found that diabetes, dialysis one session per week and the non-compliance with lifestyle and dietary rules were significantly associated with hypertension in HD (p = 0.01, 0.01 and 0.005 respectively).

Table 1. Epidemiological data.

Characteristic	Duration of disease (years)	Value
Age (years)		57.15
Sex Ratio M/F		1.21
Smoke		20 (23.25%)
Average hemodialysis (months)		48.65
Diabetes	19.2	39 (45.34%)
Cause of renal failure		
Diabetic nephropathy	21.5	33 (38.37%)
Hypertensive nephropathy	18.1	28 (32.55%)
Chronic glomerulonephritis	10.6	13 (15.11%)
Chronic Interstitial Nephritis	17.8	7 (8.13%)
Chronic kidney disease of unknown etiology	9.4	5 (5.81%)

Table 2. Clinical and laboratory features.

Parameters	Value
Pre-HD systolic BP (mm Hg)	170
Pre-HD diastolic BP (mm Hg)	87
Pre-HD mean arterial pressure (mm Hg)	123
Pre-HD mean heart rate (bpm)	76
Post-HD systolic BP (mm Hg)	132
Post-HD diastolic BP (mm Hg)	70
Post-HD mean arterial pressure (mmHg)	101
Post-HD mean heart rate (bpm)	88
PTH (pg/ml)	400
Hb (g/dl)	8.2
Albumin (g/l)	29.91
Interdialytic weight gain (Kg)	2.7
Residual renal diuresis	12 (13.95%)
Patients respecting life style and dietary rules	57 (66.27%)
Erythropoiesis stimulating agents	4 (4.65%)

4. Discussion

Hypertension is present in up to 90% of end stage renal disease (ESRD) patients irrespective of the etiology of kidney disease [3]. Hypertension is recognized as an important modifiable risk factor for progression of chronic kidney disease (CKD) to ESRD and overall cardiovascular morbidity and mortality [4].

The prevalence of hypertension in HD patients is 80% - 90% [5]. In our study, it was of the order of 70%.

Elevated pre-HD SBP was associated with the occurrence of de novo cardiac failure, coronary artery disease and left ventricular hypertrophy (LVH), while actually lower SBP was associated with increased mortality [6]. But the reduction of BP in actively treated patients was associated with lower risks of all-cause and CV mortality [7].

Clinical guidelines-derived treatment goals represent the standards for providing evidence-based treatments

Table 3. Comparison of patient's characteristics between two groups: hypertensive and not hypertensive patients.

	Hypertensive (n = 86)	CI	Not hypertensive (n = 38)	CI	p
Age (years)	57.15		54.2		0.1
Sex ratio M/F	1.21		1.11		0.1
Smoke	20 (23.25%)	[14.3% - 32.2%]	5 (13.15%)	[2.4% - 23.9%]	0.5
Respecting lifestyle and dietary rules	57 (66.27%)	[56.3% - 76.3%]	32 (84.21%)	[72.6% - 95.8%]	**0.005**
Diabetes	39 (45.34%)	[34.8% - 55.9%]	10 (26.31%)	[12.3% - 40.3%]	**0.01**
Average HD (months)	48.65		47.21		0.5
Interdialytic weight gain (Kg)	2.7		2.65		0.1
Residual renal diuresis	12 (13.95%)	[6.6% - 21.3%]	18 (47.36%)	[31.5% - 63.2%]	0.29
HD one session	13 (15.11%)	[7.5% - 22.7%]	2 (5.26%)	[−1.8% - 12.4%]	**0.01**
HD two sessions	27 (31.39%)	[21.6% - 41.2%]	8 (21.05%)	[8.1% - 34%]	0.5
HD three sessions	46 (53.48%)	[42.9% - 64%]	28 (19.15%)	[6.6% - 31.7%]	0.5
Parathyroid hormone (pg/ml)	400		458		0.21
Serum Albumin (g/l)	29.91		30.02		0.39
Hemoglobin (g/dl)	8.2		7.9		0.1
Erythropoiesis stimulating agents	4 (4.65%)	[0.2% - 9.1%]	1 (0.02%)	[−0.4% - 0.5%]	0.5

CI: Confidence interval.

for dialysis patients. Although BP levels < 140/90 mmHg are recommended by current dialysis guidelines [8].

The optimal timing and method of BP measurement has yet to be defined. Compared to predialysis or post-dialysis BP measurements, mean BP better correlates with echocardiographic LVH and with all-cause of mortality [9]-[11]. Other authors find that mean post-HD ambulatory BP correlated more strongly with left ventricular mass index (LVMI) than either mean systolic or diastolic BP [12] [13].

If ambulatory or home BP measurements are unavailable, median intradialytic midweek BP is used to define clinic BP [14].

Salt and water retention with excess extracellular fluid volume is frequent in hemodialysis patients. Overhydration is responsible for volume and pressure overload. Extracellular volume excess is an important factor in the pathogenesis of arterial hypertension, and control of volume status by ultrafiltration and achievement of dry weight is considered an essential therapeutical approach [15] [16]. Volume reduction is associated with arterial pressure reduction and with decreased LVH [17]. Reducing dietary salt intake is considered to be a fundamental intervention in this population [18] [19].

The percentage of interdialytic weight gain predicts increased pre-HD systolic BP and greater reduction in systolic BP from pre to post-HD. This is seen particularly in non-diabetics, younger patients, and those with greater estimated dry weight. We should be less aggressive with BP in older patients or those with diabetes [17].

Measurements by 24-hours ambulatory BP monitoring have shown that intensification of ultrafiltration may improve the control of hypertension in these patients [15]. But it increases the risks for arteriovenous fistula complications and CV events [20].

More frequent or longer dialysis is the ideal option for bettering BP control in HD patients. Frequent HD had significantly greater reductions in pre-HD systolic BP and number of antihypertensive medications used. A significant reduction in left ventricular (LV) mass is found with frequent HD [21] [22].

Nocturnal HD is another option suggested to improve outcomes in HD patients by offering increased dialysis time and reducing the large fluctuations in fluid shifts that occur with conventional HD. Nocturnal HD showed improvements in BP (systolic, diastolic, and mean arterial pressure) and LV mass index [23].

For our patients, we cannot ensure in the hospital 3 dialysis sessions for all. When weight gain is important, we extend the session at 5 hours. We insist on achievement of dry weight.

The RAAS has long been implicated in the etiology of hypertension in HD patients. It has been shown that ESRD patients have higher sympathetic nervous system activity. Abnormal autonomic sympathetic nervous activity can manifest as an absence of a nocturnal dip in BP. Nocturnal or diurnal dipping in BP is frequently absent in both CKD and ESRD populations and is associated with adverse outcomes [24].

Endothelial cell dysfunction involves disrupted balance of vasoconstrictors and vasodilators mediators, with as consequences, increased vasoconstriction.

Treatment with antihypertensive agents in ESRD patients was associated with improved CV events and mortality [25] [26]. The current recommendation is to employ a RAAS-blocking drug as the first-line agent in patients on HD [4]. In addition to their beneficial effect on BP, RAAS inhibitors improve LVH and pulse wave velocity. Additional antihypertensive agents are frequently needed for persistent hypertension, and calcium channel blockers and beta-blockers are some of the next recommended therapies [8].

Arterial stiffness is a pathogenetic process that occurs naturally with aging, but is accentuated in ESRD. The consequence is increased SBP and pulse pressure, which contribute to LVH.

Secondary hyperparathyroidism that accompanies CKD may contribute to the high prevalence of hypertension. Systolic and diastolic BP were significantly increased in subjects with elevated parathyroid hormone (PTH). Treatment with vitamin D significantly lowered cytosolic calcium, PTH, and mean BP [4].

More, ASE used to correct the anemia associated with ESRD are also suspected of causing increases in BP by increased sensitivity to angiotensin II and adrenergic stimuli [27]. Because of unavailability of ASE in our hospital, 4 patients only were on ASE.

It can be seen that delay in connection on the machine, needle insertion, anxiety about dialysis, are also likely to play a significant role in raising pre-HD BP [24].

5. Conclusions

Hypertension is highly prevalent in HD patients. It is associated with CV disease, the leading cause of mortality in HD patients.

Although clinical trial evidence of a target BP that improves mortality does not currently exist. The clinician is faced with a dilemma on how to evaluate blood pressure and treat this condition.

Management of hypertension in HD patients should include the establishment and maintenance of the appropriate dry weight and limitation of interdialytic sodium/fluid intake.

Pharmacologic therapy should include RAAS inhibitors as first-line agents.

We found in our study that hypertension risk factors in HD were: diabetes, dialysis one session per week and the non-compliance with lifestyle and dietary rules.

However, the two groups being compared were not homogenous. Further studies with larger numbers could be more conclusive.

Conflict of Interest

There are no conflicts of interest.

References

[1] Thompson, S., Hemmelgarn, B., Wiebe, N., Majumdar, S., Klarenbach, S., Jindal, K., *et al.* (2012) Clinical Decision Support to Improve Blood Pressure Control in Hemodialysis Patients: A Non Randomized Controlled Trial. *Journal of Nephrology*, **25**, 944-953. http://dx.doi.org/10.5301/jn.5000238

[2] Gul, A., Miskulin, D., Gassman, J., Harford, A., Horowitz, B., Chen, J., *et al.* (2014) Design of the Blood Pressure Goals in Dialysis Pilot Study. *American Journal of the Medical Sciences*, **347**, 125-130. http://dx.doi.org/10.1097/MAJ.0b013e31827daee5

[3] Agarwal, R., Nissenson, A., Battle, D., Coyne, D., Trout, J. and Warnock D. (2003) Prevalence, Treatment, and Control of Hypertension in Chronic Hemodialysis Patients in the United States. *The American Journal of Medicine*, **115**, 291-297. http://dx.doi.org/10.1016/S0002-9343(03)00366-8

[4] Van Buren, P.N. and Inrig, J.K. (2012) Hypertension and Hemodialysis: Pathophysiology and Outcomesin Adult and Pediatric Populations. *Pediatric Nephrology*, **27**, 339-350. http://dx.doi.org/10.1007/s00467-011-1775-3

[5]   Inrig, J., Oddone, E., Hasselblad, V., Gillespie, B., Patel, U.D., Reddan, D., *et al.* (2007) Association of Intradialytic Blood Pressure Changes with Hospitalization and Mortality Rates in Prevalent ESRD Patients. *Kidney International,* **71**, 454-461. http://dx.doi.org/10.1038/sj.ki.5002077

[6]   Foley, R., Parfrey, P., Darnett, J., Kent, G., Murray, D. and Barre, P. (1996) Impact of Hypertension on Cardiomyopathy, Morbidity, and Mortality in End-Stage Renal Disease. *Kidney International,* **49**, 1379-1385. http://dx.doi.org/10.1038/ki.1996.194

[7]   Heerspink, H.J., Ninomya, T., Zoungas, S., de Zeeuw, D., Grobbee, D.E., Jardine, M.J., *et al.* (2009) Effect of Lowering Blood Pressure on Cardiovascular Events and Mortality in Patients on Dialysis: A Systematic Review and Meta-Analysis of Randomised Controlled Trials. *The Lancet,* **373**, 1009-1015. http://dx.doi.org/10.1016/S0140-6736(09)60212-9

[8]   K/DOQI Workgroup (2005) K/DOQI Clinical Practice Guidelines for Cardiovascular Disease in Dialysis Patients. *American Journal of Kidney Diseases,* **45**, S1-S153.

[9]   Agarwal, R., Brim, N.J., Mahenthiran, J., Andersen, M.J. and Saha, C. (2006) Out-of-Hemodialysis-Unit Blood Pressure is a Superior Determinant of Left Ventricular Hypertrophy. *Hypertension,* **47**, 62-68. http://dx.doi.org/10.1161/01.HYP.0000196279.29758.f4

[10]   Inrig, J., Patel, U., Gillespie, B., Hasselblad, V., Himmelfarb, J., Reddan D., *et al.* (2007) Relationship between Interdialytic Weight Gain and Blood Pressure Among Prevalent Hemodialysis Patients. *American Journal of Kidney Diseases,* **50**, 108.e4-118.e4. http://dx.doi.org/10.1053/j.ajkd.2007.04.020

[11]   Agarwal, R. (2010) Blood Pressure and Mortality among Hemodialysis Patients. *Hypertension,* **55**, 762-768. http://dx.doi.org/10.1161/HYPERTENSIONAHA.109.144899

[12]   Harvey, P., Holt, A., Nicholas, J. and Dasgupta, I. (2013) Is an Average of Routine Postdialysis Blood Pressure a Good Indicator of Blood Pressure Control and Cardiovascular Risk? *Journal of Nephrology,* **26**, 94-100. http://dx.doi.org/10.5301/jn.5000119

[13]   Borsboom, H., Smans, L., Cramer, M.J., Kelder, J.C., Kooistra, M.P., Vos, P.F., *et al.* (2005) Long-Term Blood Pressure Monitoring and Echocardiographic Findings in Patients with End-Stage Renal Disease: Reverse Epidemiology Explained? *Netherlands Journal of Medicine,* **63**, 399-406.

[14]   Agarwal, R. (2012) The Controversies of Diagnosing and Treating Hypertension among Hemodialysis Patients. *Seminars in Dialysis,* **25**, 370-376. http://dx.doi.org/10.1111/j.1525-139X.2012.01092.x

[15]   Agarwal, R., Alborzi, P., Satyan, S. and Light, R.P. (2009) Dry-Weight Reduction in Hypertensive Hemodialysis Patients (DRIP): A Randomized, Controlled Trial. *Hypertension,* **53**, 500-507. http://dx.doi.org/10.1161/HYPERTENSIONAHA.108.125674

[16]   London, G.M. (2011) Ultrafiltration Intensification for Achievement of Dry Weight and Hypertension Control Is Not Always the Therapeutic Gold Standard. *Journal of Nephrology,* **24**, 395-397. http://dx.doi.org/10.5301/jn.5000006

[17]   Alborzi, P., Patel, N. and Agarwal, R. (2007) Home Blood Pressures Are of Greater Prognostic Value than Hemodialysis Unit Recordings. *Clinical Journal of the American Society of Nephrology,* **2**, 1228-1234. http://dx.doi.org/10.2215/CJN.02250507

[18]   Levin, N.W., Kotanko, P., Eckardt, K.U., Kasiske, B.L., Chazot, C., Cheung, A.K., *et al.* (2010) Blood Pressure in Chronic Kidney Disease Stage 5D-Report from a Kidney Disease: Improving Global Outcomes Controversies Conference. *Kidney International,* **77**, 273-284. http://dx.doi.org/10.1038/ki.2009.469

[19]   Charra, B. (2007) Fluid Balance, Dry Weight, and Blood Pressure in Dialysis. *Hemodialysis International,* **11**, 21-31. http://dx.doi.org/10.1111/j.1542-4758.2007.00148.x

[20]   Curatola, G., Bolignano, D., Rastelli, S., Caridi, G., Tripepi, R., Tripepi, G., *et al.* (2011) Ultrafiltration (UF) Intensification Improves Hypertension Control in Hemodialysis Patients but Increases Arterio-Venous Fistula Complications and Cardiovascular Events. *Journal of Nephrology,* **24**, 465-473. http://dx.doi.org/10.5301/JN.2011.7735

[21]   Zimmerman, D.L., Ruzicka, M., Hebert, P., Fergusson, D., Touyz, R.M. and Burns, K.D. (2014) Short Daily versus Conventional Hemodialysis for Hypertensive Patients: A Randomized Cross-Over Study. *PLoS ONE,* **9**, e97135. http://dx.doi.org/10.1371/journal.pone.0097135

[22]   Chertow, G.M., Levin, N.W., Beck, G.J., Depner, T.A., Eggers, P.W., *et al.*, The FHN Trial Group (2010) In-Center Hemodialysis Six Times per Week versus Three Times per Week. *New England Journal of Medicine,* **363**, 2287-2300. http://dx.doi.org/10.1056/NEJMoa1001593

[23]   Chan, C., Floras, J., Miller, J., Richardson, R. and Pierratos, A. (2002) Regression of Left Ventricular Hypertrophy after Conversion to Nocturnal Hemodialysis. *Kidney International,* **61**, 2235-2239. http://dx.doi.org/10.1046/j.1523-1755.2002.00362.x

[24]   Liu, M., Takashi, H., Morita, Y., Maruyama, S., Mizuno, M., Yuzawa, Y., *et al.* (2003) Non-Dipping Is a Potent Predictor of Cardiovascular Mortality and Is Associated with Autonomic Dysfunction in Haemodialysis Patients. *Neph-*

rology Dialysis Transplantation, **18**, 563-569. http://dx.doi.org/10.1093/ndt/18.3.563

[25] Heerspink, H., Ninomiya, T., Zoungas, S., de Zeeuw, D., Grobbee, D.E., Jardine, M.J., *et al.* (2009) Effect of Lowering Blood Pressure on Cardiovascular Events and Mortality in Patients on Dialysis: A Systematic Review and Meta-Analysis of Randomized Controlled Trials. *The Lancet*, **373**, 1009-1015. http://dx.doi.org/10.1016/S0140-6736(09)60212-9

[26] Agarwal, R. and Sinha, A.D. (2009) Cardiovascular Protection with Antihypertensive Drugs in Dialysis Patients: Systematic Review and Meta-Analysis. *Hypertension*, **53**, 860-866. http://dx.doi.org/10.1161/HYPERTENSIONAHA.108.128116

[27] Krapf, R. and Hulter, H.N. (2009) Arterial Hypertension Induced by Erythropoietin and Erythropoiesis-Stimulating Agents (ESA). *Clinical Journal of the American Society of Nephrology*, **4**, 470-480. http://dx.doi.org/10.2215/CJN.05040908

Abbreviations

- Blood pressure: BP
- Cardiovascular: CV
- Chronic kidney disease: CKD
- Diastolic blood pressure: DBP
- End stage renal disease: ESRD
- Erythropoiesis stimulating agents: ASE
- Hemodialysis: HD
- Left ventricular hypertrophy: LVH
- Left ventricular mass index: LVMI
- Left ventricular: LV
- National Kidney Foundation Kidney Disease Outcomes Quality Initiative: NKF-KDOQI
- New York Heart Association: NYHA
- Parathyroid hormone: PTH
- Renin-angiotensin-aldosterone system: RAAS
- Systolic blood pressure: SBP

14

Indications and Results of Kidney Biopsies in Patients over 65 Years Old

Imen Gorsane, Madiha Mahfoudhi*, Imed Helal, Taieb Ben Abdallah

Internal Medicine A Department, Charles Nicolle Hospital, Tunis, Tunisia
Email: *madiha_mahfoudhi@yahoo.fr

Abstract

Normal kidney aging is related to tissue and functional changes that make older patients very vulnerable to environmental modifications. Numerous factors can accelerate the impairment of renal function during aging. It was a single-center retrospective study extending over a period of 30 years from 1984 to 2014 and includes patients older than 65 years, hospitalized for nephropathy requiring renal biopsy and monitored in our service. There were 6 men and 7 women with an average age of 69.38 ± 4.5 years. Mean serum creatinine was 267.15 ± 124 mmol/l. Eleven patients had renal failure. Histological lesions were: Extramembranous glomerulonephritis (EMGN): 1 case, focal segmental glomerular sclerosis (FSGS): 3 cases, membranoproliferative glomerulonephritis (MPGN): 1 case, IgA nephropathy: 1 case, glomerulonephritis with IgG4 fibrillar deposits (GN IgG4): 1 case, diabetic nephropathy: 2 cases, myeloma-associated tubulopathy: 1 case, acute tubular necrosis: 1 case, acute interstitial nephritis: 1 case, vascular nephropathy: 1 case. Kidney disease will increasingly become a geriatric illness. Nephrologists are encountering a growing group of elderly patients with diminished equation for estimated glomerular filtration rate (eGFR) that require evaluation and management.

Keywords

Renal Aging, Chronic Kidney Disease, Elderly, Renal Biopsy

1. Introduction

The aging of the current population and future is recognized by all demographic studies. The health professional currently holds the age of 70 to define an old person.

The global population is aging, and the number of people above the age of 70 years is growing faster than any other age group.

---

*Corresponding author.

There is an age-related decline in kidney function; however, not all individuals will develop chronic kidney disease with advancing age.

Renal failure in the elderly is currently underestimated. Numerous factors can accelerate the impairment of renal function during aging [1]. We report our experience of care in nephrology in the elderly.

2. Material and Methods

It was a single-center retrospective study extending over a period of 30 years from 1984 to 2014 and includes patients older than 65 years, hospitalized for nephropathy requiring renal biopsy and monitored in our service.

We studied their epidemiological clinical and histological profile and the different complications.

The ethics committee had no objections against this study since it reflects our clinical work habits and did not include supplementary measures (other biological or radiological examinations).

We performed a comparative study of comorbidities between the men and women patients.

Baseline characteristics were described as means and standard deviations for continuous variables, and frequencies and proportions for categorical variables.

A study of the correlation was made between the various parameters by the statistical test CHI2. P value $\leq$ 0.05 was regarded as significant.

3. Results

There were 6 men and 7 women with an average age of 69.38 ± 4.5 years. Four patients were diabetic and 9 hypertensive whose coronary artery disease patient. Three patients had cardiac arrhythmia and 2 had stroke.

Mean serum creatinine was 267.15 ± 124 µmol/l and the mean plasma clearance of creatinine measured by MDRD was 43.60 ml/mn. Eleven patients had renal failure: Six patients in stage 3, 2 cases in stage 4 and 3 cases in stage 5.

Medium hemoglobin was 11.14 ± 0.5 g/dl and Albumin 29 ± 1.9 g/l. the mean serum cholesterol was 3.87 ± 1.06 mmol/l, the mean triglyceride level was 1.34 ± 0.7 mmol/l. The mean serum calcium was 2.33 ± 0.18 mmol/l The average phosphorus was 1.39 ± 0.17 mmol/l, and the PTH 384 ± 421 pg/ml. The mean proteinuria was 2.5 ± 0.46 g per 24 hours (**Table 1**).

A comparative study of comorbidities sex found no significant difference between the 2 groups (**Table 2**).

Indications of renal biopsy were: nephrotic syndrome in 8 cases, rapidly progressive renal failure in 4 cases and microscopic hematuria in one case.

The different histological lesions were: Extramembranous glomerulonephritis (EMGN): 1 case, focal segmental glomerular sclerosis (FSGS): 3 cases, membranoproliferative glomerulonephritis (MPGN): 1 case, IgA nephropathy: 1 case, glomerulonephritis with IgG4 fibrillar deposits (GN IgG4): 1 case, diabetic nephropathy: 2 cases, myeloma-associated tubulopathy: 1 case, acute tubular necrosis: 1 case, acute interstitial nephritis: 1 case, vascular nephropathy: 1 case (**Figure 1**).

Table 1. Patient's clinical and biochemical characteristics.

Characteristic	Value
Age (years)	69.38 ± 4.5
Sex M/F	6/7
creatinine (µmol/l)	267.15 ± 124
Hemoglobin (g/dl)	11.14 ± 0.5
Albumin (g/l)	29 ± 1.9
cholesterol (mmol/l)	3.87 ± 1.06
triglyceride (mmol/l)	1.34 ± 0.7
calcium (mmol/l)	2.33 ± 0.18
phosphorus (mmol/l)	1.39 ± 0.17
PTH (pg/ml)	384 + 421
Proteinuria (g per 24 hours)	2.5 ± 0.46

M: male, F: female, PTH: parathormone.

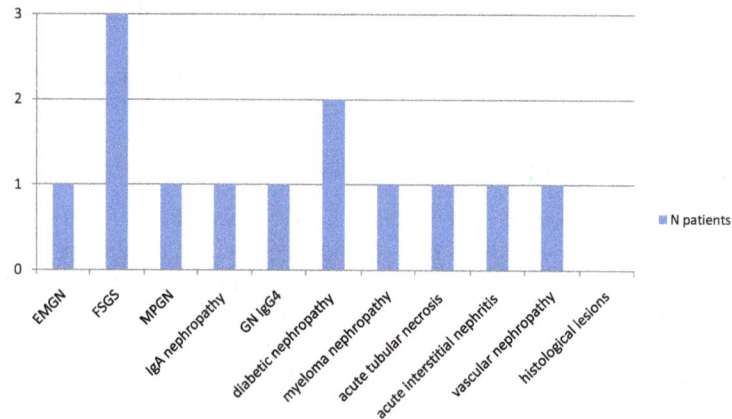

Figure 1. Graphical presentation of histological lesions of our patients.

Table 2. Comparison of comorbidities between the male and female patients.

	M (N = 6)	W (N = 7)	P
Diabetes (%)	1 (16.66)	3 (42.85)	0.12
Hypertension (%)	5 (83.33)	4 (57.14)	0.5
coronaropathy (%)	1 (16.66)	2 (28.57)	0.3
cardiac arrhythmia (%)	1 (16.66)	0 (0)	0.1
stroke (%)	1 (16.66)	15 (14.28)	0.4
poor mobility (%)	1 (16.66)	4 (57.14)	0.5

All patients had a specific treatment and the outcome was favorable for 10 patients.

The 3 patients who were immediately in stage 5 have not recovered, 2 were in hemodialysis and 1 in peritoneal dialysis.

Two patients died from severe bronchopneumopathy.

4. Discussion

From 40 years, the aging kidney results in a reduced renal mass, kidney size (−0.8%/year) and the number and the surface of the glomeruli are also observed a reduction in the length of the proximal tubule and dilatation of distal convoluted tubules. Aging functional, that is to say the change in the hemodynamic renal precedes the decreased renal mass.

Reduced mortality and morbidity, prolongation of the patient's life, and better clinical outcomes of renal replacement therapy (RRT) allowed having older patients on hospital nephrology unit for nephropathy.

The prevalence of moderate to severe Chronic Kidney Disease (CKD) increases with age [2].

Renal failure in the elderly is considered as a public health problem. Systematic application of mathematical formulae to estimate the glomerular filtration rate (GFR) of the general population, according to The Kidney Disease Outcomes Quality Initiative (KDOQI) classification of CKD, has permitted to calculate its high prevalence [3]. The MDRD Study equation is the most thoroughly validated equation in the elderly and has shown good performance for patients with all common causes of kidney disease.

Moderate reductions in eGFR can occur as the result of normal aging and should not be equated with CKD in the absence of other abnormalities or clearly defined associated risks [4] [5]. As a result, elderly patients may be mislabeled as having moderate CKD even when their eGFR corrected for age is normal [6].

Kidney biopsies are increasingly being performed in the elderly [7]. Proteinuria is the main sign of kidney injury [8]. Different spectrum of pathologies is found in old population and requires a careful assessment of risks and benefits of any potential therapeutic intervention.

Common findings are age-related kidney fibrosis related to increased collagen accumulation and advanced vascular changes, similar to chronically damaged kidneys [7] [9].

Primitive nephropathies frequently are represented by the EMGN. Regarding secondary nephropathies, vasculitis pauci immune remain largely the most frequent etiologies [10]. The kidney biopsy in the elderly remains an essential tool to establish a precise histological diagnosis and guide decision for therapeutic management.

Specific treatment of certain nephropathy based on corticosteroids and immunosuppressive with an increased risk of secondary effects in the elderly population because of their immune status related to age with increased risk of infections. Moreover, pharmacodynamics/pharmacokinetics of drugs becomes different with age and the nephrologist has to be aware of the effect of the multiple other drugs these patients are taking. This is too common in this population and is more likely to cause drug-drug interactions and serious adverse effects [11]. In our series two patients died from severe bronchopneumopathy probably due to the state of immunosuppression induced by immunosuppressive treatment.

Older patients with kidney disease often have considerable comorbidity, not only the vascular disease associated with their renal disease, but also the comorbidity found in many older people, including impaired vision, deafness, poor mobility, arthritis and cognitive dysfunction. They are often socially isolated, live in poor accommodations and may have financial problems [12] [13].

Elderly patients can use avoidance or denial based techniques. This was observed where several primitive strategies were being used, most notably denial [14]. Denial is an effective strategy in coping with illness-related stress, but may result in lower compliance with treatment [15].

The elderly patients are depressed and often avoid personal involvement, which may result in difficulties in treatment and physical rehabilitation. The role of a psychologist should be to guide elderly patients toward treatment and lifestyle that may result in substantial benefits from both the patients' and clinics' point of view [16].

However, less is known about how nephrologists prepare patients for understanding their individual prognoses and living with their kidney disease; especially when the patients are aged [17].

Our study, which recruited cases over a long period (30 years), but whose membership is low, did not draw significant conclusions; further studies with larger numbers are needed to have valid results.

5. Conclusions

Since the incidence and prevalence of kidney disease increase with advancing age, nephrologists are increasingly confronted with a population of patients who are elderly and have a large number of comorbid conditions requiring ongoing care.

A comparative study of comorbidities sex found no significant difference between the two groups probably because of the small number of our series.

Conflict of Interest

There are no conflicts of interest.

References

[1] Bolignano, D., Mattace-Raso, F., Sijbrands, E.J. and Zoccali, C. (2014) The Aging Kidney Revisited: A Systematic Review. *Ageing Research Reviews*, **14**, 65-80. http://dx.doi.org/10.1016/j.arr.2014.02.003

[2] James, M.T., Hemmelgarn, B.R. and Tonelli, M. (2010) Early Recognition and Prevention of Chronic Kidney Disease. *The Lancet*, **375**, 1296-1309. http://dx.doi.org/10.1016/S0140-6736(09)62004-3

[3] Heras, M., Fernández-Reyes, M.J., Guerrero, M.T., Sánchez, R., Muñoz, A., Macías, M.C., *et al.* (2009) Elderly Patients with Chronic Kidney Disease: What Happens after 24 Months of Follow-Up? *Nefrologia*, **29**, 343-349.

[4] Campbell, K.H. and O'Hare, A.M. (2008) Kidney Disease in the Elderly: Update on Recent Literature. *Current Opinion in Nephrology & Hypertension*, **17**, 298-303. http://dx.doi.org/10.1097/MNH.0b013e3282f5dd90

[5] Roderick, P.J., Atkins, R.J., Smeeth, L., Mylne, A., Nitsch, D.D., Hubbard, R.B., *et al.* (2009) CKD and Mortality Risk in Older People: A Community-Based Population Study in the United Kingdom. *American Journal of Kidney Diseases*, **53**, 950-960. http://dx.doi.org/10.1053/j.ajkd.2008.12.036

[6] Anderson, S., Halter, J.B., Hazzard, W.R., Himmelfarb, J., Horne, F.M., Kaysen, G.A., *et al.* (2009) Prediction, Progression and Outcomes of Chronic Kidney Disease. *Journal of the American Society of Nephrology*, **20**, 1199-1209. http://dx.doi.org/10.1681/ASN.2008080860

[7]   Moutzouris, D.A., Herlitz, L., Appel, G.B., Markowitz, G.S., Freudenthal, B., Radhakrishnan, J., *et al.* (2008) Renal Biopsy in the Very Elderly. *Clinical Journal of the American Society of Nephrology*, **4**, 1073-1082. http://dx.doi.org/10.2215/CJN.00990209

[8]   García de Vinuesa, S. (2008) Progression Factors for Chronic Kidney Disease. Secondary Prevention. *Nefrologia*, **S3**, 17-21.

[9]   Rodriguez-Puyol, D. (1998) Nephrology Forum. The Aging Kidney. *Kidney International*, **54**, 2247-2265. http://dx.doi.org/10.1038/4499994

[10]   Celik, B., Yaz, M., Bulut, T., Sahin, S., Alp, A. and Meteoglu, I. (2013) Is Focal Segmental Glomerulosclerosis Common among the Elderly? Geriatric Biopsy Results. *Saudi Medical Journal*, **34**, 760-763.

[11]   Rosner, M., Abdel-Rahman, E. and Williams, M.E. (2010) Geriatric Nephrology: Responding to a Growing Challenge. *Clinical Journal of the American Society of Nephrology*, **5**, 936-942. http://dx.doi.org/10.2215/CJN.08731209

[12]   Brown, E.A., Johansson, L., Farrington, K., Gallagher, H., Sensky, T., Gordon, F., *et al.* (2010) Broadening Options for Long-Term Dialysis in the Elderly (BOLDE): Differences in Quality of Life on Peritoneal Dialysis Compared to Haemodialysis for Older. *Nephrology Dialysis Transplantation*, **25**, 3755-3763. http://dx.doi.org/10.1093/ndt/gfq212

[13]   Foote, C., Ninomiya, T., Gallagher, M., Perkovic, V., Cass, A., McDonald, S.P., *et al.* (2012) Survival of Elderly Dialysis Patients Is Predicted by Both Patient and Practice Characteristics. *Nephrology Dialysis Transplantation*, **27**, 3581-3587. http://dx.doi.org/10.1093/ndt/gfs096

[14]   Telford, K., Kralik, D. and Koch, T. (2006) Acceptance and Denial: Implications for People Adapting to Chronic Illness: Literature Review. *Journal of Advanced Nursing*, **55**, 457-464. http://dx.doi.org/10.1111/j.1365-2648.2006.03942.x

[15]   Jadoulle, V., Hoyois, P. and Jadoul, M. (2005) Anxiety and Depression in Chronic Hemodialysis: Some Somatopsychic Determinants. *Clinical Nephrology*, **63**, 113-118. http://dx.doi.org/10.5414/CNP63113

[16]   Laudański, K., Nowak, Z. and Niemczyk, S. (2013) Age-Related Differences in the Quality of Life in End-Stage Renal Disease in Patients Enrolled in Hemodialysis or Continuous Peritoneal Dialysis. *Medical Science Monitor*, **19**, 378-385. http://dx.doi.org/10.12659/MSM.883916

[17]   Schell, J.O., Patel, U.D., Steinhauser, K.E., Ammarell, N. and Tulsky, J.A. (2012) Discussions of the Kidney Disease Trajectory by Elderly Patients and Nephrologists: A Qualitative Study. *American Journal of Kidney Diseases*, **59**, 495-503. http://dx.doi.org/10.1053/j.ajkd.2011.11.023

Abbreviations

Chronic Kidney Disease (CKD)
Equation for estimated glomerular filtration rate (eGFR)
Extramembranous glomerulonephritis (EMGN)
Focal segmental glomerular sclerosis (FSGS)
Glomerular filtration rate (GFR)
Glomerulonephritis with IgG4 fibrillar deposits (GN IgG4)
Kidney Disease Outcomes Quality Initiative (KDOQI)
Membranoproliferative glomerulonephritis (MPGN)
Modification of the Diet in Renal Disease (MDRD)
Parathyroid hormone (PTH)
Renal replacement therapy (RRT)

15

Experience of Percutaneus Kidney Biopsy from a Tertiary Care Center of Pakistan

Ali Absar[1*], Naila Asif[2], Quratulain Khan[1], Waqar Kashif[1]

[1]Aga Khan University Hospital, Karachi, Pakistan
[2]Liaquat National Hospital, Karachi, Pakistan
Email: *draliabsar@yahoo.com

Abstract

Background: Kidney biopsy is one of the most important tools in the assessment of kidney disease. Knowing the histopathology is important for immediate clinical management. It helps in predicting the long term prognosis and in planning for prevention of chronic kidney disease. Methods: This is a cross section study of percutaneus biopsies of the native kidneys of patients, who presented to the Aga Khan University Hospital Karachi Pakistan, over ten year period from 2003 to 2012. Age range was 16 to 77 years. Results: Total number of 435 biopsies were included in the study. The most common histopathological findings, regardless of the indication of biopsy were Tubulo Interstitial Nephritis in 15 percent, followed by Membranous Nephropathy in 12 percent, Focal Segmental Glomerulosclerosis in 8 percent and Membrano Proliferative Glomerulonephritis also in 8 percent. Conclusion: This study will help in better understanding the spectrum of renal disease in Pakistan. It will guide the clinician in the management and provide a data base or a starting point for the researchers for conducting the controlled and population base studies.

Keywords

Kidney, Biopsy, Pakistan

1. Introduction

Kidney biopsy is one of the essential components of the work up needed for the evaluation of the kidney disease. In an appropriate setting, it is the key investigation necessary to reach the correct diagnosis, to predict the clinical course and to institute the right treatment [1].

The common indications of biopsy of the native kidney include unexplained rise in serum creatinine, unex-

---

*Corresponding author.

plained proteinuria with or without hematuria nephrotic syndrome, and in systemic diseases like lupus nephritis for staging purposes. Biopsy of the transplanted kidney is performed most often when there is an acute rise in scrum creatinine suspecting rejection. Kidney biopsy is not indicated in diabetic patients, unless one suspects some other non diabetic pathology. With wide spread use of automatic disposable biopsy gun, the procedure is very safe. However it does not mean to relax the criteria or not to observe the standard precautions for the procedure because complications including death still do occur [2].

With rising incidence and prevalence of chronic kidney disease, now it is even more important to know the exact cause of acute and chronic kidney injury. Early intervention helps in controlling the progression of chronic kidney disease. Planning and rationing of the resources also require specific knowledge of the renal diseases in a given population. Our study will help in defining the pattern of kidney disease in Pakistan particularly in Karachi [3].

There are similar studies done in Pakistan as well as in other parts of the world. The findings of these studies are described in the discussion section latter.

2. Methods

This is a cross section study of percutaneus native kidney biopsies of patients presented to Aga Khan University Hospital Karachi Pakistan, over ten years of period from 2003 to 2012.

2.1. Inclusion Criteria

Only the biopsies performed in the premises of the Institution were included. Biopsies sent from outside for reading only were not included.

2.2. Exclusion Criteria

1) Age less than 16 years;
2) Kidney Transplant;
3) Non-Conclusive Results;
4) Poor samples *i.e.* glomeruli less than 3.

2.3. Pre-Biopsy Workup

Minimal workup included the following:
1) 24-Hours urine protein or spot urine protein/creatinine ratio;
2) Urine Detail Report;
3) Serum Urea and Creatinine;
4) Coagulation Profile;
5) Complete blood Picture (CBC);
6) Renal sonogram.

Additional tests were performed as indicated depending upon the clinical situation.

Biopsies were taken either by a nephrologist or a radiologist under ultrasound or CT scan guidance. Biopsies were read by a well trained and experienced renal histopathologist. Light microscopy included staining with Hematoxylin and Eosin (H & E), periodic acid Schiff (PAS), Massone's trichrome, and Jones silver methanamine were done. Immunofluorescence staining was also done in all the cases. Electron microscope was not available.

3. Results

Total number of 435 biopsies were included in the study.. The age range was 16 to 85 years with mean age of 40 years. There were 58% male and 42% female.

The most common histopathology, regardless of the indication of biopsy, was Tubulo Interstitial Nephritis in 67 patients (15%), followed by Membranous Nephropathy in 55 (12%) and then Focal Segmental Glomerulosclerosis in 38 (8%) and Membrano Proliferative Glomerulonephritis in 36 (8%) of biopsies.

Diabetic Nephropathy was the pathology identified in 29 out of 62 diabetic patients who were subjected to biopsy for suspecting non diabetic kidney disease. The pathological pattern of 26 lupus patients included all classes of lupus nephritis. Miscellaneous group includes those diagnosis which were only in one or two in number (**Table 1**).

4. Discussion

There are several kidney biopsy based studies available from Pakistan as well as from other countries. Most of these studies from Pakistan are from single center and usually from a teaching hospital. We are also presenting our experience from a single center, Aga Khan University Hospital Karachi, which is a tertiary care leading teaching institution attached to the medical college and University. In the following paragraphs selected representative studies from Pakistan and from other parts of the world are reviewed.

A survey of the Czech Republic registry of native kidney Biopsies from 1994-2000 included 4000 biopsies. The most frequent diagnosis was IgA nephropathy (34%) and after that minimal change disease (12%), non Ig A mesangial proliferative (11%) membranous (09%) and tubulo-Interstitial nephritis (4%) were identified [4].

An analysis of kidney biopsies done over 23 years in Korea included more than 4000 cases. In this study the most common primary glomerular disease was minimal change disease in 26% followed by IgA Nephropathy in 22% [5]. An Italian Registry data of more than 14,000 kidney biopsies from 128 centers reported IgA nephropathy, minimal disease and FSGS the highest in the list [6].

Epidemiology study from Romania reviewed 10 year data of more than 600 kidney biopsies. The most common indication for biopsy was nephrotic syndrome. The most common histopathological diagnoses were membranproliferative GN (30%) and mesangial proliferative GN (29%) among the primary glomerular diseases [7].

Table 1. Histopathological diagnosis in kidney biopsy.

Histopathological Diagnosis	Number (Percentage)
Tubulo Interstitial Nephritis	67 (15)
Membranous Nephropathy (MGN)	55 (12)
Focal Segmental Glomeruloscelosis (FSGS)	38 (8)
Membrano Proliferative Glomerulonephritis (MPGN)	36 (8)
Diabetic Glomerulosclerosis	29 (7)
Lupus Nephritis	26 (6)
Minimal Change Disease (MCD)	23 (5)
Acute Tubular Necrosis (ATN)	18 (4)
Crescentric Glomerulonephritis	17 (4)
Renal Amyloidosis	16 (4)
End Stage Renal Disease	12 (3)
Tumor	10 (2)
IgA Nephropathy	8 (1.8)
Post Infectious Glomerulonephritis	6 (1.5)
Rapidly Progressive Glomerulonephritis	7 (1.7)
Normal	7 (1.7)
Acute Cortical Necrosis	3 (0.7)
Miscellaneous	20 (5)
Non Conclusive	37 (8)
Total	**435 (100)**

Data from Spain included more than 9000 biopsies. In this study the most common disease was membranous nephropathy among nephrotic patients [8].

Study from United Arab of Emirates presented their data of 490 native kidney biopsies. In this study FSGS was diagnosed in 18% as compared to chronic proliferative Glomerulonephritis being more common in 36% [9]. An Indian group reported non IgA mesangial proliferative GN the most common primary glomerular disease in 20% followed by FSGS in 17% of patients [10].

Another study from India concluded that membranous nephropathy is the most common primary glomerular disease in elderly more than 60 years of age [11]. A study from Minnesota USA reviewed the data of 195 native kidney biopsies. Most common glomerular disease was Ig A nephropathy (22%), followed by FSGS (17%) and then membranous nephropathy (10%) [12].

A study from New York presented the biopsy review of 132 patients in which primary glomerular disease FSGS was the most common (38%) and then membranous nephropathy (16%). This study concluded that the FSGS is emerging as a most common cause of ESRD among primary glomerular diseases patients [13]. Study from San Francisco presented review of 183 native kidney biopsies. Most common diagnoses were IgA nephropathy and FSGS [14].

Jamal Q et al. from Karachi Pakistan reviewed more than 948 renal biopsies from adults. Most common diagnosis were MCD in 29%, Chronic GN in12 percent [15]. Muzzafar M et al. from Rawalpindi published data of 58 Primary Nephrotic patients. Most common three pathology in kidney biopsy were membrono glomerulo- nephritis (MPGN) in 32 percent, MCD in 24 percent and mesangial proliferative glomerulonephritis in 21 per- cent [16].

Osmani MH and Shabnam F published experience of 152 kidney biopsies from Karachi. The most common renal lesions were FSGS in 15%, Membranous in 13% and then MCD in 11 percent [17]. Khan AZ et al. from Peshawar reported experience of 130 renal biopsies. Among the patients more than 12 years the most common findings were MPGN in 22%, membranous GN in 20% and FSGS in 16 percent [18]. Kazi JI and Mubarak M from Karachi reviewed 350 biopsies from adult patients with nephritic syndrome. In this study the most com- mon diagnosis were FSGS in 36% followed by membranous GN in 24% and minimal change in 14 percent [19].

Khan SZ and Ali A published data from Peshawar. Among patients aged 60 years or above with nephrotic syndrome were studied. Most common pathology was minimal change in 40 percent followed by Membranous GN in 21 percent and crescentic GN in 19 percent [20]. Kazi JI and M Mubarak M et al. reported results of 316 kidney biopsies of nephrotic patients from Karachi. Most common pathology was focal segmental Glomerulos- clerosis (FSGS) in 40%, then membranous glomerulonephritis (MGN) in 27% followed by minimal change dis- ease [MCD) in 15 percent [21].

Mubarak M et al. from Karachi reported experience of 1793 adult patients. The most common pathology on renal biopsy was FSGN in 29%, and membranous in 23% among primary glomerular disease [11]. Abbas K et al. from Karachi presented the data of nephrotics in all ages. The three most common findings were FSGS, mi- nimal Change and membranous GN [22].

Sabir S et al. reported their experience from Karachi. Sixty biopsies were analyzed. The most common pa- thologies were FSGS in 26%, memranous GN in 16% and IgA Nephropathy in 11 percent among the primary glomerulonaephritis [23]. Choudhary M et al. from Lahore studied the histological pattern in male patients pre- sented for hematuria, proteinuria and high serum creatinine. Among the adults the most common pathology was c hronic kidney disease and end stage renal disease in 19 percent followed by mesangial proliferative GN and FSGN [24].

There are weaknesses in our study. It is a single center study. Patients may not be true representative of the population. Our study and above mentioned studies altogether is a heterogeneous group and we can not compare one study with the other. However it gives us a data base or at least starting point for the researchers interested in conducting the controlled and population base studies. Our study will help in better understanding the spec- trum of renal disease in Pakistan. In addition it will also help the clinician in decision making for the manage- ment.

5. Conclusion

TubuloInterstitial nephritis, membranous nephropathy, focal segmental glomerulosclerosis, and membrano pro- liferative glomerulonephritis were the most common histopthological diagnosis in adult patients presented to

AKU for kidney biopsy. Our data will contribute in better understanding the spectrum of renal disease in Pakistan. It will also guide the clinician in management and possibly in planning the prevention of chronic kidney disease.

References

[1] Taal, M.W., *et al.* (2011) The Renal Biopsy. In: *Brenner & Rector's The Kidney*, 9th Edition, Saunders Elsevier, Philadelphia. http://www.clinicalkey.com

[2] Johnson, R.J., *et al.* (2015) Renal Biopsy. In: *Comprehensive Clinical Nephrology*, 5th Edition, Saunders Elsevier, Philadelphia.

[3] Jafar, T.H. (2006) The Growing Burden of Chronic Kidney Disease in Pakistan. *The New England Journal of Medicine*, **354**, 995-997. http://dx.doi.org/10.1056/NEJMp058319

[4] Rychlik, I., Jancova, E., Tesar, V., Kolskey, A., Lacha, J., Stegskal, J., *et al.* (2004) The Czech Registry of Renal Biopsy. *Nephrology Dialysis Transplantation*, **19**, 3040-3049. http://dx.doi.org/10.1093/ndt/gfh521

[5] Choi, I.J., Jeong, H.J., Han, D.S., Lee, J.S., Choi, K.H., Kang, S.W., *et al.* (2001) Analysis of 4515 Cases of Renal Biopsy in Korea. *Yonseri Medical Journal*, **42**, 247-254. http://dx.doi.org/10.3349/ymj.2001.42.2.247

[6] Gesualdo, L., Di Palma, A.M., Morrone, L.F., Strippoli, G.F. and Schena, F.P. (2004) The Italian Experience of the National Registry of Renal Biopsy. *Kidney International*, **66**, 890-894. http://dx.doi.org/10.1111/j.1523-1755.2004.00831.x

[7] Covic, A., Schiller, A., Carmen, V., Gluhovschi, G., *et al.* (2006) Epidemiology of Renal Disease in Romania. *Nephrology Dialysis Transplantation*, **21**, 419-424. http://dx.doi.org/10.1093/ndt/gfi207

[8] Rivera, F., Lopez-Gomez, J. and Perez Garcia, R. (2004) Clinicopathological Correlation of Renal Pathology in Spain. *Kidney International*, **66**, 898-904. http://dx.doi.org/10.1111/j.1523-1755.2004.00833.x

[9] Yahya, T.M., Pingle, A., Boobes, Y. and Pingle, S. (1998) Analysis of 490 Kidney Biopsies: Data from United Arab Emirates Renal Disease Registry. *Journal of Nephrology*, **11**, 148-150.

[10] Narasimhan, B., Chacho, B., John, G.T., Korula, A., Kirubakaran, M.G. and Jacob, C.K. (2006) Characterization of Kidney Lesions in Indian Adults: Towards a Renal Biopsy Registry. *Journal of Nephrology*, **19**, 205-210.

[11] Prakash, J., Singh, A.K. and Sexana, R.K. (2003) Glomerular Diseases in the Elderly in India. *International Urology and Nephrology*, **35**, 283-288. http://dx.doi.org/10.1023/B:UROL.0000020429.14190.5b

[12] Swaminathan, S., Leung, N., Lager, D.J., Melton, L.J., Bergstralh, E.J., Rohlinger, A. and Fervenza, F.C. (2006) Changing Incidence of Glomerular Disease in Olmsted County, Minnesota: A 30-Year Renal Biopsy Study. *Clinical Journal of the American Society of Nephrology*, **1**, 483-487. http://dx.doi.org/10.2215/CJN.00710805

[13] Haas, M., Meehan, S.M., Karrison, T.G. and Spargo, B.H. (1997) Changing Etiologies of Unexplained Adult Nephrotic Syndrome: A Comparison of Renal Biopsy Findings from 1976-1979 and 1995-1997. *American Journal of Kidney Diseases*, **30**, 621-631. http://dx.doi.org/10.1016/S0272-6386(97)90485-6

[14] Dragovic, D., Rosenstock, J.L., Wahl, S.J., Panagopoulos, G., Devita, M.V. and Michelis, M.F. (2005) Increasing Incidence of Focal Segmental Glomerulosclerosis and an Examination of Demographic Patterns. *Clinical Nephrology*, **63**, 1-7. http://dx.doi.org/10.5414/CNP63001

[15] Jamal, Q., Jafarey, N.A. and Navi, A.J. (1988) A Review of 1508 Percutaneous Renal Biopsies. *Journal of Pakistan Medical Association*, **38**, 272-275.

[16] Muzaffar, M., Mushtaq, S., Khadim, M.T., Nabiruddin and Mamoon, N. (1997) Morphological Pattern of Glomerular Diseases in Patients with Nephrotic Syndrome in Northern Pakistan. *Pakistan Armed Forces Medical Journal*, **47**, 3-6.

[17] Osmani, M.H. and Frooqi, S. (2001) An Audit of Renal Biopsies. *Journal of Surgery Pakistan*, **6**, 28-30.

[18] Khan, A.Z., Anwar, N., Munib, M. and Shah, F. (2004) Histological Pattern of Glomerulopathies at Khyber Teaching Hospital, Peshawar. *Pakistan Journal of Medical Research*, **43**, 117-120.

[19] Kazi, J.I. and Mubarak, M. (2007) Pattern of Glomerulonephritides in Adult Nephritic Patients Report from SIUT (Letter to the Editor). *Journal of Pakistan Medical Association*, **57**, 574.

[20] Zaffar, S.A. and Ali, A. (2008) Histological Pattern of Nephrotic Syndrome in Elderly Patients. *Journal of Ayub Medical College Abbottabad*, **20**, 97-99.

[21] Mubarak, M., Kazi, J.I., Naqvi, R., Ahmed, E., Akhter, F., Naqvi, S.A. and Rizvi, S.A. (2011) Pattern of Renal Diseases Observed in Native Renal Biopsies in Adults in a Single Centre in Pakistan. *Nephrology*, **16**, 87-92. http://dx.doi.org/10.1111/j.1440-1797.2010.01410.x

[22] Abbas, K., Mubarak, M., Kaziet, J.I. and Muzaffar, R. (2009) Pattern of Morphology in Renal Biopsies of Nephritic Syndrome Patients. Correlation with Immunoglobulin and Complement Deposition and Serology. *Journal of Pakistan*

Medical Association, **59**, 540-543.

[23] Sabir, S., Mubarak, M., Ul-Haq, I. and Bibi, A. (2013) Pattern of Biopsy Proven Renal Disease at PNS SHIFA Karachi: A Cross-Sectional Survey. *Journal of Renal Injury Prevention*, **2**, 133-137.

[24] Choudhary, M., Masood, A., Rashid, F., Mand, A. and Nagi, A.H. (2014) Morphological Pattern of Glomerulonephritis in Males: A Multicenter Study. *Biomedica*, **30**, 110-114.

16

Nursing Diagnostics of Nutrition Domain of NANDA International in Hemodialysis Patients

Érida Maria Diniz Leite[1], Sama Mikaella de Oliveira[2],
Maria Isabel da Conceição Dias Fernandes[2], Maria das Graças Mariano Nunes[2],
Cyndi Fernandes de Lima[2], Ana Luisa Brandão de Carvalho Lira[2]

[1]Department of Nursing, Hospital Academic Onofre Lopes, Natal, Brasil
[2]Department of Nursing, University of Rio Grande do Norte, Natal, Brasil
Email: bebel_6@hotmail.com

Abstract

Introduction: The dialysis causes the loss of the nutrients and the elevation of catabolism, thus, patients in dialysis have at high risk for the loss of body reserves of protein and energy. Objective: To identify nursing diagnoses of nutrition domain of NANDA International in hemodialysis patients and to correlate them to the socioeconomic and clinical data. Design: Cross-sectional study. Setting: Performed in a large university hospital in northeastern Brazil. Participants: The first stage was carried out with 50 patients, selected with the following inclusion criteria: Being hospitalized and undergoing hemodialysis in that hospital; aged 18 years old or over; being conscious and oriented. Exclusion criteria were patients undergoing hemodialysis in that hospital with external service, pregnant women and patients being treated by plasmapheresis. In the second stage, participants were three nursing specialists in nephrology and nursing diagnoses. Methods: The defining characteristics of the nursing diagnoses inserted in the nutrition domain were observed in patients and then these data were judged by nurses, in order to identify diagnoses present in each patient. The Chi-square, Fisher's exact and Mann-Whitney tests were used in the analysis of the relationship of socioeconomic and clinical data, with an adopted p value of <0.05. Results: The study identified six diagnoses of nutrition domain with prevalence ≥50% in patients. Among these, the diagnosis: Risk for impaired liver function, imbalanced nutrition: More than body requirements, risk for deficient fluid volume, readiness for enhanced fluid volume were significantly associated with gender (p = 0.001), origin (p = 0.014), religion (p = 0.046) and income (p = 0.039), respectively. Conclusion: The variables that showed significant association were risk of impaired liver function and gender; imbalanced nutrition: More than body requirements and origin requirements; risk for deficient fluid volume and religion; and deficient fluid volume and income.

Keywords

Nursing, Nursing Diagnosis, Risk Groups Nutrition, Renal Dialysis

1. Introduction

The kidneys are responsible for removing harmful substances for the proper functioning of the body, reabsorbing vital nutrients, regulating the volume of fluid and electrolytes, and producing hormones [1]-[3]. However, when the kidneys become unable to perform these functions, the patient develops renal failure, resulting in body damage, such as fluid retention, electrolyte abnormalities and accumulation of toxic substances [3]. Thus, Chronic Kidney Disease (CKD) is the slow and progressive decline in renal function, causing the accumulation of metabolic waste products in the blood [4].

The need for renal replacement therapy is required when the glomerular filtration rate has a value less than 15 ml/minute/1.73 m^2 [2]. In Brazil, most people with CKD undergo outpatient hemodialysis (HD), with sessions on average three times a week and lasting three to four hours [5]. The HD is the blood's exposure of patient to extracorporeal circulation, moving through a semipermeable membrane, known as capillary dialyzer filter. The filtered blood is then returned to the patient free of excess fluids and metabolic products derived [4] [6] [7]. Thus, the HD aims to compensate for renal dysfunction through depuration of blood by removing excess fluid and metabolites [8].

The 2013 dialysis census showed that over time there has been an increase in population on dialysis, with 100,397 patients only in 2013, which was an increase of 2.8% over the year 2012, and 89.7% performed hemodialysis (HD). In addition, it was observed that the age group between 19 and 64 years old was the most affected [5].

The realization of HD led to several changes in the daily lives of patients with CKD and their families, requiring adaptation to treatment. Among the changes are highlighted food and water restrictions and limitations directed to professional activities, physical and leisure, that is why are identified feelings of revolt in these patients, as well as depressive symptoms and impotence. Thus the hemodialysis treatment, is revealed as a factor limiting the quality of life of these patients, however, in contrast, this treatment provides an improvement in their conditions of life/health. Thus, most patients evaluate the achievement of the dialysis treatment as satisfactory [9] [10].

Although prolonging the life of the patient, HD can trigger hemodynamic and nutritional complications, because during this treatment not only undesirable substances are removed, such as urea, but also important substances for the body such as amino acids, peptides, vitamins and glucose [7] [8] [11]. Besides the loss of these nutrients, the elevation of catabolism occurs during HD. Thus, the HD patients are at high risk for the loss of body reserves of protein and energy [11].

The index of morbidity and mortality is associated with nutritional status and adequacy of dialysis [8] [12]. It is stated that these rates are extremely high [13], highlighting mortality with a fee 48% [14].

In this context, the nurse is one of the agents involved in direct assistance to this population, performing an indispensable role, through the planning and provision of care, in order to prevent complications, reduce anxiety and stress [15].

Thus, the nurse is able to identify the needs of each client and prescribe a qualified and effective care through the steps of the nursing process (NP) [16] [17]. The NP stage is responsible for identifying the altered human response, called Nursing Diagnosis (ND). The ND should be identified based on taxonomy, and the most known taxonomy is the North American Nursing Association (NANDA International), composed of thirteen domains [18].

Among these, there is the nutrition domain of NANDA International in the context of patients undergoing HD [19]-[22]. Diagnostics for the intake, metabolism and hydration are included in this domain [18]. In most studies on the subject, the focus is mainly on those issues related to hydration [19]-[22]. However, problems related to overweight and malnutrition are also present and are considered relevant by its repercussions [23].

The occurrence of certain nursing problems in this clientele usually comes from different life contexts in which they live, as well as from the existing clinical variability. Malnutrition, for example, is related to depression, monthly personal income, source of income, age and low level of education [24]. Thus, the relationships between the socioeconomic or clinical variables and the nursing diagnoses help nursing professionals to focus on the best care to be provided.

Thus, in view of the above, the authors became interested in developing a study that would help the nurse in identifying problems entered into the nutrition domain present in the patient on hemodialysis linked to their socioeconomic and clinical context, given the importance of promoting safe, resolute care and supported in their own scientific knowledge. Thus, the aim of the study was to identify the nutrition domain of nursing diagnoses of NANDA International in patients undergoing hemodialysis (HD) and correlate them to the socioeconomic and clinical data.

2. Method

2.1. Design and Setting

Cross-sectional study conducted in a large teaching hospital in northeastern Brazil.

2.2. Sample Calculation and Sample

The population consisted of 210 patients, from January 2012 to January 2013. The sample was calculated based on the formula for finite populations, considering a confidence level of 95%, sample error of 12% and a conservative value for the prevalence of patients with nursing diagnoses of 50%. From this, it was identified a sample of 50 patients.

2.3. Sample Selection

Sampling was chosen by convenience of consecutive type, with the following inclusion criteria: being hospitalized and undergoing hemodialysis in that hospital; aged 18 years old or over; being conscious and oriented. Exclusion criteria were patients undergoing hemodialysis in that hospital with external service, pregnant women and patients being treated with plasmapheresis.

2.4. Data Collection and Instrument

Data collection took place from December 2013 to May 2014 during HD sessions, and was held by the researcher and four undergraduate research scholars. The collectors received six hours of training, divided into two stages: 1) lecture on the subject of study, objectives, methodology and the ND of the nutrition domain of NANDA International [25]; 2) detailed discussion of instrument and practice of physical examination.

The collection instrument was a form of history and physical examination, which was adapted from a study of nursing diagnoses in patients undergoing hemodialysis [26]. It is noteworthy that the appearance of the instrument was validated by two specialist nurses in nursing diagnoses and/or nephrology, belonging to the research group Relief and Epidemiology Practices in Health and Nursing (PAESE) of the Federal University of northeastern Brazil.

It is noteworthy that among the diagnoses that make up the nutrition domain, four were not addressed in the collection instrument, because of the profile of the studied clientele. Diagnoses were: insufficient breast milk, ineffective infant feeding pattern, neonatal jaundice and risk for neonatal jaundice.

The collected data were grouped into 50 worksheets in Microsoft Excel 2010 Officer for each patient, containing, in each of these, defining characteristics, related factors and risk related to 13 diagnoses.

2.5. Diagnostic Inference

Subsequently, the 50 worksheets were sent to specialist nurses in nursing diagnoses and/or nephrology, in order to judge the presence or absence of the 13 diagnoses in the studied clientele from the previously reported clinical indicators.

Six experts were intentionally invited to participate in the study. They underwent training, and then an evaluation of the diagnostic capacity. At that time, 12 fictitious case histories were randomly distributed to participants, who responded the clinical cases three times each, at different times, totaling 36 evaluations.

Finally, to verify the performance of experts as diagnosticians, it was applied the Kappa test to check the level of agreement of these in relation to the assessed diagnoses, and then three specialists were selected after application of the test for diagnostic inference. Kappa is an index designed to measure only the correlation between pairs. So, three diagnosticians were selected, those who obtained almost perfect agreement (0.80 - 1.00).

Therefore, to obtain only the responses of experts, these were compared and. in case of disagreement, it was applied the rule of the majority, considering the diagnosis present when two of the three diagnosticians identified it as present. This inference occurred in the period from July to August 2014.

2.6. Data Analysis

For analysis of socioeconomic and clinical data, the descriptive statistics was applied and the relative and absolute frequencies, mean, standard deviation, median, maximum and minimum were evaluated. The Kolmogorov-Smirnov test was also applied, in order to verify the normality of the data ($p < 0.05$). To analyze the statistical association between Chi-square, Fisher's exact and Mann-Whitney tests were used, and it was adopted p value < 0.05.

2.7. Ethics Approval

The research project was approved by the Research Ethics Committee of the institution responsible for the research, with opinion number 392,535 and Certificate of Presentation for Ethical Consideration number 18710613.4.00005537. It is noteworthy that patients and specialists were consulted about their interest in participating in the research and informed about the study objectives, methodological procedures, risks, making them aware of confidentiality given to information and identities. So those who expressed interest, was made the request to give consent of the study, by reading and subsequent signing of the Terms of Informed Consent.

3. Results

Most patients interviewed were female (62%), had a partner (54%), had some religion (80%), came from the country towns (76%) and underwent the classic hemodialysis type (92%). Regarding age, the average was 47.5 years old (±14.61), with a minimum of 19 and maximum of 80. With respect to years of study, there was a median of five years. The income showed a median of 1.5 minimum salaries. Concerning hemodialysis data, 86% of patients had a diagnosis of CKD, with a median of 27 months of diagnosis, 10.5 months of HD and 4 hours of dialysis duration.

Concerning the prevalence of nursing diagnoses of nutrition domain, the risk for electrolyte imbalance was present in 100% (n = 50) of patients, the risk for unstable blood glucose level and excess fluid volume was present in 90% (n = 45) readiness for enhanced fluid balance in 86% (n = 43), readiness for enhanced nutrition in 80% (n = 40), the risk for deficient fluid volume in 76% (n = 43), impaired swallowing in 50% (n = 25) risk for imbalanced fluid volume by 44% (n = 22), imbalanced nutrition: more than body requirements in 38% (n = 19), risk for impaired liver function in 34% (n = 17), imbalanced nutrition: less than body requirements in 32% (n = 16), risk for imbalanced nutrition: more than body requirements in 22% (n = 11) and deficient fluid volume in 2% (n = 1).

Regarding the association between the socioeconomic and clinical variables and the nursing diagnoses of the nutrition domain of NANDA International, imbalanced nutrition: more than body requirements was significantly associated with the variable origin ($p = 0.014$), being prevalent in patients from country towns. Diagnosis risk for impaired liver function was associated with gender ($p = 0.001$) and showed prevalence for males. Risk for deficient fluid volume had significant association with religion ($p = 0.046$), being mostly associated to individuals practicing some religion. Finally, readiness for enhanced fluid volume and family income ($p = 0.039$) showed a statistically significant association, with an income of 1.5 minimum wage, as shown in **Table 1**.

4. Discussion

Concerning the socioeconomic characterization, the study found that most HD patients were female, aged between 19 and 80 years old, had a partner, came from the country towns, had some religion, most were retired or received pension and had few years of study, with a median of five years. This data corroborate the results of research addressing a similar theme [18].

Table 1. Distribution of association between the nursing diagnoses of nutrition domain of NANDA International and the socioeconomic and clinical variables of hemodialysis patients. Natal/RN, 2016.

Nursing diagnoses	Age	Years of study	Family income	Time of RD	Time of HD	Duration of HD	Type of HD	Gender	Marital status	Religion	Origin
Impaired swallowing	0.351[1]	0.159[1]	0.194[1]	0.712[1]	0.518[1]	0.728[1]	0.695[2]	0.382[3]	0.156[3]	1.000[3]	0.508[3]
Imbalanced nutrition: more than body requirements	0.617[1]	0.770[1]	0.950[1]	0.881[1]	0.846[1]	0.085[1]	0.507[2]	0.895[3]	0.879[3]	0.579[2]	0.014[2]
Risk for imbalanced nutrition: more than body requirements	0.052[1]	0.376[1]	0.190[1]	0.972[1]	0.614[1]	0.050[1]	0.357[2]	0.405[2]	0.967[3]	0.618[2]	0.472[2]
Imbalanced nutrition: less than body requirements	0.700[1]	0.183[1]	0.896[1]	0.909[1]	0.798[1]	0.818[1]	0.091[2]	0.566[3]	0.697[3]	0.400[2]	0.120[2]
Readiness for enhanced nutrition	0.818[1]	0.353[1]	0.341[1]	0.349[1]	0.136[1]	0.880[1]	0.397[2]	0.173[2]	0.089[2]	0.349[2]	0.551[2]
Risk for impaired liver function	0.424[1]	0.992[1]	0.600	0.276	0.228	0.799	0.420[2]	0.001[3]	0.276[3]	0.461[2]	0.350[2]
Risk for unstable blood glucose level	0.706[1]	0.087[1]	0.327[1]	0.115[1]	0.296[1]	0.394[1]	0.647[2]	0.355[2]	0.578[2]	0.311[2]	0.237[2]
Risk for electrolyte imbalance	-	-	-	-	-	-	-	-	-	-	-
Readiness for enhanced fluid balance	0.891[1]	0.510[1]	0.039[1]	0.848[1]	0.827[1]	0.827[1]	0.536[2]	0.166[2]	0.407[2]	0.187[2]	0.126[2]
Deficient fluid volume	0.840[1]	0.360[1]	0.240[1]	0.880[1]	0.840[1]	0.800[1]	0.920[2]	0.620[2]	0.540[2]	0.800[2]	0.760[2]
Risk for deficient fluid volume	0.601[1]	0.775[1]	0.962[1]	0.155[1]	0.370[1]	0.500[1]	0.679[2]	0.238[2]	0.094[3]	0.046[2]	0.306[2]
Excess fluid volume	0.267[1]	0.159[1]	0.488[1]	0.683[1]	0.851[1]	0.394[1]	0.647[2]	0.638[2]	0.229[2]	0.311[2]	0.655[2]
Risk for imbalanced fluid volume	0.639[1]	0.485[1]	0.581[1]	0.468[1]	0.535[1]	0.882[1]	0.598[2]	0.121[3]	0.522[3]	0.216[2]	0.393[2]

[1]Mann-Whitney U test; [2]Fisher's exact test; [3]Chi-square test.

On the income, the study reveals that this is directly related to the clinical treatment of the patient. Thus, patients with monthly personal income below one minimum wage are more likely to develop malnutrition, and are 1.5 to 4.2 more likely to have this diagnosis than those who earn more than one minimum wage. In terms of occupation, the retired patients are 1.3 to 5.9 more likely to acquire malnutrition than those who had other sources as main income. And finally, regarding education, illiterates were more likely to develop malnutrition compared those with complete/incomplete higher education [24].

The percentage of malnourished patients in the final stages of the disease is between 40% and 70% according to a study on the topic [27]. The percentage of this problem was identified in a smaller amount, 32% in this study. This variation is due to the use of different methods used for nutritional assessment and population characteristics, being related, among others, loss of appetite, dysgeusia, impaired digestion and absorption, metabolic acidosis and emotional stress [27].

Malnutrition can also be explained by considering the hemodialysis treatment, where smaller molecules like urea, glucose, sodium and potassium, present in the blood pass through the membrane of the dialyser is removed, larger molecules also are removed, substances essential to the body, and amino acids, peptides and vitamins [7] [8].

Thus, the HD procedure interferes with protein metabolism by loss of amino acids from 6 to 12 grams per hemodialysis, which comes to be reduced between 20% and 50% after each HD [28]. Low albumin levels are associated with increased mortality for patients on hemodialysis. Thus, dietary changes to promote greater protein intake to improve the nutritional status of these patients should be suggested [29].

Are also lost glucose molecules whose molecular weight is too small, facilitating your displacement of the membrane of capillary [30]. These losses can vary from 15grams to 30 grams of glucose per hemodialysis, which entails energy loss, as evidenced per episodes of hypoglycemia [31] [32]. To control hypoglycemia are needed as nursing measures: monitor blood glucose levels and provide simple carbohydrates at the time of dialysis [33].

The risk for unstable blood glucose level was present in 90% of the sample. Thus, a study on complications during dialysis showed a frequency of 62.37% of hypoglycemia compared to other complications [31]. In contrast, a survey showed a low rate for this diagnosis: only 9% of patients had risk for unstable blood glucose level

[34]. However, despite the low prevalence of association between diabetes and hypoglycemia in some studies, it is important to consider it because of the large number of hemodialysis patients with diabetes.

Furthermore, research shows that many of these individuals are sedentary [35], which contributes to the increase in obesity, factors directly related to insulin resistance, thereby contributing to the onset of this nursing diagnosis in the patients studied, which have a greater tendency to changes in blood glucose level [36].

Added to this, are highlights the feelings of loss, frustration and limitations of treatment and disease that are related to mental and emotional aspects. The burden of treatment may be expressed by feelings of worthlessness, devaluation and depression evidenced by impairment of quality of life of these patients [37]. Thus, renal failure patients on hemodialysis experience psychological stress situations that may affect the blood glucose levels. This perspective, the nurse must be alert to stressful situations experienced by these patients, as well as monitoring of blood glucose levels [31].

The diagnosis of risk for electrolyte imbalance was present in 100% of patients in this study and therefore it was not possible to apply statistical tests. Similar result was identified in a survey conducted in HD units in Belo Horizonte [34]. In this respect, it is observed that the kidney patient commonly has glomerular, tubular and endocrine functions of kidneys impaired. These organs do not perform effectively blood filtration, triggering an imbalance in electrolytes rate [1]. Thus, it is assumed that these patients have a higher risk for the development of electrolyte imbalance.

In this context, effective measures are needed performed by the nurses for the control of electrolytes, especially sodium, in these individuals. In study about the self-care measures undertaken by HD patients to manage restrictions of sodium and fluids in the diet, indicates as main measures: Avoid instant products and Asian food, do not put salt on the table, reduction of salt the food cooking, to avoid foods with very salt [38].

The excess fluid volume was prevalent in most of the studied clientele, corroborating study on the prevalence of this diagnosis with similar clientele, which showed an 82% rate. That research also highlighted as main clinical symptoms linked to this diagnosis: edema, weight gain, pulmonary congestion and abnormal breath sounds [19]. For this nursing problem the following nursing activities must be performed: monitor the intake and output of fluids, checking vital signs and to weight the pacient before and after hemodialysis [33].

The presence of the nursing diagnoses readiness for enhanced fluid balance and readiness for enhanced nutrition, which had prevalence of 86% and 80%, respectively, can be directly related to the guidelines provided by health professionals to these patients. A survey conducted in 12 dialysis clinics noted that all guidance provided to patients were directed to the water and nutrient restriction, and that 49.9% of subjects reported following these recommendations [24]. In this context, educational activities performed by nurses are essential for the patient to understand their health-disease process and consequently have a good acceptance and adherence to treatment [39].

The risk for deficient fluid volume had a percentage of 76%, but, in the literature, nothing was found to justify the presence of this diagnosis. Thus, its high prevalence may be related to the presence of risk factors such as deficiency of knowledge, failure of regulatory mechanisms and fluid loss by abnormal pathways [25]. Among the nursing activities that can be applied to this diagnosis are: monitoring the intake and output of fluids, monitor water loss, check vital signs, measure weight, position the patient in the Trendelenburg position when hypotension, and guide the patient and/or family on measures for the treatment of hypovolemia [33].

Thus, with regard to diagnoses identified in this study with frequencies greater than 50%, they were found in studies with similar population [22] [34] [40].

In this study, we could also see some significant statistical associations. One of those was between the ND risk for impaired liver function and gender, in which male was dominant in this clientele. In this aspect, a cross-sectional study conducted in an Occupational Health Care Service at a public university found that males had the highest rates for the standard group of risk and harmful alcohol consumption and probable alcohol dependence, with a percentage of 65.9%% [41]. This may have contributed to the emergence of this diagnosis.

Another association occurs between the ND imbalanced nutrition: More than body requirements and the variable origin, in which most individuals come from country towns. This association may be related to the cultural issue, since these individuals usually have higher calorie eating habits and have little access to information about appropriate diet. In addition, a study indicated that this ND is linked to physical inactivity and poor eating habits. It is the nurse's role to guide the patient regarding diet according to the possibilities and customs of each patient [42].

For this problem of nursing, nursing interventions listed are: control of eating disorders, performing the following activities: consult a nutritionist to determine daily caloric intake required to achieve and/or maintain ideal weight, teach and reinforce patient information on good nutrition, to monitoring of daily intake of high-calorie foods, offer support to the patient as part of new eating habits and monitor the patient's weight routine. Another positive intervention for weight loss would be do exercises, with the following activities: encourage the person to get exercise, assist the patient to establish short and long term goals for your exercise program, report on the health benefits and physiological effects of exercise, counseling on the frequency, duration and intensity of exercise and monitor patient compliance [33].

Regarding the diagnosis risk for deficient fluid volume, this was associated with religion, and most of the individuals had some religion. Study claims that religion is an important issue for the health of hemodialysis patient, because it is related to increased quality of life and better coping with the disease [43].

Finally, there was association between readiness for enhanced fluid balance and family income, but it was not found in the literature any justification for such an association.

Given the above, it is up to the nurse to remain attentive to the clinical indicators of this population and their relationship with socioeconomic and clinical factors, in order to solve health problems, especially with regard to nutritional changes involving this clientele.

5. Conclusions

This study identified the diagnoses of the domain nutrition of NANDA International with higher prevalence in patients undergoing hemodialysis, namely: Risk for electrolyte imbalance, risk for unstable blood glucose level, excess fluid volume, readiness for enhanced fluid balance, readiness for enhanced nutrition and risk for deficient fluid volume.

It is noteworthy that the ND: Risk for impaired liver function, imbalanced nutrition: More than body requirements, risk for deficient fluid volume, and readiness for enhanced fluid balance were significantly associated with gender, origin, religion and income respectively.

From the above, it is evident that there is a high prevalence of this domain in patients undergoing hemodialysis, and that a relationship exists between these diagnoses and the socioeconomic and clinical variables. Therefore, it is imperative that nurses recognize these problems in their social and clinical context, with a view to elucidating them efficiently.

Thus, the conduction of studies that deal with the identification of specific nursing diagnoses for certain clientele favors the decision making performed by nurses in clinical practice, so that the diagnostic inference is fast and accurate front to the individual's needs.

This study was limited by the shortage of studies on the nutrition domain and HD patients. Thus, it is suggested the development of more studies on this domain of NANDA International, keeping in view the importance and impact of nursing diagnoses included in this domain.

References

[1]   Bastos, M.G., Bregman, R. and Kirsztajn, G.M. (2010) Doença renal crônica: Frequente e grave, mas também prevenível e tratável. *Revista Associação Médica Brasileira*, **56**, 248-253.
       http://dx.doi.org/10.1590/S0104-42302010000200028

[2]   National Kidney Foundation (2013) KDIGO, Kidney Disease Improving Global Outcomes: Clinical Practice Guideline for the Evaluation and Management of Chronic Kidney Disease. *American Journal of Kidney Diseases*, **3**, 1-24.

[3]   Zatz, R., Seguro, A.C. and Malnic, G. (2011) Bases fisiológicas da nefrologia. Atheneu, São Paulo.

[4]   Riella, M.C. (2010) Princípios de nefrologia e distúrbios hidroeletrolíticos. 5th Edition, Guanabara Koogan, São Paulo.

[5]   Sociedade Brasileira de Nefrologia (SBN) (2014) Censo de Diálise 2013. São Paulo.
       http://www.sbn.org.br/pdf/censo_2013-14-05.pdf

[6]   Fermi, M.R.V. (2011) Manual de Diálise para Enfermagem. 2nd Edition, Medsi, Rio de Janeiro.

[7]   Reddenna, L., Basha, S.A. and Reddy, K.S.K. (2014) Dialysis Treatment: A Comprehensive Description. *International Journal of Pharmaceutical Sciences Review and Research*, **3**, 1-13.

[8]   Riella, M.C. and Martins, C. (2013) Nutrição e o Rim. 2nd Edition, Guanabara Koogan, Rio de Janeiro.

[9]   Rudnicki, T. (2014) Doença renal crônica: Vivência do paciente em tratamento de hemodiálise. *Contextos Clínicos*, **7**, 105-116. http://dx.doi.org/10.4013/ctc.2014.71.10

[10] Silva, A.S., Silveira, R.S., Fernandes, G.F.M., Lunardi, V.L. and Backes, V.M.S. (2011) Percepções e mudanças na qualidade de vida de pacientes submetidos à hemodiálise. *Revista Brasileira de Enfermagem*, **64**, 839-844. http://dx.doi.org/10.1590/S0034-71672011000500006

[11] Associação Médica Brasileira: Conselho Federal de Medicina (2011) Projeto diretrizes para terapia nutricional para pacientes em hemodiálise crônica. São Paulo.

[12] Li, T., Liu, J., An, S., Dai, Y. and Yu, Q. (2014) Body Mass Index and Mortality in Patients on Maintenance Hemodialysis: A Meta-Analysis. *International Urology and Nephrology*, **46**, 623-631. http://dx.doi.org/10.1007/s11255-014-0653-x

[13] Jablonski, K.L. and Chonchol, M. (2014) Recent Advances in the Management of Hemodialysis Patients: A Focus on Cardiovascular Disease. F1000Prime Reports, **6**, 1-10.

[14] Siviero, P.C.L., Machado, C.J. and Cherchiglia, M.L. (2014) Insuficiência renal crônica no Brasil segundo enfoque de causas múltiplas de morte. *Caderno de Saúde Coletiva*, **22**, 75-85. http://dx.doi.org/10.1590/1414-462X201400010012

[15] Smeltzer, S.C. and Bare, B.G. (2011) Brunner & Suddarth: Tratado de Enfermagem Médico-Cirúrgica. 12th Edition, Guanabara Koogan, Rio de Janeiro.

[16] Frazão, C.M.F.Q., Ramos, V.P. and Lira, A.L.B.C. (2011) Qualidade de vida de pacientes submetidos à hemodiálise. *Revista Enfermagem UERJ*, **19**, 577-582.

[17] Silva, E.G.C., Oliveira, V.C., Neves, G.B.C. and Guimarães, T.M.R. (2011) El conhecimento do enfermeiro sobre a Sistematização da Assistência de Enfermagem: da teoria à prática. *Revista da Escola de Enfermagem da USP*, **45**, 1380-1386. http://dx.doi.org/10.1590/S0080-62342011000600015

[18] Herdman, T.H. and Kamitsuru, S. (2014) NANDA International Nursing Diagnoses: Definitions & Clasification, 2015-2017. 10th Edition, Wiley Blackwell, Oxford.

[19] Fernandes, M.I.C.D., Medeiros, A.B.A., Macedo, B.M., Vitorino, A.B.F., Lopes, M.V.O. and Lira, A.L.B.C. (2014) Prevalência do diagnóstico de enfermagem Volume de líquidos excessivo em pacientes submetidos à hemodiálise. *Revista da Escola de Enfermagem da USP*, **48**, 446-453. http://dx.doi.org/10.1590/S0080-623420140000300009

[20] Frazão, C.M.F.Q., Medeiros, A.B.A., Silva, F.B.B.L., Sá, J.D. and Lira, A.L.B.C. (2014) Diagnósticos de enfermagem em pacientes renais crônicos em hemodiálise. *Acta Paulista de Enfermagem*, **27**, 40-43. http://dx.doi.org/10.1590/1982-0194201400009

[21] Poveda, V.B., Alves, J.S., Santos, E.F. and Moreira, A.G.E. (2014) Diagnósticos de enfermagem em pacientes submetidos à hemodiálise. *Enfermería Global*, **34**, 70-81.

[22] Dallé, J. and Lucena, A.F. (2012) Diagnósticos de enfermagem identificados em pacientes hospitalizados durante sessões de hemodiálise. *Acta Paulista de Enfermagem*, **25**, 504-510. http://dx.doi.org/10.1590/S0103-21002012000400004

[23] Stefanelli, C., Andreoti, F.D., Quesada, K.R. and Detregiachi, C.R.P. (2010) Avaliação nutricional de pacientes em hemodiálise. *Journal of the Health Sciences Institute*, **28**, 268-267.

[24] Oliveira, G.T.C., Andrade, E.I.G., Acurcio, F.A., Cherchiglia, M.L. and Correia, M.I.T.D. (2011) Avaliação nutricional de pacientes submetidos à hemodiálise em centros de Belo Horizonte. *Revista da Associação Médica Brasileira*, **58**, 240-247. http://dx.doi.org/10.1590/S0104-42302012000200022

[25] Herdman, T.H. (2013) Diagnósticos de Enfermagem da NANDA: Definições e classificação—2012/2014. 2nd Edition, Artmed, Porto Alegre.

[26] Frazão, C.M.F.Q. (2012) Diagnósticos de enfermagem em pacientes submetidos à hemodiálise: Semelhanças entre o Modelo de Adaptação e a NANDA Internacional. Dissertação, Universidade Federal do Rio Grande do Norte, Natal.

[27] Sahay, M., Sahay, R. and Baruah, M.P. (2014) Nutrition in Chronic Kidney Disease. *Journal of Medical Nutrition and Nutraceuticals*, **3**, 11-18. http://dx.doi.org/10.4103/2278-019X.123437

[28] Garibotto, G., Sofia, A., Saffioti, S., Bonanni, A., Mannucci, I. and Verzola, D. (2010) Amino Acid and Protein Metabolism in the Human Kidney and in Patients with Chronic Kidney Disease. *Clinical Nutrition*, **29**, 424-433. http://dx.doi.org/10.1016/j.clnu.2010.02.005

[29] Lukawsky, L.R., Kheifets, L., Arah, O.A., Nissenson, A.R. and Kalantar-Zadeh, K. (2014) Nutritional Predictors of Early Mortality in Incident Hemodialysis Patients. *International Urology and Nephrology*, **46**, 129-140. http://dx.doi.org/10.1007/s11255-013-0459-2

[30] Abe, M., Okada, K., Ikeda, K., Matsumoto, S., Soma, M. and Matsumoto, K. (2011) Characterization of Insulin Adsorption Behavior of Dialyzer Membranes Used in Hemodialysis. *Artificial Organs*, **35**, 398-403. http://dx.doi.org/10.1111/j.1525-1594.2010.01112.x

[31] Leite, E.M.D., Araújo, A.R.A., Lira, A.L.B.C., Fernando, S.F.S., Oliveira, A.C.F. and Lima, C.F. (2013) Perfil clínico de pacientes submetidos à hemodiálise. *Paraninfo Digital*, **19**, 1-8.

[32] Pedersen, E.B., Ardal, B., Bech, J.N., Lauridsen, T.G., Larsen, N.A., Mikkelsen, L., *et al.* (2011) The Effect of Glucose Added to the Dialysis Fluid on Blood Pressure, Vasoactive Hormones and Energy Transfer during Hemodialysis in Chronic Renal Failure. *Open Journal of Nephrology*, **1**, 5-14. http://dx.doi.org/10.4236/ojneph.2011.12002

[33] Docheterman, J.M. and Bulechek, G.M. (2010) Classificação das Intervenções de Enfermagem (NIC). Artmed, Porto Alegre.

[34] Guimarães, G.L., Mendoza, I.Y.Q., Goveia, V.R., Baroni, F.C.A. and Godoy, S.C.B. (2014) Diagnósticos de Enfermagem em Hemodiálise fundamentados na teoria de Horta. *REUOL*, **8**, 3444-3451.

[35] Nunes, F.A., Nunes, S.A., Lorena, Y.G., Novo, N.F., Juliano, Y. and Schnaider, T.B. (2014) Autoestima, depressão e espiritualidade em pacientes portadores de doença renal crônica em tratamento hemodialítico. *Revista do Médico Residente*, **16**, 18-26.

[36] Negritti, C.D., Mesquita, P.G.M. and Baracho, N.C.V. (2014) Perfil Epidemiológico de pacientes renais crônicos em tratamento conservador em um hospital escola do Sul de Minas. *Revista Ciências em Saúde*, **4**, 1-12.

[37] Coutinho, N.P.S., *et al.* (2010) Qualidade de vida de pacientes renais crônicos em hemodiálise. *Revista de Pesquisa em Saúde*, **11**, 13-17.

[38] Cristóvão, A.F.A.J. (2015) Eficácia das restrições hídrica e dietética em pacientes renais crônicos em hemodiálise. *Revista Brasileira de Enfermagem*, **68**, 842-850. http://dx.doi.org/10.1590/0034-7167.2015680622i

[39] Santana, J.C.B., Fortes, N.M., Monteiro, C.L.A., Carvalho, I.M., Leonardo, L.M.U. and Albuquerque, P.G. (2012) Assistência de enfermagem em um serviço de terapia renal substitutiva: Implicações no processo do cuidar. *Enfermagem Revista*, **15**, 161-178.

[40] Bezerra, M.L.R., Ribeiro, P.R.S., Sousa, A.A., Costa, A.I.S. and Batista, T.S. (2012) Diagnósticos de Enfermagem conforme a Teoria do Autocuidado de Orem para pacientes em Tratamento Hemodialítico. *Revista Ciência em Extensão*, **8**, 60-81.

[41] Brites, R.M.R. and Abreu, A.M.M. (2014) Padrão de consumo de bebidas alcoólicas entre os trabalhadores e perfil socioeconômico. *Acta Paulista de Enfermagem*, **27**, 93-99. http://dx.doi.org/10.1590/1982-0194201400018

[42] Ximenes, S.S.R.F. (2013) Diagnósticos de enfermagem no cuidado clínico a pessoas com hipertensão e doença cardiovascular. Dissertação, Universidade Estadual do Ceará, Fortaleza.

[43] Nepomuceno, F.C.L., Melo Jr., I.M.D., Silva, E.D.A. and Lucena, K.D.T.D. (2014) Religiosidade e qualidade de vida de pacientes com insuficiência renal crônica em hemodiálise. *Saúde em Debate*, **38**, 119-128.

17

The Relationship between Thyroid Hormone Levels and Corrected QT Interval and QT Dispersion in Non-Diabetic Hemodialysis Patients

Heo-Yeong Kim, Ji Soo Kim, Seung Eun Suh, Yu Kyung Hyun,
Kyeong Mi Park, Hyung-Jong Kim*

Department of Internal Medicine, Bundang CHA Medical Center, CHA University, Seongnam, South Korea
Email: *khj@.cha.ac.kr

Abstract

Background: Cardiovascular disease and sudden cardiac death are common in hemodialysis patients. These cardiac complications are often associated with prolonged QTc interval (QTc) and QTc dispersion (QTcd). Subclinical hypothyroidism (SH) can alter autonomic modulation of heart rate and cause increased inhomogeneity of ventricular recovery time. We aimed to evaluate the relationship between thyroid hormone levels and QTc and QTcd in non-diabetic hemodialysis patients. Methods: We enrolled 29 non-diabetic hemodialysis patients without thyroid disease. After each hemodialysis session, a 12-lead ECG was recorded. Before each hemodialysis session, routine laboratory tests and measurement of thyroid hormone levels were performed. Patients were divided into 2 groups according to QTc (group 1 QTc < 430 ms, group 2 QTc ≥ 430 ms). We examined the relationship between QTc or QTcd and thyroid hormone in the respective groups and then compared the results from the 2 groups. Results: The mean age was 54.06 ± 14.72 years and the means of QTc and QTcd were 433.82 ± 22.03 ms, 59.10 ± 28.29 ms, respectively. Homocysteine levels were significant higher in group 2 than group 1 ($p < 0.05$) and QTcd was comparable between groups. In group 1, QTc and QTcd were not significant correlated with TSH, T3, fT4 and biochemical parameters. In group 2, QTc was significant positively correlated with TSH ($p < 0.05$) and QTcd was not significant correlated with thyroid hormone levels. Conclusion: The results of this study showed that TSH is associated with prolonged QTc interval and hyperhomocysteinemia in non-diabetic hemodialysis patients. Moreover, we suggest that SH may be associated with prolonged QTc in non-diabetic hemodialysis patients. However, further studies are required to elucidate the role of the L-thyroxine doses and TSH target levels in hemodialysis patients.

---

*Corresponding Author.

Keywords

Thyroid Hormone; Hemodialysis; Cardiovascular Disease

1. Introduction

Cardiovascular disease and sudden cardiac death are common in hemodialysis patients. The cause of cardiovascular death in advanced renal disease is variable. Acute myocardial infarction is relatively rare. More commonly, death is developed suddenly and due to progressive heart failure [1]. Therefore, determinants of sudden cardiac death such as arrhythmia, left ventricular hypertrophy, prolonged QTc interval (QTc) and increased QTc dispersion (QTcd) are of great importance.

Subclinical hypothyroidism (SH) is an asymptomatic condition defined by slightly increased serum thyrotrophin (thyroid stimulating hormone; TSH) concentrations, but normal serum free T3 (fT3) and free T4 (fT4) hormone levels. Altered serum lipid levels and abnormal vascular reactivity in patients with SH may confer a higher risk for cardiovascular disease [2] [3]. SH is associated with a risk of heart failure, other cardiovascular events, and death [4]. Clinical studies have shown that SH can influence autonomic modulation of the heart rate and cause increased inhomogeneity of ventricular recovery times in patients with normal renal function. These previous studies also reported that early L-thyroxine treatment may be recommended not only to prevent progression to overt hypothyroidism but also to improve abnormal cardiac autonomic function and ventricular repolarization inhomogeneity [5].

We hypothesized that SH may be associated with cardiovascular disease and sudden cardiac death in hemodialysis patients. In the present study, we aimed to evaluate the relationship between thyroid hormone levels and QTc and QTcd in non-diabetic hemodialysis patients.

2. Materials and Method

Total 29 hemodialysis patients (13 men and 16 women; mean age 54.06 ± 14.72 years) without thyroid disease were enrolled in this study. Dialysis was performed in a standard setting with synthetic membranes, for the duration of 180 to 240 minutes, for 3 times per week. All patients are under went by standard bicarbonate dialysis.

After each hemodialysis session, a simultaneous 12-lead ECG was recorded using a 12-channel electrocardiograph at a paper speed of 25mm/s. RR and QT intervals were measured with a magnifying ruler on the ECG tracing. QT interval was measured from the beginning of the QRS complex to the end of the downslope of the T wave (crossing of the isoelectric line). When T waves were inverted, the end was considered as the point where the trace returned to the isoelectric line. When U waves were present, the end of the T wave was considered as the nadir between the T and the U wave. If the end of the T wave was not clearly identifiable, the lead was not included in the analysis.

QT intervals were corrected for the previous cardiac cycle length according to Bazett's formula: QTc (ms) = $QT/\sqrt{RR}$. QTc was considered to be prolonged when it was >440 ms, in accordance with the criteria commonly used in the literature [6] [7].

QTcd was calculated as the maximum QT interval minus the minimum QT interval in any of the leads. As QTcd does not depend on the heart period unlike the QT interval, it was not corrected using Bazett's formula [8].

Before each hemodialysis session, routine laboratory tests (plasma concentration of potassium, sodium, magnesium, calcium, phosphorus, chloride, urea, creatinine, albumin, bicarbonate, cholesterol, and homocysteine) and measurement of TSH, fT4, and T3 levels were performed.

Patients were divided into 2 groups according to QTc (group 1: QTc < 430 ms; group 2: QTc ≥ 430 ms). We examined the relationship between QTc or QTcd and thyroid hormone in the respective groups and then compared the results from the 2 groups.

All data are expressed as mean ± S.D. and compared using the one-way analysis of variance (ANOVA) among groups. Linear correlation analysis was used to assess the relationships between variables. Differences were considered significant when $P < 0.05$.

3. Results

Of the 29 patients, 13 were men and 16 were women. The mean age was 54.06 ± 14.72 at commencement of the study. Underlying renal diseases included hypertension (HTN) (55.2%), glomerulonephritis (GN) (20.7%), ADPKD (10.3%), and unknown (13.7%). The mean hemodialysis duration, Kt/V, nPCR, and BMI were 63.72 ± 42.78 months, 1.48 ± 0.20, 0.88 ± 0.22 g/kg/d, and 23.03 ± 3.93 kg/m^2, respectively. Moreover, TSH, T3, and fT4 were 4.66 ± 10.85 uIU/mL, 1.09 ± 0.16 ng/mL, and 0.99 ± 0.83 ng/dL respectively in group 1. And 2.50 ± 2.52 uIU/mL, 1.06 ± 0.20 ng/mL, and 0.96 ± 0.16 ng/dL respectively in group 2. TSH levels were significantly higher in group 2 patients than in group 1 patients ($P < 0.05$), whereas T3 and fT4 were comparable between groups.

There were no significant differences between the two groups, except for homocysteine levels. The mean homocysteine levels were 14.70 ± 4.26 umol/L in group 1 and 18.47 ± 3.84 umol/L in group 2 (**Table 1**).

Table 1. Clinical characteristics and biochemical parameters of patients (N = 29).

	Total (N = 29)	Group 1 (N = 13)	Group 2 (N = 16)
Age (years)	54.06 ± 14.72	53.23 ± 13.92	54.75 ± 15.02
Sex (M:F)	13:16	5:8	8:8
Cause of ESRD N (%)			
Hypertension	16 (55.2)	7 (53.8)	9 (56.3)
Chronic GN	6 (20.7)	5 (38.5)	1 (6.3)
Polycystic kidney	3 (10.3)	0	3 (18.8)
Unknown	4 (13.7)	1 (7.7)	3 (18.8)
BMI (kg/m2)	23.02 ± 3.93	22.37 ± 3.13	23.55 ± 3.80
Kt/V	1.48 ± 0.20	1.48 ± 0.21	1.48 ± 0.20
nPCR (g/kg/day)	0.88 ± 0.22	0.85 ± 0.24	0.90 ± 0.20
HD duration (months)	63.72 ± 42.78	70.15 ± 45.95	58.50 ± 40.78
CRP (mg/dL)	0.35 ± 0.46	0.35 ± 0.56	0.34 ± 0.38
Calcium (mg/dL)	9.26 ± 0.88	9.26 ± 0.64	9.27 ± 1.05
Phosphorus (mg/dL)	5.22 ± 1.44	5.33 ± 1.34	5.13 ± 1.55
Ca × P product	48.54 ± 14.52	49.58 ± 13.82	47.69 ± 15.46
Uric acid (mg/dL)	8.10 ± 1.73	7.87 ± 1.36	8.28 ± 2.02
Protein (mg/dL)	6.83 ± 0.47	6.73 ± 0.41	6.91 ± 0.51
Albumin (mg/dL)	3.94 ± 0.36	3.98 ± 0.42	3.91 ± 0.31
Pre-albumin (mg/dL)	27.20 ± 7.48	27.10 ± 7.28	27.27 ± 7.87
tCO$_2$ (mEq/L)	20.96 ± 2.43	20.70 ± 2.55	21.17 ± 2.40
Hemoglobin (g/dL)	9.61 ± 2.12	9.66 ± 2.49	9.56 ± 1.86
Total Chol. (mg/dL)	130.79 ± 37.69	137.23 ± 48.32	125.56 ± 26.81
Triglyceride (mg/dL)	100.48 ± 53.56	107.30 ± 59.98	94.93 ± 49.02
HDL-Chol. (mg/dL)	37.60 ± 8.57	37.62 ± 6.68	37.59 ± 10.07
LDL-Chol. (mg/dL)	75.17 ± 20.99	76.46 ± 21.16	74.12 ± 21.48
TSH (uIU/mL)	3.69 ± 8.18	2.50 ± 2.52	4.66 ± 10.85
fT4 (ng/dL)	0.97 ± 0.12	0.96 ± 0.16	0.99 ± 0.08
T3 (ng/mL)	1.08 ± 0.18	1.06 ± 0.20	1.09 ± 0.16
Homocysteine (umol/L)	16.78 ± 4.39	14.70 ± 4.26	18.47 ± 3.84[*]
HOMA-IR	6.58 ± 5.32	6.64 ± 7.48	6.54 ± 2.84
QTc (ms)	433.82 ± 22.03	414.46 ± 6.15	449.56 ± 16.93[*]
QTcd (ms)	59.10 ± 28.29	51.65 ± 28.08	65.15 ± 27.86

Mean ± SD, [*]P < 0.05 vs. group 1. *Abbreviations*: ESRD; end stage renal disease, GN; glomerular nephropathy, BMI; body mass index, HD; hemodialysis, nPCR; normalized protein catabolic rate, CRP; C-reactive protein, Chol.; cholesterol, HDL; high density lipoprotein, LDL; low density lipoprotein, TSH; thyroid stimulating hormone, HOMA-IR; homeostasis model assessment method of insulin resistance.

In group 1, QTc and QTcd were not significantly correlated with TSH, T3, or fT4 and biomedical parameters (data not shown). In group 2, QTc was significantly positively correlated with nPCR and TSH (p < 0.05) (**Table 2**), but was not significantly correlated with thyroid hormone levels (**Figure 1**).

4. Discussion

Cardiovascular disease is the leading cause of death in patients with progressive renal disease and is responsible for up to 50% of deaths among patients underlying hemodialysis [9]. The cardiovascular risk of patients with progressive renal disease is up to 20 times that of the general population, and cardiovascular mortality in patients underlying dialysis is up to 10 times that of the general population [10]. These cardiac complications are often associated with prolonged QTc and QTcd.

QTc reflects the total duration of ventricular depolarization and repolarization [5]. QTc is an index of inhomogeneity of ventricular repolarization [11]. Experimental and clinical studies have shown that increased QTcd and reduced heart rate variability correlate with an increased risk of ventricular arrhythmias and cardiac mortality [12]-[14]. In ESRD patients, many factors can contribute to QTc prolongation, such as electrolyte abnormalities, associated conditions (including diabetes, heart failure, left ventricular hypertrophy and autonomic neuropathy) and medications. SH has also been reported to influence autonomic modulation of the heart rate and cause increased inhomogeneity of ventricular recovery times [5].

In the present study, our results showed that TSH is associated with prolonged QTc in non-diabetic hemodialysis patients. Prolonged QTc has been reported to be corrected when TSH levels of >10 mIU/L returned to normal after L-thyroxine therapy [15]. We suggest that the administration of L-thyroxine may be decreases the death rate associated with cardiovascular disease in hemodialysis patients without hypothyroid symptoms who have prolonged QTc as assessed by EKG. Further studies are required to elucidate QTc criterion, L-thyroxine dose and TSH target level.

In the present study, QTcd was not significantly correlated with TSH, T3, or fT4. An increase in QTcd is associated with repetitive and life-threatening ventricular arrhythmias and has been shown to be an independent risk factor for sudden death [16]-[23]. Several factors can affect QTcd, such as age, gender, myocardial ischemia, cardiac failure, diabetes, hypertension, electrolyte imbalance, certain drugs, and the circadian pattern of QTcd making its clinical use difficult to assess. The relationship between SH and QTcd in non-diabetic dialysis patients remains controversial, and our results in this regard were inconclusive. In addition, because, our study did not include patients with a long QTcd of >80 ms, further research is needed involving this group of patients.

A high level of homocysteine (Hcys) has been proposed as an independent risk factor for cardiovascular dis-

Table 2. The correlation of QTc with other study parameters in group 2 (QTc ≥ 430 ms).

	Bivariate analysis (N = 16)	
	Correlation coefficient	P value
BMI (kg/m^2)	0.450	0.080
Kt/V	−0.375	0.152
nPCR (g/kg/day)	0.609	0.012*
CRP (mg/dL)	0.088	0.747
Albumin (mg/dL)	−0.001	0.996
Pre-albumin (mg/dL)	0.367	0.162
tCO$_2$ (mEq/L)	−0.166	0.538
TSH (uIU/mL)	0.505	0.046*
fT4 (ng/dL)	−0.338	0.201
T3 (ng/mL)	−0.172	0.523
Homocysteine (umol/L)	0.018	0.947
HOMA-IR	0.202	0.453

Abbreviations: BMI; body mass index, Kt/V; dialyzer clearance of urea × dialysis time/volume of distribution of urea, approximately equal to patient's total body water, nPCR; normalized protein catabolic rate, CRP; C-reactive protein, HOMA-IR; homeostasis model assessment method of insulin resistance.

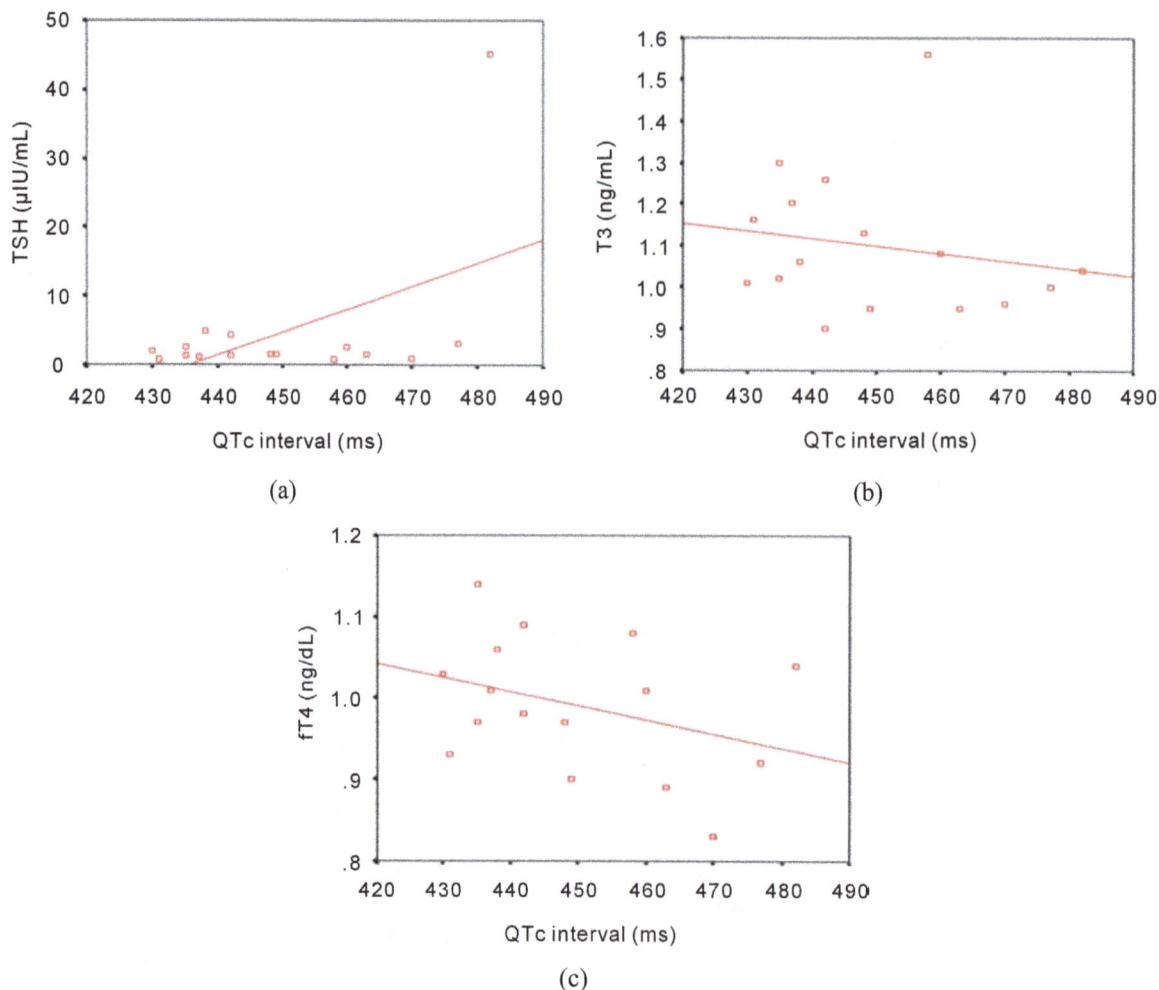

(a)

(b)

(c)

Figure 1. In group 2, QTc was significantly correlated with TSH (A) (P < 0.05), and not correlated with T3 (B) and fT4 (C) (P > 0.05).

ease. Plasma Hcys levels can be affected by several life-style and physiological factors and are elevated in renal failure [24]. There are consistent reports demonstrating that thyroid status is an important determinant of the plasma concentration of Hcys [25] [26]. Elevated plasma Hcys levels have been reported in overt hypothyroidism, and have been proposed as an independent risk factor for cardiovascular disease [27]. However, it remains unclear whether individuals with SH also have increased Hcys concentrations and whether this elevation can explain the increased prevalence of cardiovascular disease in this condition. A recent study reported that SH is not associated with hyperhomocysteinemia and Hcys does not appear to contribute to the increased risk for atherosclerotic disease in patients with SH [28] [29].

In contrast, in the present study, the SH group showed a higher plasma Hcys level than the control group. We suggest that the administration of L-thyroxine could prevent the development of cardiovascular disease in hemodialysis patients who have hyperhomocysteinemia and high TSH levels.

5. Conclusion

Prolonged QTc, QTcd and SH are reported to be associated with cardiovascular disease and sudden cardiac death. The results of this study showed that TSH is associated with prolonged QTc and hyperhomocysteinemia in non-diabetic hemodialysis patients. Moreover, we suggest that SH may be associated with prolonged QTc in non-diabetic hemodialysis patients. However, further studies are required to elucidate the role of the L-thyroxine doses and TSH target levels in hemodialysis patients.

References

[1]   Jardine, A.G. and McLaughlin, K. (2001) Cardiovascular Complications of Renal Disease. *Heart*, **86**, 459-466. http://dx.doi.org/10.1136/heart.86.4.459

[2]   Althaus, B.U., Staub, J.J., Ryff-De Leche, A., Oberhansli, A. and Stahelin, H.B. (1988) LDL/HDL-Changes in Subclinical Hypothyroidism: Possible Risk Factors for Coronary Heart Disease. *Clinical Endocrinology (Oxford)*, **28**, 157-163. http://dx.doi.org/10.1111/j.1365-2265.1988.tb03651.x

[3]   Monzani, F., Caraccio, N., Kozakowa, M., Dardano, A., Vittone, F., Virdis, A., *et al.* (2004) Effect of Levothyroxine Replacement on Lipid Profile and Intima-Media Thickness in Subclinical Hypothyroidism: A Double-Blind, Placebo-Controlled Study. *The Journal of Clinical Endocrinology & Metabolism*, **89**, 2099-2106. http://dx.doi.org/10.1210/jc.2003-031669

[4]   Hak, A.E., Pols, H.A., Visser, T.J., Drexhage, H.A., Hofman, A. and Witteman, J.C. (2000) Subclinical Hypothyroidism Is an Independent Risk Factor for Atherosclerosis and Myocardial Infarction in Elderly Women: The Rotterdam Study. *Annals of Internal Medicine*, **132**, 270-278. http://dx.doi.org/10.7326/0003-4819-132-4-200002150-00004

[5]   Galetta, F., Franzoni, F., Fallahi, P., Rossi, M., Carpi, A., Rubello, D., *et al.* (2006) Heart Rate Variability and QT Dispersion in Patients with Subclinical Hypothyroidism. *Biomedicine & Pharmacotherapy*, **60**, 425-430. http://dx.doi.org/10.1016/j.biopha.2006.07.009

[6]   Schouten, E.G., Dekker, J.M., Meppelink, P., Kok, F.J., Vandenbroucke, J.P. and Pool, J. (1991) QT interval Prolongation Predicts Cardiovascular Mortality in an Apparently Healthy Population. *Circulation*, **84**, 1516-1523. http://dx.doi.org/10.1161/01.CIR.84.4.1516

[7]   Schwartz, P.J. and Wolf, S. (1978) QT Interval Prolongation as Predictor of Sudden Death in Patients with Myocardial Infarction. *Circulation*, **57**, 1074-1077. http://dx.doi.org/10.1161/01.CIR.57.6.1074

[8]   Batchvarov, V. and Malik, M. (2000) Measurement and Interpretation of QT Dispersion. *Progress in Cardiovascular Diseases*, **42**, 325-344. http://dx.doi.org/10.1053/pcad.2000.0420325

[9]   Port, F.K. (1994) Morbidity and Mortality in Dialysis Patients. *Kidney International*, **46**, 1728-1737. http://dx.doi.org/10.1038/ki.1994.475

[10] Brown, J.H., Hunt, L.P., Vites, N.P., Short, C.D., Gokal, R. and Mallick, N.P. (1994) Comparative Mortality from Cardiovascular Disease in Patients with Chronic Renal Failure. *Nephrology Dialysis Transplantation*, **9**, 1136-1142.

[11] Zaidi, M., Robert, A., Fesler, R., Derwael, C. and Brohet, C. (1997) Dispersion of Ventricular Repolarisation: A Marker of Ventricular Arrhythmias in Patients with Previous Myocardial Infarction. *Heart*, **78**, 371-375.

[12] Algra, A., Tijssen, J.G., Roelandt, J.R., Pool, J. and Lubsen, J. (1993) Heart Rate Variability from 24-Hour Electrocardiography and the 2-Year Risk for Sudden Death. *Circulation*, **88**, 180-185. http://dx.doi.org/10.1161/01.CIR.88.1.180

[13] Tsuji, H., Larson, M.G., Venditti Jr., F.J., Manders, E.S., Evans, J.C., Feldman, C.L., *et al.* (1996) Impact of Reduced Heart Rate Variability on Risk for Cardiac Events. The Framingham Heart Study. *Circulation*, **94**, 2850-2855. http://dx.doi.org/10.1161/01.CIR.94.11.2850

[14] Balanescu, S., Galinier, M., Fourcade, J., Dorobantu, M., Albenque, J.P., Massabuau, P., *et al.* (1996) Correlation between QT Interval Dispersion and Ventricular Arrhythmia in Hypertension. *Archives des Maladies du Coeur et des Vaisseaux*, **89**, 987-990.

[15] Bakiner, O., Ertorer, M.E., Haydardedeoglu, F.E., Bozkirli, E., Tutuncu, N.B. and Demirag, N.G. (2008) Subclinical Hypothyroidism Is Characterized by Increased QT Interval Dispersion among Women. *Medical Principles and Practice*, **17**, 390-394. http://dx.doi.org/10.1159/000141503

[16] Hii, J.T., Wyse, D.G., Gillis, A.M., Duff, H.J., Solylo, M.A. and Mitchell, L.B. (1992) Precordial QT Interval Dispersion as a Marker of Torsade de Pointes. Disparate Effects of Class Ia Antiarrhythmic Drugs and Amiodarone. *Circulation*, **86**, 1376-1382. http://dx.doi.org/10.1161/01.CIR.86.5.1376

[17] Yunus, A., Gillis, A.M., Duff, H.J., Wyse, D.G. and Mitchell, L.B. (1996) Increased Precordial QTc Dispersion Predicts Ventricular Fibrillation during Acute Myocardial Infarction. *American Journal of Cardiology*, **78**, 706-708. http://dx.doi.org/10.1016/S0002-9149(96)00405-5

[18] Zareba, W., Moss, A.J. and le Cessie, S. (1994) Dispersion of Ventricular Repolarization and Arrhythmic Cardiac Death in Coronary Artery Disease. *American Journal of Cardiology*, **74**, 550-553. http://dx.doi.org/10.1016/0002-9149(94)90742-0

[19] Naas, A.A., Davidson, N.C., Thompson, C., Cummings, F., Ogston, S.A., Jung, R.T., *et al.* (1998) QT and QTc Dispersion Are Accurate Predictors of Cardiac Death in Newly Diagnosed Non-Insulin Dependent Diabetes: Cohort Study. *BMJ*, **316**, 745-746. http://dx.doi.org/10.1136/bmj.316.7133.745

[20] Kweon, K.H., Park, B.H. and Cho, C.G. (2007) The Effects of L-Thyroxine Treatment on QT Dispersion in Primary Hypothyroidism. *Journal of Korean Medical Science*, **22**, 114-116. http://dx.doi.org/10.3346/jkms.2007.22.1.114

[21] de Bruyne, M.C., Hoes, A.W., Kors, J.A., Hofman, A., van Bemmel, J.H. and Grobbee, D.E. (1998) QTc Dispersion Predicts Cardiac Mortality in the Elderly: The Rotterdam Study. *Circulation*, **97**, 467-472. http://dx.doi.org/10.1161/01.CIR.97.5.467

[22] Okin, P.M., Devereux, R.B., Howard, B.V., Fabsitz, R.R., Lee, E.T. and Welty, T.K. (2000) Assessment of QT Interval and QT Dispersion for Prediction of All-Cause and Cardiovascular Mortality in American Indians: The Strong Heart Study. *Circulation*, **101**, 61-66. http://dx.doi.org/10.1161/01.CIR.101.1.61

[23] Somberg, J.C. and Molnar, J. (2002) Usefulness of QT Dispersion as an Electrocardiographically Derived Index. *American Journal of Cardiology*, **89**, 291-294. http://dx.doi.org/10.1016/S0002-9149(01)02230-5

[24] Lien, E.A., Nedrebo, B.G., Varhaug, J.E., Nygard, O., Aakvaag, A. and Ueland, P.M. (2000) Plasma Total Homocysteine Levels during Short-Term Iatrogenic Hypothyroidism. *The Journal of Clinical Endocrinology & Metabolism*, **85**, 1049-1053.

[25] Nedrebo, B.G., Nygard, O., Ueland, P.M. and Lien, E.A. (2001) Plasma Total Homocysteine in Hyper- and Hypothyroid Patients before and during 12 Months of Treatment. *Clinical Chemistry*, **47**, 1738-1741.

[26] Chadarevian, R., Bruckert, E., Leenhardt, L., Giral, P., Ankri, A. and Turpin, G. (2001) Components of the Fibrinolytic System Are Differently Altered in Moderate and Severe Hypothyroidism. *The Journal of Clinical Endocrinology & Metabolism*, **86**, 732-737. http://dx.doi.org/10.1210/jcem.86.2.7221

[27] Welch, G.N. and Loscalzo, J. (1998) Homocysteine and Atherothrombosis. *The New England Journal of Medicine*, **338**, 1042-1050. http://dx.doi.org/10.1056/NEJM199804093381507

[28] Cakal, B., Cakal, E., Demirbas, B., Ozkaya, M., Karaahmetoglu, S., Serter, R., *et al.* (2007) Homocysteine and Fibrinogen Changes with L-Thyroxine in Subclinical Hypothyroid Patients. *Journal of Korean Medical Science*, **22**, 431-435. http://dx.doi.org/10.3346/jkms.2007.22.3.431

[29] Turhan, S., Sezer, S., Erden, G., Guctekin, A., Ucar, F., Ginis, Z., *et al.* (2008) Plasma Homocysteine Concentrations and serum Lipid Profile as Atherosclerotic Risk Factors in Subclinical Hypothyroidism. *Annals of Saudi Medicine*, **28**, 96-101. http://dx.doi.org/10.4103/0256-4947.51750

Before the Jury Is out on Cinacalcet's Cardiovascular Effects in Hemodialysis Patients: Is Troponin a Missing Link?

Samra Abouchacra[1], Ahmed Chaaban[1], Mohammad Budruddin[1], Fares Chedid[2], Mohamad Hakim[1], Mohamad Ahmed[1], Nicole Gebran[3], Farida Marzouki[1], Muhy Eddin Hassan[4], Faiz Al Abbacheyi[1]

[1]Department of Medicine, Tawam Hospital, Abu Dhabi, UAE
[2]Department of Pediatrics, Tawam Hospital, Abu Dhabi, UAE
[3]Department of Pharmacology, Tawam Hospital, Abu Dhabi, UAE
[4]SEHA Dialysis Services, Tawam Hospital, Abu Dhabi, UAE
Email: drbudruddin@gmail.com

Abstract

Raised levels of the cardiac biomarker, Troponin I, are frequently encountered in hemodialysis patients and appear to be prognostic indicators for cardiovascular risk. Though evidence suggests that control of secondary hyperparathyroidism may reduce cardiac endpoints, the effect of the calcimimetic agent, cinacalcet, remains controversial. This retrospective study aimed at evaluating troponin levels in hemodialysis patients with severe secondary hyper parathyroidism (SHPT) who are on cinacalcet vs controls on conventional treatment. In addition, clinical outcomes including all-cause, cardiovascular morbidity and mortality were compared among both groups. A decline in Troponin I levels was observed in the cinacalcet group, this however was not translated clinically into improved survival. In fact, all-cause and cardiac mortality was similar in the two groups. Conversely, comparison of the incidence of cardiovascular events revealed lower rates in the cinacalcet group including cardiac, cerebral and peripheral vascular complications. Given some of our study limitations, further long-term, placebo-controlled trials are necessary to definitively establish the effect of cinacalet on cardiac biomarkers and ultimately its impact on clinical outcomes.

Keywords

Calcimimetics; Secondary Hyperparathyroidism; Parathyroid Hormone; Cinacalcet; Chronic Kidney Disease; Cardio Vascular Disease; End Stage Renal Disease; Troponin I; C-Reactive Protein; Parathyroidectomy; Acute Coronary Syndrome;

Peripheral Vascular Disease; Atherogenesis; Myocardial Infraction

1. Introduction

Increased cardiovascular morbidity and mortality are observed in chronic kidney disease (CKD) patients that have been attributed to traditional and uremia-related risks. The latter includes secondary hyperparathyroidism (SHPT) associated factors with multiple potential mechanisms, most notably related to vascular calcification [1] induced by abnormalities in calcium phosphate balance. This may directly lead to myocardial ischemia, finally culminating in overt cardiac disease, as secondary hyperparathyroidism progresses. Moreover, clinical observations support the etiologic role for parathyroid hormone (PTH) in the development of cardio vascular disease, whereby lowering its levels by parathyroidectomy, for instance, is associated with reduced vascular event rates and mortality in dialysis patients [2]. It has therefore been postulated that alternate measures to control SHPT and calcium-phosphate imbalance may impact myocardial ischemia and cardiac outcomes [3]. Most promising in its treatment is the emergence of the calcimimetic agent cinacalcet, which in addition to improving the biochemical parameters, has been anticipated to potentially impact cardiovascular outcomes [3].

On the other hand, since early detection is key to preemptive cardiovascular intervention, it follows that cardiac biomarkers' use is of tremendous clinical value, especially in CKD patients on dialysis. Though several cardiac peptides are available, troponin I appears more specifically for myocardial ischemia [4]-[7] and even serves as a prognostic indicators in dialysis patients [8]. It would hence be plausible that following troponin I trends may serve as possible markers of cinacalcet treatment effect on cardiac risk in these patients.

The aim of our study was to assess the effect of cinacalcet treatment on cardiac biomarker troponin I levels in patients on hemodialysis with severe SHPT. We also investigated the associated clinical outcomes in these patients compared to matched historical controls. The outcome measures included, in addition to overall and CV mortality, the composite CV event rates of myocardial infarction (MI), acute coronary syndrome (ACS), congestive heart failure (CHF), arrhythmia as well as cerebrovascular events (CVA) and peripheral vascular disease (PVD) complications.

2. Study Design & Methods

This was a retrospective review of 246 hemodialysis patients in our center. The study was conducted between March 2012 until September 2013. Included were 71 adults with end stage renal disease on regular dialysis for >6 months with severe SHPT who had been on cinacalcet for at least 6 months. The control group was a historical matched cohort also with secondary hyperparathyroidism but of moderate severity who were maintained on vitamin D analogs and not receiving cinacalcet. Severe secondary hyperparathyroidism was defined as levels of PTH more than six times the upper limit of normal. Excluded were unstable patients and those in pediatric age group.

Baseline PTH, calcium, phosphate, C-Reactive Protien and Troponin I levels were retrieved and tracked over the two year period of the study. In our unit, PTH and troponin levels are routinely measured every three months. For the cinacalcet group, these parameters were obtained at baseline prior to starting the treatment with cinacalcet. Morbidity and mortality outcomes were followed for 6 months beyond the follow up period and included composite rates (MI, ACS, CHF, arrhythmia), CVA and PVD complications as well as sepsis-related admissions and overall mortality.

3. Statistical Analysis

Quantitative data were presented as mean (SD) or median (P25-P75) as appropriate, categorical data were presented as proportions. The basic characteristics, the laboratory results and the outcome variables were compared between the Cinacalcet group and the historical control with the two independent samples t test or Mann Whitney U test for measured data and Chi square tests or Fisher Exact test for nominal data. Changes in laboratory values in the Cinacalcet group overtime from baseline to 12 and 18 months were analyzed with repeated measure ANOVA when the assumptions of the test were met or the Friedman analysis of variance by ranks when the assumptions were not met (Troponin I levels). Further comparison PTH, Tropinin I, calcium and phosphorus between baseline and 18 months in patients of the Cinacalcet group who suffered a cardiac event was performed using with paired t test and its non-parametric alternative the Wilcoxin Sign Rank test as appropriate. All reported P values were 2-sided and deemed significant when they reached a 5% level. Statistical analysis was conducted using the PASW 19.0 statistical package (IBM SPSS, Chicago, Illinois).

4. Results

Out of 71 adult hemodialysis patients with severe secondary hyperparathyroidism who were on cinacalcet, we retrospectively reviewed 63 adult patients (30 Male; 33 Female) with complete data. Their mean age was 55.4 ± 16 years with duration on HD ranging between 12 and 243 months averaging 74 ± 58 months. Associated co-morbidities, shown in (**Table 1**), included hypertension 78%, diabetes 44%, ischemic heart disease (IHD) 33%. The control cohort was comprised of 40 adult patients (23 Male: 17 Female) with end stage renal disease on regular hemodialysis with moderately severe secondary hyperparathyroidism who were on Vitamin D or analogs but not receiving cinacalcet treatment. Their mean age was 60.4 ± 15 years and mean duration on HD of 46 ± 89 months with the following comorbid conditions: hypertension 80%, diabetes 53%, IHD 35% (**Table 1**). None of the differences in baseline demographics achieved statistical significance except for dialysis vintage which was significantly longer in patients on cinacalcet (p < 0.01).

PTH Levels decreased from baseline at 12 and 18 months, but the difference only achieved statistical significance with the latter interval. Similarly, although Troponin I levels tended to decrease at 12 months, a statistically significant decrement was noted only at 18 months. Conversely, calcium x phosphate product decreased significantly at both time periods however, C-reactive protein values decreased by 23% and 53% at 12 and 18 months respectively, but the difference did not reach statistical significance (**Table 2**).

Further statistical analysis was undertaken, where patients were paired serving as their own controls during follow up over the designated time periods. Data as shown in (**Table 3**) revealed a decrease in PTH levels at 12 and 18 months, the difference from baseline significant only at 18 months (p = 0.026). In parallel, a statistically significant decrease of Troponin I was noted at 12 months (p 0.045), this however was not sustained at 18 months. CRP values decreased by 30% and 73%, at 12 and 18 months respectively but the difference was not significant. One way repeated measure ANOVA comparing Calcium x Phosphate product at baseline, 12 and 18 months revealed a significant drop at both time points (p < 0.001).

Comparison of clinical outcome measures between patients receiving cinacalcet and the control group, revealed similar incidence of all-cause mortality of 10% in each. Cardiac mortality accounted for 50% in both groups, with no between group statistical difference. A comparison of the incidence of composite cardiac events revealed 33% in the cinacalcet group versus 68% in the control group as shown in (**Table 4**). This increased event rate in the controls was also observed for CVA and PVD complications although the latter approached yet did not achieve statistical significance (p = 0.07). Episodes of sepsis were similar in both groups averaging 20%.

5. Clinical Outcomes/End Points

Further subgroup analysis of patients on cinacalcet who suffered the cardiac events (**Table 5**) indicated a significantly higher troponin I levels at baseline and 18 months, the latter highly significant (p < 0.009). PTH levels on the other hand, were statistically more increased at baseline in these patients but this difference was not maintained at 18 months, likely demonstrating cinacalcet treatment effect.

6. Discussion

Our results demonstrated an association between reduction in PTH levels induced by cinacalcet and a decline in levels of Troponin I. This was observed in patients with severe secondary hyper parathyroidism after a relatively short period on treatment and with only modest improvement in their biochemical profiles. Moreover, the calcimimetic treatment was initiated late in the course of the disease and its dosing was not maximized (average daily dose 45 mg). Despite this, the findings suggest a possible link between cinacalcet-induced PTH reduction and a possible cardioprotective effect reflected by decreased troponin levels. There is supportive evidence in the literature for the role of PTH. Secondary hyper parathyroidism, increased the cardio vascular risk, seen in chronic kidney disease (CKD) with a number of plausible mechanisms [9]-[14]. These include direct effects on atherogenesis via vascular calcification and remodeling, induction of LVH, cardiac calcification and fibrosis, in addition to its key regulatory role on   factors involved in mineral metabolism and homeostasis such as hypercalcemia, hyperphosphatemia, vitamin D deficiency, which may individually have direct detrimental myocardial effects [11] [15]-[19]. Interestingly, PTH has also been implicated with predicting cardiovascular (CV) mortality even in normal individuals with plasma levels well within normal range [9].

Additionally, indirect evidence for the contributions of secondary hyperparathyroidism to cardiac disease comes from the noted association between serum alkaline phosphatase levels and coronary artery calcification in HD patients [11]. Moreover, measures which lower PTH levels, such as parathyroidectomy, have been associated with reduced vascular event rates and mortality in dialysis patients [2]. Similar findings have been reported with renal transplantation [20]. In addition, a lowered incidence of CV disease has also been observed with calcimimetics use, not only in patients with secondary hyperparathyroidism but also in those with primary hyperparathyroidism [18] [21]. The effects of calcimimetics remain controversial however, with some studies like the ADVANCE [22] showing promising results with reduced vascular calcification scores in HD patients, whereas others demonstrating no outcomes benefit as will be discussed. In the recently published metaanaysis by

Table 1. Basic characteristics of the cohort.

	Cinacalcet N = 63	Control N = 40
Age: mean (SD) (yrs)	55.4 (16.5)	60.4 (15)[*]
Female: n (%)	33 (52.4)	17 (42.5)[*]
Duration of dialysis: mean (SD) months	74 (58)	46 (89)[†]
Hypertension: n (%)	49 (77.8)	35 (80)[*]
Diabetes: n (%)	28 (44.4)	21 (52.5)[*]
Ischemic heart diseases: n (%)	21 (33.3)	14 (35)[*]

[*]P values NS [†]p value < 0.05.

Table 2. Variation of parameters over the study duration.

	baseline	12 Month	18 month
Mean PTH **(pmol/l)**	95.45 ± 62	88.06 ± 68[*]	71.91 ± 48[†]
Troponin I (ng/ml)	0.05 ± 0.11	0.036 ± 0.2[*]	0.025 ± 0.03[†]
CRP **(mg/l)**	16.24 ± 19	12.55 ± 11[*]	7.7 ± 9[*]
Ca (mg/L) x Ph (mg/L) Mean (SD)	3.89 (1.28)	2.87 (2.03)[††]	1.91(1.97)[††]
Cinacalcet dose (mg)	0	37.9±19	40.26±23

p value vs baseline [*]NS; [†]p value ≤ 0.05; [††]P value < 0.001.

Table 3. Changes of studied parameters over time after pairing patients as their own control.

Baseline	12 months	18 months
PTH **(pmol/l)** Mean (SD) 105.2 (70.1)	95.7(72.7) **(pmol/L)**[*]	76.9 (50.7)[†] **(pmol/L)**
Troponin I **(ng/ml)** Median (P25-P75) 0.02 (0.01 - 0.04)	0.01 (0.01 - 0.03)[†] **(ng/ml)**	0.02 (0.01-0.02)[†] **(ng/ml)**
CRP **(mg/l)** Median (P25-P75) 10.5 (5 - 20)	7 (3.75 - 17.25)[*] **(mg/l)**	4 (2 - 12.5)[*] **(mg/l)**
Cinacalcet dose (mg) 30 mg 86.9% >60 mg 13.1%	79.6% 20.4%	81.6% 18.4%

p value vs baseline. [*]NS; [†]p value < 0.05.

Table 4. Rate of complications in cinacalcet versus control group.

	Cinacalcet N = 63 n (%)	Control N = 40 n (%)
Overall mortality	6 (9.5)	4 (10)[*]
Cardiac related mortality	3 (4.8)	2 (5)[*]
Cardiac events	21 (33.3)	27 (67.5)[†]
CVA	1 (1.6)	8 (20)[†]
PVD	4 (6.3)	7 (17.5)[±]
Sepsis	12 (19)	8 (20)[*]

[*]P value NS, [†]pvalue = 0.001 [±]p = 0.07.

Before the Jury Is out on Cinacalcet's Cardiovascular Effects in Hemodialysis...

131

Table 5. Subgroup analysis of subjects with cardiovascular events.

	CV Events N = 48	No CV Events N = 55
Troponin at baseline ng/ml	0.05 ± 0.11	0.01 ± 0.026[†]
Troponin at 18 months ng/ml	0.04 ± 0.03	0.023 ± 0.03[†]
PTH at baseline pmol/L	95.45 ± 62	49.76 ± 44[†]
PTH at 18 months pmol/L	71.91 ± 48[*]	51.37 ± 78[*]

[*]P value NS, [†]p value ≤ 0.05.

Zhang, 15 large studies in end-stage renal disease patients with secondary hyperparathyroidism were reviewed [12]. This trial demonstrated effective improvement of biochemical parameters by cinacalcet without increasing all-cause of mortality or adverse events but conversely no advantages were noted either. However, a major limitation of this trial was the few number of studies available as well as the small number of subjects and short duration of follow-up.

Similar findings were reported by Palmer [23] in another large meta-analysis with data from 18 trials, whereby the use of cinacalcet conferred no significant benefit for all-cause mortality in patients with stage 5D Chronic Kidney Disease. Nevertheless, the investigators reported "uncertain" effects on cardio vascular outcomes. The results are hence inconclusive since in addition as with all metaanalysis, their generalizability is limited by protocol herterogeneity and differences in study population. We must therefore seek evidence from randomized clinical trials, though there has been few.

Nonetheless, the long awaited EVOLVE trial [24] showed these same findings with similar mortality outcomes in patients on cinaclacet compared to those on conventional treatment. There were however, some limitations to this well designed and executed trial. These included a high dropout rate of 20% and an additional 20% of patients in placebo group who were actually receiving commercially available cinacalcet [25]. As importantly, the difference in age though small, may have had great importance in dialysis patients [25]. Hence post hoc secondary analysis might actually be signaling some benefits [25]. Namely after adjusting for age and other comorbidities, a significant reduction of 12% was observed in the composite end point of death or major CV events [25]. Furthermore, censoring of data at 6 months after drug discontinuation found 15% reduction in primary composite and 17% in mortality with cinacalcet [25]. It therefore remains speculative whether the EVOLVE trial may in fact be marginally positive in favor of cinacalcet.

In our study, we noted a similar lack of cinacalcet treatment impact on all -cause and cardiac mortality. Interestingly however, our data demonstrated significantly lower cardiovascular event rates in the cinacalcet-treated group versus controls. This was seen despite longer dialysis vintage in the former which was not in their favor. There are some demographic variables in our study which may be potential confounders of the witnessed results, namely the older age of the control cohort and the higher proportion with diabetes. None of these differences however, achieved statistical significance. On the other hand, the cinacalcet group had more severe SHPT reflected by higher PTH levels which along with their longer duration on dialysis, may actually predispose to increased CV risk.

Moreover, it appears that the subgroup of patients with cardiac events had higher baseline troponin levels vs their non-cardiac events counterparts. Since troponin I is a specific biomarker for myocardial ischemia, this may explain in part their increased CV risk. It would hence be plausible that following troponin I trends may serve not only as possible marker of cinacalcet treatment effect on cardiac risk but suggests its utility as an overall prognostic indicator.

Finally, the paired group analysis showed an early drop in Troponin I levels at 12 months with non-significant changes in PTH levels, perhaps suggesting PTH-independent effects on the cardiac biomarker levels. The role of inflammation is possible, given the strong association described between chronic inflammatory markers (CRP) and disturbance of bone mineral metabolism in chronic hemodialysis patients [26]. This however, was not confirmed by our findings with no significant time variation in CRP levels. Unexplained in addition, is the nonsustained decline in troponin levels in this subgroup at 18 months, a time when PTH levels dropped significantly. These observations may be explained by additional unrelated factors or may have little clinical significance possibly due to our small sample size. All in all, given our study limitations which include the short duration, its retrospective nature, suboptimal cinacalcet dosing as well as late initiation, these findings require confirmation with appropriately designed prospective trials.

7. Conclusion

Our results suggest an association between reduction in PTH levels induced by cinacalcet and a decline in levels of Troponin I with demonstrably lower cardiovascular event rates. This however was not linked to an observed mortality benefit in the treated group. There are some potential confounders which may account for our findings including possible selection bias, however, clearly the pathophysiologic mechanisms are plausible and observations are warranting further investigation. Moreover, the raised baseline troponins in the subgroup of cinacalcet-treated patients with cardiac events may suggest utility of this biomarker in risk stratification. Large long-term placebo-controlled prospective trials are needed to explore this further and establish the clinical implications of calcimimetic treatment of secondary hyperparathyroidism on cardiovascular outcomes before the jury is out on cinacalcet.

Acknowledgements

We have no conflict of interest to disclose.

References

[1]   Salgueira, M., del Toro, N., Moreno-Alba, R., Jimenez, E., Areste, N., et al. (2003) Vascular Calcification in the Uremic Patient: A Cardiovascular Risk? Kidney International, **Supl**, S119-S121.

[2]   Costa-Hong, V., Jorgetti, V., Gowdak, L.H., Moyses, R.M., Krieger, E.M. and De Lima, J.J. (2007) Parathyroidectomy Reduces the Cardiovascular Events and Mortality in Renal Hyperparathyroidism. Surgery, **142**, 699-703. http://dx.doi.org/10.1016/j.surg.2007.06.015

[3]   Block, G.A., Zaun, D., Smits, G., Persky, M., Brillhart, S., et al. (2010) Cinacalcet Hydrochloride TNT Significantly Improves All Cause and Cardiovascular Survival in a Large Cohort of Hemodialysis Patients. Kidney International, **78**, 578-599.

[4]   Gaiki, M.R., Devita, M.V., Michelis, M.F., Panagopoulos, G. and Rosenstock, J.L. (2012) Troponin I as a Prognostic Marker of Cardiac Events in Symptomatic Hemodialysis Patients Using a Sensitive Trop I Assay. International Urology and Nephrology, **44**, 1841-1845.

[5]   Artunc, F., Mueller, C., Breidthardt, T., Twerenbold, R., Peter, A., Thamer, C., Weyrich, P., Haering, H.U. and Friedrich, B. (2012) Sensitive Troponins Which Suits Better for Hemodialysis Patients? Associated Factors and Prediction of Mortality. PLOS One, **7**, Article ID: e47610.

[6]   Flisinski, M., Strozecki, P., Stefanska, A., Zarzycka-Lindner, G., Brymora, A. and Manitius, J. (2007) Cardiac Troponin I in Patients with Chronic Kidney Disease Treated Conservatively or Undergoing Long-Term Haemodialysis. Kardiologia Polska, **65**, 1068-1078.

[7]   Kalaji, F.R. and Albitar, S. (2012) Predictive Value of Cardiac Troponin T and I in Hemodialysis Patients. Saudi Journal of Kidney Disease and Transplantation, **23**, 939-945. http://dx.doi.org/10.4103/1319-2442.100868

[8]   Geerse, D.A., Van Berkel, M., Vogels, S., Kooman, J.P., Konings, C.J. and Scharnhorst, V. (2012) Moderate Elevation of High Sensitivity Cardiac Troponin I and B Type Natriuretic Peptide in Chronic Hemodialysis Patients Are Associated with Mortality. Clinical Chemistry and Laboratory Medicine, **10**, 1-8.

[9]   Hagstrom, E., Hellman, P., Larsson, T.E., Ingelsso, E., Berglund, L., Sundstrom, J., Meihus, H., Held, C., Lind, L., Michaelsson, K. and Aenlov, J. (2009) Plasma Parathyroid Hormone and the Risk of Cardiovascular Mortality in the Community. Circulation, **119**, 2765-2771. http://dx.doi.org/10.1161/CIRCULATIONAHA.108.808733

[10] Weiner, D.E., Tabatabai, S., Tighiouart, H., Elsayed, E., Bansal, N., et al. (2006) Cardiovascular Outcomes and All-Cause Mortality: Exploring the Interaction between CKD and Cardiovascular Disease. American Journal of Kidney Diseases, **48**, 392-401. http://dx.doi.org/10.1053/j.ajkd.2006.05.021

[11] Shantouf, R., Kovesdy, C.P., Kim, Y., Ahmadi, N., Luna, A., Luna, C., Rambod, M., Nissenson, A.R., Budoff, M.J. and Kalantar-Zadeh, K. (2009) Association of Serum Alkaline Phosphatise with Coronary Artery Calcification in Maintenance Hemodialysis Patients. Clinical Journal of the American Society of Nephrology, **6**, 1106-1114. http://dx.doi.org/10.2215/CJN.06091108

[12] Zhang, Q., Li, M., You, L., Li, H.M., Ni, L., Gu, Y., Hao, C.M. and Chen, J. (2012) Effects and Safety of Calcimimetics in End Stage Renal Disease Patients with Secondary Hyperparathyroidism: A Meta-Analysis. PLoS One, **7**, Article ID: e48070. http://dx.doi.org/10.1371/journal.pone.0048070

[13] Block, G.A., Martin, K.J., de Francisco, A.L., Turner, S.A., Avram, M.M., et al. (2004) Cinacalcet for Secondary Hyperparathyroidism in Patients Receiving Hemodialysis. The New England Journal of Medicine, **350**, 1516-1525.

[14] Fukagawa, M., Yumita, S., Akizawa, T., Uchida, E., Tsukamoto, Y., et al. (2008) Cinacalcet (KRN1493) Effectively

Decreases the Serum Intact PTH Level with Favourable Control of the Serum Phosphorous and Calcium Levels in Japanese Dialysis Patients. *Nephrology Dialysis Transplantation*, **23**, 328-335.

[15] Saleh, F.N., Schirmer, H., Sundsfjord, J. and Jorde, R. (2003) Parathyroid Hormone and Left Ventricular Hypertrophy. *European Heart Journal*, **24**, 2054-2060. http://dx.doi.org/10.1016/j.ehj.2003.09.010

[16] Johnson, D.W., Craven, A.M. and Isbel, N.M. (2007) Modification of Cardiovascular Risk in Hemodialysis Patients: An Evidence-Based Review. *Hemodialysis International*, **11**, 1-14.

[17] Goodman, W.G., Goldin, J., Kuizon, B.D., Yoon, C., Gales, B., *et al.* (2000) Coronary Artery Calcification in Young Adults with End Stage Renal Disease Who Are Undergoing Dialysis. *The New England Journal of Medicine*, **342**, 1478-1483.

[18] Andersson, P., Rydberg, E. and Willenheimer, R. (2004) Primary Hyperparathyroidism and Heart Disease: A Review. *European Heart Journal*, **25**, 1776-1787. http://dx.doi.org/10.1016/j.ehj.2004.07.010

[19] Giovannucci, E., Liu, Y., Hollis, B.W. and Rimm, E.B. (2008) 25-Hydroxyvitamin D and Risk of Myocardial Infarction in Men: A Prospective Study. *Archives of Internal Medicine*, **168**, 1174-1180. http://dx.doi.org/10.1001/archinte.168.11.1174

[20] Wolfe, R.H., Ashby, V.B., Milford, E.L., Ojo, A.O., Ettenger, R.E., Agodoa, L.Y., Held, P.J. and Port, F.K. (1999) Comparison of Mortality in all Patients on Dialysis, Patients on Dialysis Awaiting Transplantation and Recipients of a First Cadaveric Transplant. *The New England Journal of Medicine*, **341**, 1725-1730. http://dx.doi.org/10.1056/NEJM199912023412303

[21] Cunninghm, J., Danese, M., Olson, K., Klassen, P. and Chertow, G.M. (2005) Effects of the Calcimimetic Cinacalcet HCl on Cardiovascular Disease, Fracture, and Health Related Quality of Life in Secondary Hyperparathyroidism. *Kidney International*, **68**, 1793-1800. http://dx.doi.org/10.1111/j.1523-1755.2005.00596.x

[22] Raggi, P., Chertow, G.M., Torres, P.U., Csiky, B., Naso, A., *et al.* (2011) The ADVANCE Study: A Randomised Study to Evaluate the Effects of Cinacalcet Plus Low Dose Vitamin D on Vascular Calcification in Patients on Hemodialysis. *Nephrology Dialysis Transplantation*, **26**, 1327-1339.

[23] Palmer, S.C., Nistor, I., Craig, J.C., Pellegrini, F., Messa, P., Tonelli, M., Covic, A. and Strippoli, G.F.M. (2013) Cinacalcet in Patients with Chronic Kidney Disease: A Cumulative Meta-Analysis of Randomised Controlled Trials. *PLOS Medicine*, **10**, Article ID: e1001436. http://dx.doi.org/10.1371/journal.pmed.1001436

[24] Glenn, M.C., Geoffrey, A.B., Ricardo, C.R., Tilman, B.D., Jurgen, F., willim, G.G., Charles, A.H., Yumi, K., Gerard, M.L., Kenneth, W.M., Christian, T.H., Sharon, M.M., Marie, L.T., David, C.W. and Patrick, S.P. (2012) Evaluation of Cinacalcet Hydrochloride Therapy to Lower Cardio Vascular Events. *The New England Journal of Medicine*, **2**, 898-905.

[25] The Evolve Trial Investigators (2012) Effects of Cinacalcet on Cardiovascular Disease in Patients Undergoing Dialysis. *The New England Journal of Medicine*, **367**, 2482-2494. http://dx.doi.org/10.1056/NEJMoa1205624

[26] Lee, C.T., Tsai, Y.C., Ng, H.Y., Su, Y., Lee, W.C., Lee, L.C., Chiou, T.T., Liao, S.C. and Hsu, K.T. (2009) Association between C-Reactive Protein and Biomarkers of Bone and Mineral Metabolism in Chronic Hemodialysis Patients: A Cross-Sectional Study. *Journal of Renal Nutrition*, **19**, 220-227.

19

Infections Following Kidney Transplant in Children: A Single-Center Study

Alexandre Fernandes[1*], Liliana Rocha[2], Teresa Costa[2], Paula Matos[2], Maria Sameiro Faria[2], Laura Marques[1], Conceição Mota[2], António Castro Henriques[3]

[1]Pediatric Infectious Diseases and Immunodeficiency Department, Centro Hospitalar do Porto, Oporto, Portugal
[2]Pediatric Nephrology Department, Centro Hospitalar do Porto, Oporto, Portugal
[3]Kidney Transplant Department, Centro Hospitalar do Porto, Oporto, Portugal
Email: [*]xanofernandes@gmail.com

Abstract

Introduction: Infections are a major cause of morbidity and mortality in pediatric patients undergoing kidney transplantation (KT). Aim and Methods: To determine the patterns of infectious complications during the first 6 months post transplantation, we report our single center experience with data from pediatric kidney recipients transplanted between 2006 and 2011. Results: Thirty-two children (20 males) were submitted to KT. The most common cause of end-stage renal disease (ESRD) was congenital anomalies of the kidney and urinary tract (CAKUT) accounting for 62%. Over the first 6 months post-transplant period, twenty-eight (87.5%) children developed a total of 77 infections, mainly urinary tract infections (UTI) (64.9%). CAKUT etiology of ESRD and UTI before KT increased the risk to develop more than one episode of UTI [71.4% vs. 14.3% and 81.8% vs. 18.2%, respectively; $p < 0.05$]. Twenty-three (29.9%) viral infections occurred. Cytomegalovirus (CMV) was the most common opportunistic pathogen, occurred in 11 patients and was more frequently in those with a donor (D)+/recipient (R)− CMV sero-status [74.5% vs. 25.5% ($p < 0.05$)]. A polyomaviruses (BKV) disease with nephropathy and meningitis was registered. The majority of infectious episodes had mild or moderate severity. No deaths occurred. Conclusion: A significant number of patients presented infectious complications during the first 6 months post transplantation. UTI are the most common type of infection, followed by viral infections, particularly CMV. Recognition, prevention and early treatment of infections are of major importance.

Keywords

CMV Infection, Immunosuppression, Kidney Transplantation, Urinary Tract Infections

---

[*]Corresponding author.

1. Introduction

Kidney transplantation (KT) is the treatment of choice for end-stage renal disease (ESRD) in children [1] [2]. Despite improvements on immunosuppressive therapy and surgical techniques, infections remain important complications and have been associated with increased morbidity and graft rejection [3] [4]. Indeed, infection is the predominant reason for hospitalization post transplantation and in the last few decades the successive emergence of new viral infections has been observed [5]. Specifically, cytomegalovirus (CMV) infections have been prominent in kidney transplant recipients since the 1980s, followed by Ebstein-Barr virus (EBV)-induced post transplantation lymphoproliferative disorder (PTLD) since the 1990s, and BK-virus-associated allograft nephropathy (BKVAN) in the last 10 years [5]. Infections are not only a significant source of morbidity and hospitalization but an important source of patient mortality and graft loss.

The immunosuppressive regimens currently in use are accompanied by a well-defined temporal sequence of infections [6]. During the first post-transplant month, the most frequent categories of infection are related to technical problems (including surgical site infections), urinary tract infections, vascular access infections, and pulmonary infections [7]. During this period, more than 90% of all infections are caused by bacteria and fungi and opportunistic infections are unusual [7] [8]. The greatest risk of life-threatening infection occurs between 1 and 6 months post transplantation, when the effects of immunosuppressive therapy peak [8] [9]. During this period, most common infections are opportunistic agents: virus like cytomegalovirus (CMV), polyomaviruses (BKV), Epstein-Barr Virus (EBV) and fungi (aspergillus). These opportunistic infections can occur with minimal epidemiological exposure and are related to the immunosuppression [7] [10]. CMV is the most common opportunistic organism encountered during this period [6] [9], and causes significant morbidity by direct infection and its immunomodulatory effects predispose to other infectious complications [5].

Although rejection rates have significantly decreased with the introduction of more potent immunosuppressive regimens, infections became a major problem in the transplant recipients [3] [10]. Death-censored graft loss from infectious complications is on the rise [7]. Similar to rejection rates, infection rates should be analyzed periodically in order to improve post transplantation outcome.

The purpose of this study was to analyze the patterns of infectious complications during the first 6 months post transplantation in our department.

2. Material and Methods

2.1. Design and Study Protocol

A retrospective study was performed to review the infectious complications over the first six months post transplantation, in children undergoing KT between January 2006 and December 2011. Two patients were excluded from the analysis because they experienced early graft loss, not related to infection.

Data were collected by clinical files review and included: all infectious episodes, clinical signs associated to these episodes, severity, renal function when infections occurred, pharmacological treatment, kidney and patient survival. We also divided the post transplant follow-up into two periods: less than 1 month and from 1 to 6 months.

2.2. Anti-Infectious Prophylaxis

In all patients prophylaxis consisted of intravenous 50 mg/kg cefoxitin (single dose, maximum 1000 mg) before the transplantation surgery and trimethoprim-sulfamethoxazole orally for *Pneumocystis jirovecci* prophylaxis for the first 6 months. Oral nystatin was added in the first month as antifungal prophylaxis. For CMV prophylaxis, oral valgancyclovir (3.5 × body surface area × creatinine clearance) was given for the first 6 months in all recipients, except D(−)/R(−) sero-CMV status. Intravenous CMV immunoglobulin (1 mL/Kg, weekly) was administered to D+/R− CMV within the first month after transplantation.

2.3. Immunosuppressive Therapy

The protocol in use in our institution included induction with antibodies anti-T cell (antithymocyte globulin or daclizumab), calcineurin inhibitors, mycophenolate mofetil and prednisolone, associated to maintenance immunosuppressive therapy with low doses of mofetil mycofenolate (300 mg/m^2; bid); tacrolimus (target-levels range of 8 - 10 ng/ml in the first month) and very low corticosteroids doses.

2.4. Definitions

UTI was diagnosed in the presence of a positive urine culture (more than 10^5 colony-forming units). A second UTI was diagnosed if between first and second episode there was a time free of symptoms and with a negative urine culture.

CMV infection was considered to be present if one or more of the following findings was noted: detection of one or more cells positive for CMV pp65 antigen per 10^5 leukocytes; seroconversion with the appearance of anti-CMV IgM antibodies; a fourfold increase in preexisting anti-CMV IgG titers; detection of CMV-DNAemia by molecular techniques; and/or isolation of the virus by culture of the throat, buffy coat, or urine. CMV disease requires clinical signs and symptoms, such as fever, leucopenia, or organ involvement.

Acute rejection was defined as an acute rejection episode treated either based upon clinical presumption or biopsy confirmed.

Graft dysfunction was defined as an episode when serum creatinine rise more than 0.5 mg/dl of previous values.

Infection with mild or moderate severity was defined when there was no need for hospitalization or when there was hospitalization only for anti-infectious intravenous therapy (without other organ dysfunction).

2.5. Surveillance

During the post transplant period, the patients were closely monitored for infections. Urine culture was performed in all outpatient visits and whenever symptoms suggestive of UTI or unexplained fever. CMV antigenemia (pp65 assays) was performed in the first month and every two months or when clinical suspicion of infection. BK virus in urine (by nucleic acid detection) was also monitored monthly: if BKV positive in urine a quantitative PCR BKV in plasma was also performed. Any fever (temperature higher than 38°C) was investigated systematically with white blood count and C-reactive protein serum level.

2.6. Treatment of Infections

Empirical UTI treatment was performed with antimicrobials covering the common gram-negative organisms or based on the susceptibility of the last pathogen identified. Upon identification of the etiologic agent, specific antimicrobial therapy was prescribed according to the microorganism susceptibility.

Therapeutic doses of valgancyclovir were given in the presence of a CMV infection and Intravenous gancyclovir was administered in CMV disease.

Preemptive reduction in immunosuppression was always done in BKV infection.

2.7. Statistical Analyses

Results were reported as mean, median and range for the quantitative variables and percentages for the categorical variables. Patients that presented infections were compared with those that do not had infections using the Fisher's exact test for categorical variables and differences between means were analyzed by Student t test or Mann-Whitney U test. P-values of 0.05 or less were considered statistically significant. All the statistical analyses were performed using SPSS version 20.0 (SPSS Inc., Chicago, IL, USA).

3. Results

Thirty-two patients underwent KT between January 2006 and December 2011, 20 (62.5%) male, with a mean patient age at KT of 11.5 years (range from 2 to 17 years). Twenty seven (84.4%) received KT from deceased donors and the remaining 5 (15.6%) from living related donors. CAKUT were the most common cause of renal disease accounting for 62%. The distribution of primary renal diseases is shown in **Table 1**. Fifteen (46.9%) children had UTI before undergoing KT. The donor (D)/recipient (R) sero-CMV status was: D(+)/R(−): 10 (31.3%); D(−)/R(+): 8 (25%); D(+)/R(+): 9 (28.1%); D(−)/R(−): 5 (15.6%). The immunossupressive therapy included induction with antibodies (84.4% with antithymocyte globulin and 15.6% with basiliximab) associated with a triple regimen with tacrolimus, mycophenolate mofetil and low doses of prednisolone. The mean post-transplant hospitalization time was 12.9 days (range: 7 to 37 days).

Twenty-eight (87.5%) children developed a total of 77 infection episodes (2.7 infections /patient) over the first 6 months post-transplant. The types of infections in our population are shown in **Table 2**. Seventy-eight percent of these infectious episodes occurred between 1 and 6 months and 22% in the first month post transplantation. There was a predominance of UTI (64.9%), followed by viral infections (29.8%). Four children had bacterial infections related to surgical procedure (1 surgical site infections, 1 peritonitis and 2 infected lymphocele). There had been no invasive fungal or mycobacterial infections. The infection episodes distribution in the first month and between 1 - 6 months post-transplant is shown in **Figure 1**.

UTI was the main infection occurring during this period (50 episodes in 21 (66%) patients) with an incidence of 2.4 episodes/child with UTI. Eleven (34.4%) patients had more than one UTI episode. More than one episode of UTI was more frequent in patients with CAKUT etiology of ESRD and UTI before KT [71.4% vs. 14.3% and 81.8% vs. 18.2%, respectively ($p < 0.05$)].

Fourteen (28%) episodes of UTI were febrile. Children with UTI before KT had higher risk to develop febrile UTI [100% vs. 0% ($p < 0.05$)]. UTI were mainly caused by Gram-negative bacteria (86%); *Klebsiella pneumonia* (40%) and *Escherichia coli* (32%) were the most common agents (**Table 3**). A multi-drug resistant microorganism was isolated in 12 (24%) UTI episodes in 7 patients; these microorganisms were more frequent in patients with CAKUT etiology of ESRD [100% vs. 0% ($p < 0.05$)] and were more frequently identified in febrile UTI [80% vs. 18.8% ($p < 0.05$)].

Table 1. Demographic characteristics and etiology of ESRD of 32 children submitted to kidney transplantation; ESRD: End-stage renal disease; CAKUT: Congenital anomalies of the kidney and urinary tract.

Demographic characteristics	
Male	20 (62.5%)
Age at transplantation	Mean: 11.5 years
	(Minimum: 2 years; Maximum: 17 years)
Caucasian	32 (100%)
Infections pre-KT	21 (65.6%)
UTI	15 (46.9%)
Peritonitis	6 (18.8%)
Causes of ESRD	
CAKUT	20 (62.5%)
Posterior urethral valves	6
Neurogenic bladder	5
Renal dysplasia	4
Reflux nephropathy	2
Other	3
Glomerular	4 (12.5%)
Cystic disease	3 (9.4%)
Other	3 (9.4%)
Unknown	2 (6.2%)

Table 2. Infections occurred during the first 6 months after kidney transplantation [UTI—urinay tract infection; CMV—Cytomegalovirus; Bk—Polyomavirus; *Rhinovirus, Influenza].

Pos Transplant infection	
Number of infections	77—occurred in 28 children
Number of infections per child	2.4
Type of Infections	
Bacterial infections	54 (70.1%)
UTI	50—occurred in 21 children
Other bacterial infections	4
Viral infections	23 (29.9%)—occurred in 19 children
CMV	11
Bk virus	3
Herpes simplex 1	4
Herpes zoster	1
Epstein Barr	1
Miscelaneous*	3
Invasive fungal infections	0

Table 3. Urinary tract infections occurred in the first 6 months after kidney transplantation [UTI—urinay tract infection; KT—Kidney transplantation].

	Number (%)
Episodes of UTI	50
Patients with UTI during first month after KT	14 (43.8%)
Episodes of febrile UTI	14 (28%)
Gram-negative bacteria	
Escherichia coli	16 (32%)
Klebsiella	20 (40%)
Proteus	1 (2%)
Pseudomonas	4 (8%)
Citrobacter freundii	2 (4%)
Gram-positive bacteria	
Enterococcus	7 (14%)

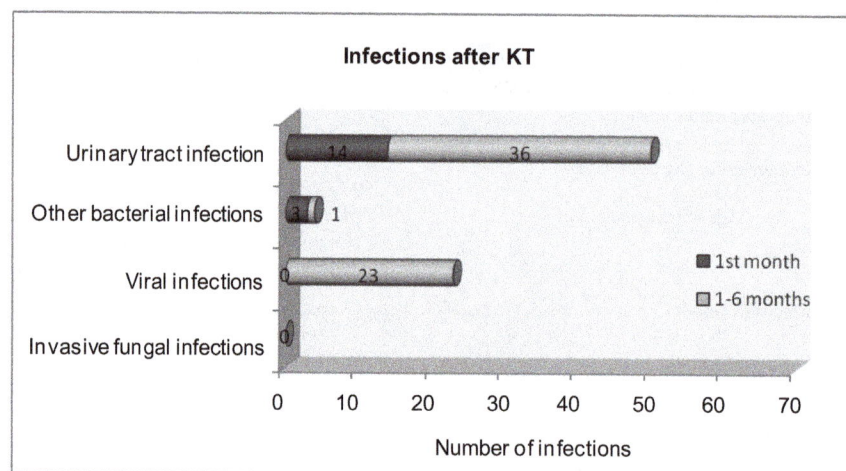

Figure 1. Infections occurred after kidney transplantation divided in 2 periods: 1st month and between 1 - 6 months.

CMV infection was recorded in 11 patients (34.4%), one of these with symptomatic infection (e.g., CMV disease). This infection occurred more frequently in patients with a D(+)/R(−) CMV sero-status [74.5% vs. 25.5% (p < 0.05)]. Three children had BKV infection one of them with special severity with nephropathy and meningitis.

During the observation period one patient had an acute rejection episode successfully treated with 3-day course of intravenous methylprednisolone (10 mg/Kg/day).

Two patients presented serious infections: one urosepsis with shock requiring admission to intensive care unit and one BKV disease with meningitis. All the other infections were of mild or moderate severity.

Eighteen (23.4%) infection episodes were associated with acute reversible graft dysfunction. None of the patients died during this period.

4. Discussion

Renal transplantation is the treatment of choice for children with ESRD and frequently restores the potential for normal growth and development with improved morbidity and mortality rates compared to dialysis. Short-term renal graft survival rates have improved with the use of newer immunosuppressive medications but carry the risk of increased infectious complications [11].

In this group, twenty-eight (87.5%) children developed a total of 77 infection episodes over the first 6 months post-transplant. The majority of these infectious episodes occurred between 1 and 6 months (78%) and the remaining in the first month post transplantation. As previously described, UTI and others bacterial infections (related to surgery) predominate in the first month and opportunistic infections were unusual; between 1 and 6 months post transplantation a high frequency of UTI persisted and viral infections occurred, in particular CMV and BKV infections, matching the typical infection patterns described [6] [7] [9].

According to the literature UTI is the most common form of bacterial infection in renal transplant and the data presented demonstrate that prevalence. Multiple episodes of UTI were more frequent in urologic causes of ESRD [5] [6] [8] [12]. Urinary tract abnormalities, bladder pathology with abnormal urodynamic assessment and a significant post-micturition residue requiring urinary catheterization is frequent. In our population CAKUT were the main cause of ESRD, accounting for 62.5%, and we observed in these patients a greater risk to develop more than 1 UTI episode. The presence of UTI episodes before KT is also associated with a greater risk to develop multiple UTI episodes post transplantation.

In our study, the prevalence of febrile UTI was 28% which was in agreement with previous reports in pediatric renal transplantation studies that range between 15% and 33% [1] [2]. Febrile UTI after KT may lead to kidney damage, negatively affecting long-term graft survival by scarring and interstitial injury, although precise data for the pediatric population are scarce. Therefore, in order to prevent allograft damage induced by febrile UTI, aggressive and specific treatment is mandatory [2]. In our patients antibiotic therapy was frequently initiated if bacteriuria was present and severe infections were infrequently found.

The most frequent organisms causing UTI in our population were *Klebsiella* species followed by *Escherichia coli*. *Escherichia coli* was isolated less frequently than in the general pediatric population, where it is found up to 80% [13]. This epidemiologic change may be due to underlying immunosuppression, colonization and mainly to the higher prevalence of bladder malformations in this population [8]. Unusual organisms such as *Pseudomonas* species were isolated in 8% of the children in this study and multiple antibiotic resistances were also seen in patients with abnormal lower urinary tract and neurogenic bladder.

The incidence of other bacterial infections related to surgery was low in the present study, as in other recent studies [14] [15]. The lower incidences of those infections in recent years may be partly due to improvements in surgical transplant techniques and prophylaxis strategies.

Viral infections are an important concern between the 1 - 6 months post-transplantation in recipients' kidney transplants. CMV infection is one of the most common infections after transplantation, only preceded by UTI as reported in other studies [9]. The major determinants of CMV infection are an active or latent CMV agent in the donor or recipient and the dose, duration and type of immunosuppressive therapies [16]. The induction with lymphocyte depletion is also associated with an increase of CMV infections [16] [17]. In our cohort about a third of patients had CMV infection although only one presented CMV disease. CMV infections were more frequent in D(+)/R(−) positive donors as previously reported [5] [12]. The widespread use of prophylactic and/or preemptive antiviral therapy has greatly reduced the incidence of CMV disease and can explain the low rate of CMV disease in our population. Without preventive therapy, the incidence of symptomatic CMV infection in such recipients would be about 50% to 65% [5]. Literature documents a relation between CMV infection and acute rejection [5] [12]; in our cohort, only one KT recipient had an acute rejection episode, during the observation period.

In kidney transplant recipients, BKV can be responsible to allograft nephropathy [5] and its incidence in pediatric KT ranges from 3% to 8%; risk factors include aggressive immunosuppression and recent treatment for acute rejection [5]. We identified 3 children with BK infection, one case with nephropathy and BK meningitis. The cornerstone of the treatment of BKV infection is to decrease the immunosuppressive therapy. In our patient with a disseminated disease we also administered cyprofloxacin, cidofovir and intravenous immunoglobulin with a successful outcome [18].

The use of induction immunosuppression with polyclonal antibodies (84.4%) in our population probably increased the risk of infection [17]. On the other hand, a very low number of acute rejection episodes were observed and no additive anti-rejection therapy was needed. Although a potent induction antibody was often used in our institution for pediatric recipients from deceased donors, the cumulative immunosuppression is not considered too burden.

The risk of non Hodgkin lymphoma (PTLD) was associated to Epstein Barr virus infection, and in children was commonly attributed to primary EBV infections from an EBV-positive renal graft [19]. In our series no PTLD was registered during the observation period. However a longer follow-up period is needed.

Study limitations: the data collected from files may not have all information. Indeed, some mild infections (like could infection) could be treated at home with no records in clinical files. Our study only considered infections occurred during first 6 months after KT and not assessed infections occurred after this period.

5. Conclusion

The current opinion is that the optimal approach to preserving renal allograft function is to minimize the immunosuppressive burden, thereby achieving a balance between the risk of rejection and infections complications. The antimicrobial prophylaxis protocol, close monitoring and an early treatment of infections could justify the mild or moderate severity of the almost all infections over the observation period in our pediatric kidney recipients. The long term care of transplant recipients should include all preventive measures; close monitoring for any subtle infections and immunosuppression must be prudently managed and adjusted to the patients to reach a favorable outcome.

References

[1]   Esezobor, C.I., Nourse, P. and Gajjar, P. (2012) Urinary Tract Infection Following Kidney Transplantation: Frequency, Risk Factors and Graft Function. *Pediatric Nephrology*, **27**,651-657 http://dx.doi.org/10.1007/s00467-011-2044-1

[2]   Ulrike, J.M. and Kemper, J. (2009) Urinary Tract Infections in Children after Renal Transplantation. *Pediatric Nephrology*, **24**,1129-1136 http://dx.doi.org/10.1007/s00467-007-0690-0

[3]   Green, M. and Michaels, M.G. (2012) Infections in Pediatric Solid Organ Transplant Recipients. *Journal of the Pediatric Infectious Diseases Society*, **1**,144-151 http://dx.doi.org/10.1093/jpids/pir001

[4]   Allen, U. and Green, M. (2010) Prevention and Treatment of Infectious Complications after Solid Organ Transplantation in Children. *Pediatric Clinics of North America*, **57**, 459-479. http://dx.doi.org/10.1016/j.pcl.2010.01.005

[5]   Neu, A. and Dharnidharka, V. (2008) Prevention and Treatment of Infectious Complications in Pediatric Renal Allograft Recipients. In: Geary, D.F. and Schaefer, F., Eds., *Comprehensive Pediatric Nephrology*, Mosby-Elsevier, Philadelphia, 967-973

[6]   Rubin, R. (1993) Infectious Disease Complications of Renal Transplantation. *Kidney International*, **44**, 221-236. http://dx.doi.org/10.1038/ki.1993.234

[7]   Parasuramana, R., Samarapungavana, D. and Venkatb, K.K. (2010) Updated Principles and Clinical Caveats in the Management of Infection in Renal Transplant Recipients. *Transplantation Reviews*, **24**, 43-51. http://dx.doi.org/10.1016/j.trre.2009.09.001

[8]   Mencarelli, F. and Marks, S. (2012) Non-Viral Infections in Children after Renal Transplantation. *Pediatric Nephrology*, **27**, 1465-1476. http://dx.doi.org/10.1007/s00467-011-2099-z

[9]   Charfeddine, K., Zaghden, S., Kharrat, M., Kamoun, K., Jarraya, F. and Hachicha, J. (2005) Infectious Complications in Kidney Transplant Recipients, A Single-Center Experience. *Transplantation Proceedings*, **37**, 2823-2825. http://dx.doi.org/10.1016/j.transproceed.2005.05.009

[10] Fishman, J. (2007) Infection in Solid-Organ Transplant Recipients. *The New England Journal of Medicine*, **357**, 2601-2614. http://dx.doi.org/10.1056/NEJMra064928

[11] Dharnidharka, V.R.1., Caillard, S., Agodoa, L.Y. and Abbott, K.C. (2006) Infection Frequency and Profile in Different Age Groups of Kidney Transplant Recipients. *Transplantation*, **81**, 1662-1667. http://dx.doi.org/10.1097/01.tp.0000226068.66819.37

[12] Ranchin, B., Hees, L., Stamm, D., Bertholet-Thomas, A., Billaud, G., Lina, G., Cochat, P. and Gillet, Y. (2011) Transplantation rénale et infection chez l'enfant. *Néphrologie & Thérapeutique*, **7**, 608-610 http://dx.doi.org/10.1016/j.nephro.2011.11.006

[13] Jodal, U. and Winberg, J. (1987) Management of Children with Unobstructed Urinary Tract Infection. *Pediatric Nephrology*, **1**, 647-656. http://dx.doi.org/10.1007/BF00853603

[14] Gargah, T., Labessi, A., Ounissi, M., Derouiche, A., Chokri, Z., Abdallah, T., Chebil, M. and Lakhoua, M.R. (2011) Early Infections in Children Following Renal Transplantation. *La Tunisie Médicale*, **89**, 26-30.

[15] Maraha, B., Bonten, H., van Hooff, H., Fiolet, H., Buiting, A.G. and Stobberingh, E. (2001) Infectious Complications and Antibiotic Use in Renal Transplant Recipients during a 1-Year Follow-Up. *Clinical Microbiology and Infection*, **7**, 619-625. http://dx.doi.org/10.1046/j.1198-743x.2001.00329.x

[16] Conceição, M., Lassalete, M., Costa, T., Leonidio, D., Almeida, M., Santos, J., Sameiro Faria, M., Castro Henriques, A. and Almeida, R. (2010) Nineteen Years of Experience Utilizing Anti-T-Lymphocyte Globulin Induction in Pediatric kidney Transplantation. *Annals of Transplantation*, **15**, 84-91.

[17] Issa, N. and Fishman, J. (2009) Infectious Complications of Antilymphocyte Therapies in Solid Organ Transplantation. *Clinical Infectious Diseases*, **48**, 772-786. http://dx.doi.org/10.1086/597089

[18] Rocha, A., Faria, S., Costa, T., Marques, L., Freitas, C. and Mota, C. (2013) BK Virus Nephropathy Complicated with Meningoencephalitis after Kidney Transplantation. *Pediatric Transplantation*, **18**, E48-E51.

http://dx.doi.org/10.1111/petr.12209

[19] Opelz, G., Daniel, V., Naujokat, C. and Döhler, B. (2009) Epidemiology of Pretransplant EBV and CMV Serostatus in Relation to Posttransplant Non-Hodgkin Lymphoma. *Transplantation*, **88**, 962-967.
http://dx.doi.org/10.1097/TP.0b013e3181b9692d

Abbreviations

BKV: Polyomaviruses; CAKUT: Congenital Anomalies of the Kidney and Urinary Tract; CMV: Cytomegalovirus; D/R: Donor/Recipient; EBV: Epstein-Barr Virus; ESRD: End-Stage Renal Disease; Ig: Immunoglobulin; KT: Kidney Transplantation; PTLD: Post-Transplant Lymphoproliferative Disorder; UTI: Urinary Tract Infections

20

Urinary Neutrophil Gelatinase Associated Lipocalin as a Marker of Tubular Damage in Type 2 Diabetic Patients with and without Albuminuria

Abeer A. Al-Refai[1], Safaa I. Tayel[1], Ahmed Ragheb[2], Ashraf G. Dala[2], Ahmed Zahran[2]*

[1]Biochemistry Department, Faculty of Medicine, Menofia University, Shibin El Kom, Egypt
[2]Internal Medicine Department, Faculty of Medicine, Menofia University, Shibin El Kom, Egypt
Email: *ahmed173@hotmail.com

Abstract

Background: Neuttrophil gelatinase associated lipocalin (NGAL) was shown to be a good marker for predicting acute kidney injury (AKI). Some recent reports demonstrated that NGAL may be an early biomarker for kidney affection in diabetic patients. The aim of this work is to investigate urinary NGAL (UNGAL) in type 2 diabetic patients with and without albuminuria. Methods: This study included 46 type 2 diabetic patients and 15 healthy age and sex matched individuals as the control group. Diabetic patients were divided into three groups according to urinary albumin excretion (UAE), normoalbuminuria, microalbuminuria and macroalbuminuria. UNGAL was measured in all populations and corrected to urinary creatinine to account for day to day variation in urine volume and transformed log. Comparison between 4 groups (control, normoalbuminuria, microalbuminuria and macroalbuminuria) was done. Results: Log UNGAL/Creatinine ratio showed significant difference when comparing control group (0.70 ± 0.58) versus normoalbuminuria (1.71 ± 1.06), microalbuminuria (1.57 ± 0.72) and macroalbuminuria (1.92 ± 0.63), however, there was no significant difference among diabetic groups. Pearson's correlation showed that log UNGAL/Creatinine ratio positively correlated with glycated hemoglobin (HbA1c) and inversely with estimated glomerular filtration rate (eGFR). Regression analysis showed that HbA1c, urinary creatinine and eGFR were the independent predictors of log UNGAL/Creatinine ratio. Conclusion: Tubular markers like UNGAL may be early elevated in type 2 diabetic patients even before the incidence of glomerular injury detected by microalbuminuria and it can be used as an early marker for detection of kidney involvement in diabetic patients.

---

*Corresponding author.

Keywords

Neutrophil Gelatinase Associated Lipocalin (NGAL); Diabetic Nephropathy; Albuminuria; Tubular Markers

1. Introduction

Diabetes mellitus is the leading cause of chronic kidney disease (CKD), and the rapidly increasing prevalence of diabetes worldwide virtually assures that the proportion of CKD attributable to diabetes will continue to rise [1]. Diabetic kidney disease is associated with enhanced morbidity and mortality, particularly with accelerated cardiovascular disease [2]. The earliest clinical evidence of nephropathy is elevated urine albumin level ≥ 30 mg/ 24hours [3]. Microalbuminuria is generally considered as the earliest non-invasive marker for the development of diabetic nephropathy [4], however, microalbuminuria is diagnosed once significant glomerular damage has occurred [5]. Although glomerular dysfunction is thought to be a major factor for the development and progression of diabetic nephropathy, tubulointerstitial damage might also play an important role in the pathogenesis of diabetic nephropathy [6]. It has been suggested that an early increase in urinary albumin excretion is relevant to proximal tubular damage or dysfunction in addition to glomerular permeability [7]. Several different markers of tubular damage have been widely investigated in the areas related to acute kidney injury (AKI) and have presented promising data as early predictive biomarkers of AKI [8] [9]. Recently, some investigators have demonstrated that these tubular markers have clinical importance as biomarkers of diabetic nephropathy [10] [11]. NGAL is an ubiquitous protein of 178 amino acids with a molecular mass of approximately 25 kDa. It belongs to the family of lipocalins, which is a family of proteins that have been associated with many biological processes, such as inflammation, the transport of pheromones and the synthesis of prostaglandins [12] [13]. NGAL was initially identified by Allen and Venge in 1989 from human neutrophils, and it is now known that it is expressed at low levels in several human tissues, including kidney, trachea, lungs, stomach and colon [14], However, its precise role has been clarified by Paragas *et al.* who found that the timing and the intensity of NGAL mRNA and protein were correlated and dependent on the degree of kidney damage in an experimental model of mouse with induced AKI and they found that its production was located in the distal convoluted tubule and the collecting duct while the proximal tubule was involved in the process of NGAL reabsorption [15]. NGAL is produced and secreted into the urine in response to ischemic kidney damage and is therefore a promising early indicator of tubulointerstitial damage [16]. Several recent reports showed that NGAL is an important biomarker and is elevated in DKD [10] [11] [17]. The aim of this work is to evaluate the UNGAL in patients with type 2 diabetes with and without albuminuria.

2. Patient and Methods

This study included 46 type 2 diabetic patients on either oral anti diabetic or insulin therapy. In addition, 15 apparently healthy, non-diabetic, without CKD, age and gender matched subjects were included in this study as a control group. All the patients were recruited from outpatient clinic, Internal Medicine Department, Menofia University hospital. The protocol for this study followed the ethical standards and approved by the ethical committee of our institution and all subjects gave informed consent to participate in this study. All patients fulfilled the following inclusion criteria, Type 2 Diabetes mellitus (DM) more than one year, older than 18 years old with stable kidney function defined as stable serum creatinine with less than 10% change in last three months. The following patients were excluded, Type 1 DM, unstable kidney function or kidney disease other than diabetic nephropathy, pregnancy, malignancy, infections or any inflammatory conditions. Patients were divided according urinary albumin excretion (UAE) which was measured by spot morning urine sample for albumin to creatinine ratio (UACR) into 3 groups diabetic with normoalbuminuria (UACR less than 30 mg/gm), diabetic with microalbuminuria (UACR between 30 - 299 mg/gm) and diabetic with macroalbuminuria (UACR equal or more than 300 mg/gm). All subjects underwent full history taking and clinical examination, including weight, height and measuring blood pressure. Mean arterial pressure (MAP) was calculated as $\{(2 \times \text{diastolic blood pressure (mmHg)} + \text{systolic blood pressure (mmHg)}\}/3$. BMI Was calculated as weight $(Kg)/\{\text{Height (m)}\}^2$ and GFR was estimated using Modification of Diet in Renal Disease Abbreviated Equation (MDRD): [GFR = 186 × (serum Cr)$^{-1.154}$ × (age)$^{-0.203}$ × (0.742 if female) × (1.210 if African American)] [18].

3. Laboratory Assessment

Venous blood samples were collected following an overnight fasting for measurements of fasting plasma glucose, glycosylated hemoglobin (HbA1c), creatinine and serum urea. A whole blood was obtained by using EDTA containing tube for measurement of glycosylated hemoglobin (HbA1c). Fasting plasma glucose was determined by enzymatic colorimetric test, using Spinreact kit, SPAIN [19]. Serum and urine creatinine concentration was assessed by a kinetic Jaffe´ method [20] and serum urea by enzymetic colorimetry methods [21]. Glycosylated hemoglobin was assayed by quantitative colorimetric measurement of glycohemoglobin as percent of total hemoglobin using kits supplied by Teco Diagnostics, Lakeview Ave, Anaheim, CA, USA [22]. The Urinary albumin concentration was measured by a commercially available solid phase enzyme linked immunosorbent assay kit provided by DRG International Inc., USA; cat no EIA-2361], according to manufacturer s instructions from early morning spot urine collections [23] and adjusted for urinary creatinine which has been found to be an accurate measure of urinary albumin excretion per 24 hours [24]. Urinary NGAL was measured in one morning spot urine sample collected in labeled sterile container and thereafter was immediately centrifuged at 4°C for 10 min at 4000 rpm to obtain supernatant. Supernatant of urine were stored at −20°C till analysis. Urine-NGAL was measured using an ELISA method according to manufacturer s instructions and provided by [Ray Biotech, Inc. Norcross, GA; Cat#: ELH-Lipocalin2-001] and adjusted for urine creatinine to account for day-today variation in urine volume, as 24-h urine samples were not available [25]. It was expressed as Pg/mg.

4. Statistical Evaluations

We used the statistical package of social signs (SPSS, version 16) to perform the analysis. Categorical data were presented as number and percentages and continuous variables as means ± standard deviation (SD). One way ANOVA test or Kruskalwalis test was used as appropriate for comparison of quantitative variables more than two independent groups. Chi-Square test was used for categorical variables and Fischer exact test was used if one cell less than 5. T-test or Mann-Whitney test was used as appropriate for comparison between two quantitative variables. The Kolmogorov-Smirnov test was done to determine the distribution of data. Log transformation of UNGAL/Creatinine ratio was done improve interpretability and data scatter. The correlations between the variables were analyzed using Pearson's correlation. Regression analysis was performed to detect the possible predictor of log UNGAL/Creatinine ratio as a marker of tubular injury. Receiving operation characteristic (ROC) curve was constructed to detect cut off value of log UNGAL/Creatinine ratio at which tubular injury can occur comparing normal group with whole diabetic patients. P value ≤ 0.05 was considered significant.

5. Results

This study included 46 patients with type 2 diabetes mellitus with 15 healthy persons as a control group. The diabetic patients were divided into 3 groups according (UACR). So the whole cohort was divided into 4 groups. Group 1: Control group consists of 15 health persons 11(73.3%) male and 4(26.7%) female; Group 2: Diabetic patients with normoalbuminuria (UACR < 30 mg/gm) consists of 16 patients, 12 (75%) males and 4 (25%) females; Group 3: Diabetic patients with microalbuminuria (UACR between 30 - 299 mg/gm) consists of 14 patients, 8 (57.1%) males and 6 (42.9%) females; Group 4: Diabetic patients with macroalbuminuria (UACR > 300 mg/gm) consists of 16 patients, 7 (43.8%) males and 9 (56.2%) females. All groups were matched regarding age, sex and BMI. Base line characteristics and comparison between studied groups are shown in **Table 1**. All groups were compared together using ANOVA or Kruskalwalis test as appropriate then each two groups were compared together using student t test or Mann-Whitney test as appropriate. There was significant difference among the studied groups regarding log UNGAL/Creatinine ratio with P value 0.0001. Analysis between each two groups showed that there was a significant difference between group 1 (Control group) and each group separately while the diabetic groups did not show significant difference among themselves (**Figure 1**). Correlation between log UNGAL/Creatinine ratio with HbA1c, eGFR, Duration of diabetes in years and UACR showed significant positive correlation with HbA1c with r value + 0.4 and P value 0.01 and significant negative correlation with eGFR with r value - 0.4 and P value 0.02 while it did not show significant correlation with UACR and duration of diabetes mellitus (**Figure 2**) Regression analysis demonstrated that HbA1c, urinary creatinine and

Table 1. Demographics and comparison between the studied groups.

Variable	(Group 1) Control group UACR (mg/gm) 4.93 ± 2.26 (n = 15)	(Group 2) Diabetics with normoalbuminuria UACR (mg/gm) 6.38 ± 8.42 (n= 16)	(Group 3) Diabetics with microalbuminuria UACR (mg/gm) 113.21 + 51.83 (n = 14)	(Group 4) Diabetics with macroalbuminuria UACR (mg/gm) 1812.6 + 2074.5 (n = 16)	P Value
Age in years	50.67 ± 5.70	48.63 ± 16.78	56.21 ± 11.11	54.94 ± 7.42	>0.05$^\$$
Sex (M/F) (No and %)	11/4 (73.3/26.7)	12/4 (75/25)	8/6 (57.1/42.9)	7/9 (43.8/56.2)	>0.05$^\#$
Duration of DM (years)	-	7.69 ± 4.66	10.36 ± 2.82	15.19 ± 5.32	0.01$^\$$ (<0.05$^{\#\#,+}$) (>0.05$^\#$)
BMI (kg/m^2)	29.2 + 3.39	27.96 ± 7.34	28.53 ± 2.12	28.24 ± 3.45	>0.05$^\$$
MAP (mmHg)	88.00 ± 6.88	100.21 ± 11.66	100.36 ± 10.24	100.52 ± 5.19	0.001$^\$$ (<0.05$^{*,**,***,\#\#}$) (>0.05$^{\#,+}$)
Fasting blood glucose (mg/dl)	92.40 ± 2.47	147.12 ± 30.13	181.12 ± 49.83	166.31 ± 46.74	0.0001$^\$$ (<0.05$^{*,**,***,\#}$) (>0.05$^{\#\#,+}$)
HbA1c %	4.88 ± 0.82	9.22 ± 3.50	6.82 ± 1.99	7.76 ± 3.60	0.001$^\$$ (<0.05$^{*,**,***,\#}$) (>0.05$^{\#\#,+}$)
Creatinine (mg/dl)	0.7 ± 0.13	1.58 ± 0.88	1.98 ± 1.01	3.94 ± 1.84	0.0001$^\$$ (<0.05$^{**,***,\#\#,+}$) (>0.05$^{*,\#}$)
Urea (mg/dl)	21.00 ± 2.20	37.56 ± 30.99	42.64 ± 28.89	74.81 ± 40.49	0.0001$^\$$ (<0.05$^{***,\#\#,+}$) (>0.05$^{*,**,\#}$)
Urinary creatinine (mg/dl)	100.24 ± 29.42	76.87 ± 27.21	79.14 ± 24.85	75.63 ± 31.79	0.0001$^\$$ (<0.05*,**,***) (0.05$^{\#,\#\#,+}$)
eGFR (ml/min/1.73m^2)	93.89 ± 16.79	72.73 ± 59.84	46.32 ± 30.26	20.17 ± 16.01	0.0001$^\$$ (<0.05$^{*,**,***,\#\#,+}$) (>0.05$^\#$)
Log UNGAL/Creatinine ratio (Pg/mg)	0.70 ± 0.58	1.71 ±1.06	1.57 ± 0.72	1.92 ± 0.63	0.0001$^\$$ (<0.05*,**,***) (>0.05$^{\#,\#\#,+}$)

$^\$$: All groups together, *: Control VS Normoalbuminuria, **: Control VS Microalbuminuria, ***: Control VS Macroalbuminuria, $^\#$: Normoalbuminuria VS Microalbuminuria, $^{\#\#}$: Normoalbuminuria VS Macroalbuminuria, $^+$: Microalbuminuria VS Macroalbuminuria. ACR: Albumin creatinine ratio, M/F: Male/Female, BMI: Body mass index, MAP: Mean arterial pressure, HbA1c: Glycated hemoglobin, eGFR: estimated glomerular filtration rate, Log U NGAL/Creatinine: Logarithm Urinary neutrophil gelatinase associated lipocalin/Creatinine.

eGFR were the independent predictors of Log UNGAL/Creatinine ratio (**Table 2**). ROC curve was constructed to detect cut off value of Log UNGAL/Creatinine ratio considering control group as status variable. It showed a best cut off value at 1.035 Pg/mg with good area under the curve (AUC) of 0.87 and sensitivity of 80.4% and specificity of 80% (**Figure 3** and **Table 3**).

6. Discussion

Diabetic nephropathy is currently the leading cause of CKD. It is also one of the most significant long-term complications in terms of morbidity and mortality for individual patients with diabetes [26]. Serum and urinary NGAL are arguably the most promising emerging biomarkers for early detection of AKI [27]. Several recent studies also have defined the role of NGAL in CKD and showed serum and UNGAL levels are markers of kidney disease and severity in CKD [10] [11] [28] [29]. The aim of this work is to evaluate the UNGAL in type 2

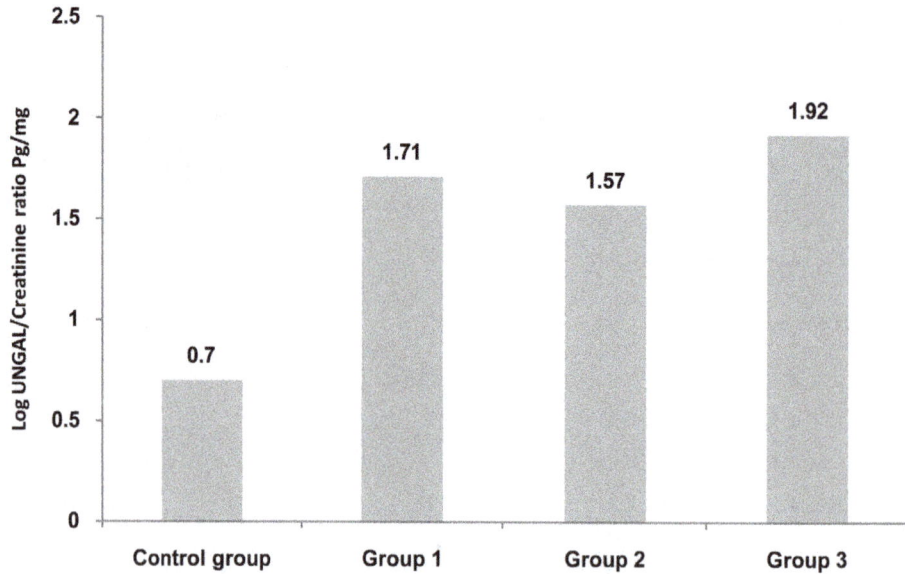

Figure 1. Comparison between studied groups as regard Log UNGAL/Creatinine ratio Pg/mg. Logarithm Urinary Neutrophil Gelatinase Associated lipocaline.

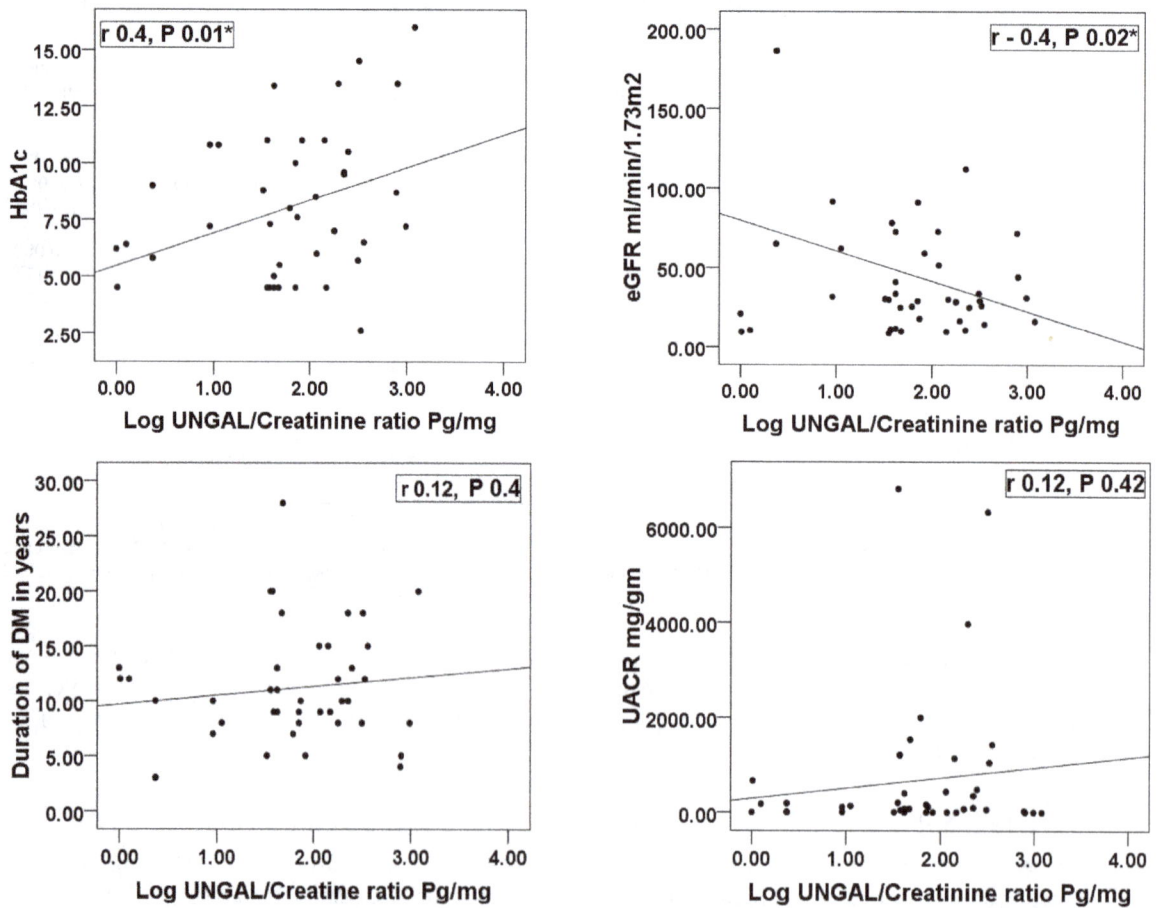

Figure 2. Correlation between log UNGAL/Creatinine ratio with, HbA1c, eGFR ml/min/1.73 m^2, duration of diabetes in years and UACR mg/gm. UNGAL; Urinary neutrophil gelatinase associated lipocalin, Log; Logarithm, UACR; Urinary albumin creatinine ratio, eGFR; Estimated glomerular filtration rate, DM; Diabetes Mellitus, *Significant difference.

Table 2. linear regression analysis to detect the predictors of Log UNGAL/Creatinine ratio.

	Log UNGAL/Creatinine ratio Pg/mg	
	β	P
Duration of DM in years	−0.115	0.52
Mean blood pressure	0.013	0.92
HbA1c	0.411	0.003[*]
Fasting blood glucose	−0.22	0.98
UACR mg/gm	−0.103	0.47
Creatinine	0.15	0.94
Urea	−0.022	0.98
Urine creatinine	−0.548	0.001[*]
eGFR ml/min/1.73m^2	−0.434	0.014[*]

Log UNGAL/Creatinine: Logarithm urinary neutrophil gelatinase associated lipocaline/Creatinine ratio, DM: Diabetes mellitus, HbA1c: Glycated hemoglobin, UACR: Urinary albumin creatinine ratio, eGFR: Estimated glomerular filtration rate, [*]Significant difference.

Table 3. AUC, sensitivity and specificity of cut off value of log UNGAL/creatnine ratio.

AUC	SE	Asymptomatic Significance	Asymptomatic 95% Confidence Interval		Sensitivity	Specificity	Cut off point
			Lower bond	Upper bond			
0.87	0.045	0.0001	0.779	0.957	80.4 %	80 %	1.035

AUC: Area under the curve, SE: Standard error.

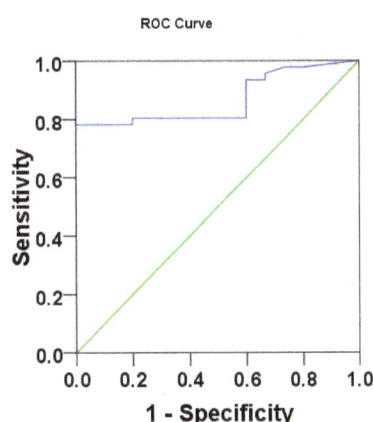

Figure 3. Receiving operation characteristic curve of UNGAL/Creatinine ratio Pg/mg to detect cut off value of raising log UNGAL/Creatinine ratio considering control group as status variable.

di-abetic patients with albuminuria (microalbuminuria and macroalbuminuria) and those without (Normoalbuminuria). Also a control group without diabetes and CKD was compared with all diabetic groups. In our study we found that there was a significant difference among the studied 4 groups (Control, Normoalbuminuria, Microalbuminuria and Macroalbuminuria) regarding log UNGAL/Creatinine ratio while comparison of each 2 groups separately showed that there was significant difference between the control group with each group separately while the diabetic groups did not show significant difference among themselves. It means that UNGAL increased in diabetic patients without albuminuria when compared with control group suggesting that UNGAL as a marker of tubular injury precede the appearance of microalbuminuria as a marker of glomerular injury. In accordance with our results, Bolignano D. *et al.* who evaluated serum and UNGAL in diabetic patients with albuminuria and found that serum and UNGAL was significantly elevated in diabetic patients in respect to control group, Also like our results he found elevated levels in diabetic patients without early signs of glomerular damage (Normoalbuminuria) [10]. Nauta FL *et al.* demonstrated that NGAL is 1.5 fold significantly elevated in diabetic patients with normoalbuminuria compared to non-diabetic control group [11]. In an experimental animal study, Miller ML *et al.* found that urinary biomarkers including UNGAL were elevated in an established rat model of diabetic nephropathy and concluded that these biomarkers appeared even before the classical biomarkers of diabetic nephropathy such as albuminuria [30]. Another study by Lacquaniti A. *et al.* concluded that NGAL increases in patients with type 1 diabetes, even before diagnosis of microalbuminuria representing an early biomarker of normoalbuminuric diabetic nephropathy with a good sensitivity and specificity. NGAL measurement could be useful for the evaluation of early renal involvement in the course of diabetes [31]. Also in children some reports showed that serum and UNGAL were elevated in diabetic children without albuminuria and concluded that Normal-range albuminuria does not exclude diabetic nephropathy defined as increased serum and UNGAL concentration and NGAL measurement can be more sensitive than microalbumin and may become a useful tool for evaluating renal involvement in diabetic children [32]. Some other studies showed inconsistency with our results. Kim S.S. *et al.* found that UNGAL was elevated in diabetic patients with macroalbuminuria compared to control, normoalbuminuria and microalbuminuria groups, however he did not find any significant difference between control group and normoalbuminuria group [33]. Although Nielsen S.E. *et al.* found that UNGAL is elevated in diabetic patients with and without albuminuria similar to our results, however in contrast to our results he found that UNGAL increases significantly with increasing albuminuria [34]. Also WU J. *et al.* was observed that baseline level of urinary NGAL was significantly elevated and correlated with the severity of albuminuria in patients with diabetes and during the follow up, the urinary level of NGAL was observed to be significantly correlated with a rapid decline in the eGFR [35]. In our study log UNGAL/Creatinine ratio showed significant positive correlation with HbA1c and significant negative correlation with eGFR, while it did not show any correlation with UACR and duration of diabetes. Some studies found significant inverse correlation between UNGAL and eGFR like our finding however in contrast to our results they found also significant correlation with albuminuria [10] [36]. Similar to our results Woo *et al.* found inverse correlation between UNGAL with eGFR while he did not find any correlation with albuminuria [37]. In contrast to our results, Zachwieja J. *et al.* found correlation between UNGAL and UAE while he did not find any correlation with eGFR and HbA1c [32]. In our study, linear regression analysis demonstrated that independent predictors of log UNGAL/Cr ratio were HbA1c, urine creatinine and eGFR. It means that UNGAL as a marker of tubular damage is highly associated with uncontrolled diabetes and decline of kidney function detected by decreased urinary creatinine and eGFR. We could not find any association between tubular damage detected by log UNGAL/Creatine ratio and glomerular damage detected by microalbuminnria as albuminuria could not predict log UNGAL/Creatinine ratio and also log UNGAL/Creatinine ratio could not predict development of microalbuminuria (Data not shown). So according our data both tubular and glomerular damage occur simultaneously in diabetic patients and we could not decide if the underlying mechanisms are the same or different. We could not find any study determined the independent predictors of urinary NGAL. Most of the studies addressed the value of UNGAL as a predictor of acute kidney injury [38]-[40]. We constructed a ROC curve to detect the cut off value of log UNGAL/Creatinine ratio to determine the normal value of log UNGAL/Creatinine ratio and it was found 1.035 Pg/ml with good AUC, sensitivity and specificity. There are some limitations of our work. First the small number of patients, second it is an observational study and we did not address the pathophysiology and underlying mechanisms for tubular injury and if there is an interplay between tubular and glomerular damage, third we did not follow up the patients to see the effect of tight control of diabetes on regression of UNGAL to confirm the role of uncontrolled diabetes on pathogenesis of tubular injury.

7. Conclusion

Tubular damage and tubular markers are highly associated with diabetic kidney disease patients. Tubular damage may precede glomerular injury. Tubular markers like UNGAL may be an early marker for detection of kidney involvement in diabetes, and it can be early elevated even before early signs of glomerular injury detected by microalbuminuria. More studies are needed to confirm our results and to detect the underlying mechanisms of tubular injury in diabetic patients.

References

[1]   KDOQI (2012) KDOQI Clinical Practice Guideline for Diabetes and CKD: 2012 Update. *American Journal of Kidney Diseases*, **60**, 850-886. http://dx.doi.org/10.1053/j.ajkd.2012.07.005

[2]   Sarnak, M.J., Levey, A.S., Schoolwerth, A.C., Coresh, J., Culleton, B., Hamm, L.L., McCullough, P.A., Kasiske, B.L.,

Kelepouris, E., Klag, M.J., Parfrey, P., Pfeffer, M., Raij, L., Spinosa, D.J. and Wilson, P.W. (2003) Kidney Disease as a Risk Factor for Development of Cardiovascular Disease: A Statement from the American Heart Association Councils on Kidney in Cardiovascular Disease, High Blood Pressure Research, Clinical Cardiology, and Epidemiology and PREVENTION. *Hypertension*, **42**, 1050-1065. http://dx.doi.org/10.1161/01.HYP.0000102971.85504.7c

[3]   American Diabetes Association (2004) Position Statement: Nephropathy in Diabetes. *Diabetes Care Supplement*, **27**, 79-83.

[4]   Narita, T., Hosoba, M., Kakei, M. and Ito, S. (2006) Increased Urinary Excretions of Immunoglobulin G, Ceruloplasmin, and Transferrin Predict Development of Microalbuminuria in Patients with Type 2 Diabetes. *Diabetes Care*, **29**, 142-146. http://dx.doi.org/10.2337/diacare.29.01.06.dc05-1063

[5]   Barratt, J. and Topham, P. (2007) Urine Proteomics: The Present and Future of Measuring Urinary Protein Components in Disease. *CMAJ*, **177**, 361-369. http://dx.doi.org/10.1503/cmaj.061590

[6]   Bangstad, H.J., Seljeflot, I., Berg, T.J., and Hanssen, K.F. (2009) Renal Tubulointerstitial Expansion Is Associated with Endothelial Dysfunction and Inflammation in Type 1 Diabetes. *Scandinavian Journal of Clinical & Laboratory Investigation*, **69**, 138-144. http://dx.doi.org/10.1080/00365510802444080

[7]   Thomas, M.C., Burns, W.C. and Cooper, M.E. (2005) Tubular Changes in Early Diabetic Nephropathy. *Advances in Chronic Kidney Disease*, **12**, 177-186. http://dx.doi.org/10.1053/j.ackd.2005.01.008

[8]   Haase, M., Bellomo, R., Devarajan, P., Schlattmann, P. and Haase-Fielitz, A. (2009) Accuracy of Neutrophil Gelatinase-Associated Lipocalin (NGAL) in Diagnosis and Prognosis in Acute Kidney Injury: A Systematic Review and Meta-Analysis. *American Journal of Kidney Diseases*, **54**, 1012-1024. http://dx.doi.org/10.1053/j.ajkd.2009.07.020

[9]   Peres, L.A., Cunha Júnior, A.D., Schäfer, A.J., Silva, A.L., Gaspar, A.D., Scarpari, D.F., Alves, J.B., Girelli Neto, R. and Oliveira, T.F. (2013) Biomarkers of Acute Kidney Injury. *Jornal Brasileiro de Nefrologia*, **35**, 229-236. http://dx.doi.org/10.5935/0101-2800.20130036

[10]   Bolignano, D., Lacquaniti, A., Coppolino, G., Donato, V., Fazio, M.R. and Nicocia, G. (2009) Neutrophil Gelatinase-Associated Lipocalin as an Early Biomarker of Nephropathy in Diabetic Patients. *Kidney and Blood Pressure Research*, **32**, 91-99. http://dx.doi.org/10.1159/000209379

[11]   Nauta, F.L., Boertien, W.E., Bakker, S.J., van Goor, H., van Oeveren, W. and de Jong, P.E. (2011) Glomerular and Tubular Damage Markers Are Elevated in Patients with Diabetes. *Diabetes Care*, **34**, 975-981. http://dx.doi.org/10.2337/dc10-1545

[12]   Tesch, G.H. and Lim, A.K. (2011) Recent Insights into Diabetic Renal Injury from the db/db Mouse Model of Type 2 Diabetic Nephropathy. *American Journal of Physiology. Renal Physiology*, **300**, 301-310. http://dx.doi.org/10.1152/ajprenal.00607.2010

[13]   Stanton, R.C. (2011) Oxidative Stress and Diabetic Kidney Disease. *Current Diabetes Reports*, **11**, 330-336. http://dx.doi.org/10.1007/s11892-011-0196-9

[14]   Lim, A.K. and Tesch, G.H. (2012) Inflammation in Diabetic Nephropathy. *Mediators of Inflammation*, **2012**, Article ID: 146154. http://dx.doi.org/10.1155/2012/146154

[15]   Paragas, N., Qiu, A., Zhang, Q., Samstein, B., Deng, S.X., Schmidt-Ott, K.M., Viltard, M., Yu, W., Forster, C.S., Gong, G., Liu, Y., Kulkarni, R., Mori, K., Kalandadze, A., Ratner, A.J., Devarajan, P., Landry, D.W., D'Agati, V., Lin, C.S. and J. Barasch, (2011) The NGAL Reporter Mouse Detects the Response of the Kidney to Injury in Real Time. *Nature Medicine*, **17**, 216-222. http://dx.doi.org/10.1038/nm.2290

[16]   Ding, H., He, Y., Li, K., Yang, J., Li, X. and Lu, R. (2007) Urinary Neutrophil Gelatinase-Associated Lipocalin (NGAL) Is an Early Biomarker for Renal Tubulointerstitial Injury in IgA Nephropathy. *Clinical Immunology*, **123**, 227-234. http://dx.doi.org/10.1016/j.clim.2007.01.010

[17]   Nielsen, S.E., Hansen, H.P., Jensen, B.R., Parving, H.H. and Rossing, P. (2011) Urinary Neutrophil Gelatinase-Associated Lipocalin and Progression of Diabetic Nephropathy in Type 1 Diabetic Patients in a Four-Year Follow-up Study. *Nephron Clinical Practice*, **118**, 130-135. http://dx.doi.org/10.1159/000320615

[18]   Levey, A.S., Coresh, J., Greene, T., Stevens, L.A., Zhang, Y.L. and Hendriksen, S. (2006) Using Standardized Serum Creatinine Values in the Modification of Diet in Renal Disease Study Equation for Estimating Glomerular Filtration Rate. *Annals of Internal Medicine*, **145**, 247-254. http://dx.doi.org/10.7326/0003-4819-145-4-200608150-00004

[19]   Burtis, E., Santos-Rosa, M., Bienvenu, J. and Whicher, J. (2006) Role of the Clinical Laboratory in Diabetes Mellitus. In: C. Bruit and E. Ashwood, Eds., *Tietz Textbook of Clinical Chemistry Chapter* 25, 4th Edition, Mosby, St. Louis, 837-903.

[20]   Larsen, K. (1972) Creatinine Assay by a reaCtion-Kinetic Principle. *Clinica Chimica Acta*, **41**, 209-217. http://dx.doi.org/10.1016/0009-8981(72)90513-X

[21]   Talke, H. and Schubert, G.E. (1965) Enzymatic Determination of Urea Using the Coupled Urease-GLDH Enzyme System. *Mediators of Inflammation*, **43**, 174-176. http://dx.doi.org/10.1007/BF01484513

[22] Gonen, B. and Rubenstein, A.H. (1978) Determination of Glycohemoglobin. *Diabetologia*, **15**, 1-5.
http://dx.doi.org/10.1007/BF01219319

[23] Rowe, D.J.F., Dawnay, A. and Watts, G.F. (1990) Microalbuminuria in Diabetes Mellitus: Review and Recommendations for the Measurement of Albumin in Urine. *Annals of Clinical Biochemistry*, **27**, 297-312.
http://dx.doi.org/10.1177/000456329002700404

[24] Rodby, R.A., Rohde, R.D., Sharon, Z., Pohl, M.A., Bain, R.P. and Lewis, E.J. (1995) The Urine Protein to Creatinine
Ratio as a Predictor of 24-Hour Urine Protein Excretion in Type 1 Diabetic Patients with Nephropathy. The Collaborative Study Group. *American Journal of Kidney Diseases*, **26**, 904-909.
http://dx.doi.org/10.1016/0272-6386(95)90054-3

[25] Brunner, H.I., Mueller, M., Rutherford, C., Passo, M.H., Witte, D. and Grom, A. (2006) Urinary Neutrophil Gelatinase-Associated Lipocalin as a Biomarker of Nephritis in Childhood-Onset Systemic Lupus Erythematosus. *Arthritis &
Rheumatology*, **54**, 2577-2584. http://dx.doi.org/10.1002/art.22008

[26] Gray, S.P. and Cooper, M.E. (2011) Diabetic Nephropathy in 2010: Alleviating the Burden of Diabetic Nephropathy.
Nature Reviews Nephrology, **7**, 71-73. http://dx.doi.org/10.1038/nrneph.2010.176

[27] Mishra, J., Dent, C., Tarabishi, R., Mitsnefes, M.M., Ma, Q., Kelly, C., Ruff, C., S.M., Zahedi, K., Shao, M., Bean, J.,
Mori, K., Barasch, J. and Devarajan, P. (2005) Neutrophil Gelatinase-Associated Lipocalin (NGAL) as a Biomarker for
Acute Renal Injury after Cardiac Surgery. *Lancet*, **8**, 1231-1238. http://dx.doi.org/10.1016/S0140-6736(05)74811-X

[28] Bolignano, D., Coppolino, G., Campo, S., Aloisi, C., Nicocia, G., Frisina, N. and Buemi, M. (2008) Urinary Neutrophil
Gelatinase-Associated Lipocalin (NGAL) Is Associated with Severity of Renal Disease in Proteinuric Patients. *Nephrology Dialysis Transplantation*, **23**, 414-416. http://dx.doi.org/10.1093/ndt/gfm541

[29] Bolignano, D., Lacquaniti, A., Coppolino, G., Donato, V., Campo, S., Fazio, M.R., Nicocia, G. and Buemi, M. (2009)
Neutrophil Gelatinase-Associated Lipocalin (NGAL) and Progression of Chronic Kidney Disease. *Clinical Journal of
the American Society of Nephrology*, **4**, 337-344. http://dx.doi.org/10.2215/CJN.03530708

[30] Alter, M.L., Kretschmer, A., Von Websky, K., Tsuprykov, O., Reichetzeder, C., Simon, A., Stasch, J.P. and Hocher, B.
(2012) Early Urinary and Plasma Biomarkers for Experimental Diabetic Nephropathy. *Clinical Laboratory*, **58**, 659-
671.

[31] Lacquaniti, A., Donato, V., Pintaudi, B., Di Vieste, G., Chirico, V., Buemi, A., Di Benedetto, A., Arena, A. and Buemi,
M. (2013) "Normoalbuminuric" Diabetic Nephropathy: Tubular Damage and NGA. *Acta Diabetologica*, **50**, 935-942.
http://dx.doi.org/10.1007/s00592-013-0485-7

[32] Zachwieja, J., Soltysiak, J., Fichna, P., Lipkowska, K., Stankiewicz, W., Skowronska, B., Kroll, P. and Lewandows-
ka-Stachowiak, M. (2010) Normal-Range Albuminuria Does Not Exclude Nephropathy in Diabetic Children. *Pediatric
Nephrology*, **25**, 1445-1451. http://dx.doi.org/10.1007/s00467-010-1443-z

[33] Kim, S.S., Song, S.H., Kim, J.J., Yang, J.Y., Lee, J.G., Kwak, I.S. and Kim, Y.K. (2012) Clinical Implication of Urinary Tubular Markers in the Early Stage of Nephropathy with Type 2 Diabetic Patients. *Diabetes Research and Clinical Practice*, **97**, 251-257. http://dx.doi.org/10.1016/j.diabres.2012.02.019

[34] Nielsen, S.E., Schjoedt, K.J., Astrup, A.S., Tarnow, L., Lajer, M., Hansen, P.R., Parving, H.H. and Rossing, P. (2010)
Neutrophil Gelatinase-Associated Lipocalin (NGAL) and Kidney Injury Molecule 1 (KIM1) in Patients with Diabetic
Nephropathy: A Cross-Sectional Study and the Effects of Lisinopril. *Diabetic Medicine*, **27**, 1144-1150.
http://dx.doi.org/10.1111/j.1464-5491.2010.03083.x

[35] Wu, J., Ding, Y., Zhu, C., Shao, X., Xie, X., Lu, K. and Wang, R. (2013) Urinary TNF-α and NGAL Are Correlated
with the Progression of Nephropathy in Patients with Type 2 Diabetes. *Experimental and Therapeutic Medicine*, **6**,
1482-1488.

[36] Fu, W.J., Xiong, S.L., Fang, Y.G., Wen, S., Chen, M.L., Deng, R.T., Zheng, L., Wang, S.B., Pen, L.F. and Wang, Q.
(2012) Urinary Tubular Biomarkers in Short-Term Type 2 Diabetes Mellitus Patients: A Cross-Sectional Study. *Endocrine*, **41**, 82-88.

[37] Woo, K.S., Choi, J.L., Kim, B.R., Kim, J.E., An, W.S. and Han, J.Y. (2012) Urinary Neutrophil Gelatinase-Associated
Lipocalin Levels in Comparison with Glomerular Filtration Rate for Evaluation of Renal Function in Patients with Diabetic Chronic Kidney Disease. *Diabetes & Metabolism Journal*, **36**, 307-313.
http://dx.doi.org/10.4093/dmj.2012.36.4.307

[38] Liebetrau, C., Dörr, O., Baumgarten, H., Gaede, L., Szardien, S., Blumenstein, J., Rolf, A., Möllmann, H., Hamm, C.,
Walther, T., Nef, H. and Weber, M. (2013) Neutrophil Gelatinase-Associated Lipocalin (NGAL) for the Early Detection of Cardiac Surgery Associated Acute Kidney Injury. *Scandinavian Journal of Clinical & Laboratory Investigation*,
73, 392-399. http://dx.doi.org/10.3109/00365513.2013.787149

[39] Makris, K., Markou, N., Evodia, E., Dimopoulou, E., Drakopoulos, I., Ntetsika, K., Rizos, D., Baltopoulos, G. and Ha-
liassos, A. (2009) Urinary Neutrophil Gelatinase-Associated Lipocalin (NGAL) as an Early Marker of Acute Kidney

Injury in Critically Ill Multiple Trauma Patients. *Clinical Chemistry and Laboratory Medicine*, **47**, 79-82. http://dx.doi.org/10.1515/CCLM.2009.004

[40] Wagener, G., Gubitosa, G., Wang, S., Borregaard, N., Kim, M. and Lee, H.T. (2008) Urinary Neutrophil Gelatinase-Associated Lipocalin and Acute Kidney Injury after Cardiac Surgery. *American Journal of Kidney Diseases*, **52**, 425-433. http://dx.doi.org/10.1053/j.ajkd.2008.05.018

21

Page Kidney: A Case of Acute or Chronic Renal Failure & Refractory HTN Presenting after Renal Biopsy

Stephen Meyer, Aswin Nukala, Nikita Maniar*, Waldo Herrera

Department of Internal Medicine, Mt. Sinai Hospital, Chicago, USA
Email: *nikita.maniar@sinai.org

Abstract

Page Kidney is a relatively rare cause of Acute Renal Failure (ARF) presenting as accelerated and uncontrolled hypertension secondary direct compression of the renal parenchyma by an extrinsic source. This case report describes a 44-year-old male with advanced acute renal failure requiring hemodialysis, hypertension, and initial suspicion for thrombotic thrombocytopenic purpura who developed a case of Page Kidney following retroperitoneal hematoma following a renal biopsy. The patient was medically managed with intravenous nifedipine until blood pressure stabilized after improvement of the hematoma. Usually hematomas are self-resolving, however rarely they can result in the Page phenomenon—extrinsic compression of the affected kidney by the hematoma resulting in a picture that is similar to acute renal failure (ARF). This case highlights the importance of early medical management of blood pressure control after renal compression has been identified.

Keywords

Page Kidney, Acute Renal Failure, Refractory Hypertension

1. Introduction

Page kidney is a relatively rare cause of ARF and accelerated hypertension secondary to compression of the renal parenchyma often by intra-capsular hematoma leading to activation of the RAAS. Page kidney was first discovered in a canine experiment in which Irvin Page wrapped kidneys in cellophane and noted the induction of hypertension by peri-nephritis and compression of the renal parenchyma [1]. The pathophysiology of Page Kidney

---

*Corresponding author.

involves external compression of the renal parenchyma by a mass often resulting from trauma. This leads to persistent activation of the renin-aldosterone system resulting in accelerated hypertension that tends to be refractory [2]. This injury has been reported in the literature as presenting after trauma from Motor Vehicle Accidents, sports injuries, or after renal biopsies. As is seen in cases of renal artery stenosis, when perfusion to the kidney is diminished, the renin-angiotensin pathway is activated resulting in an elevation in blood pressure to increase renal perfusion [3]. In Page Kidney, this pathway is persistently activated resulting in acute onset accelerated hypertension.

2. Case Report

A 44-year-old African American male with past medical history of migraine headaches, ARF requiring hemodialysis, hypertension, and recent suspicion thrombotic thrombocytopenic purpura (TTP) not responding to weekly plasmapheresis presented to our institution as a transfer from an LTAC facility due to down-trending platelet counts and further workup of recently suspected TTP. Five months prior to admission, the patient had presented to an outside hospital with complaints of headache. At that time he was found to have ARF and uncontrolled hypertension which required ICU admission and hemodialysis. The patient had a prolonged hospitalization during which there was a suspicion of TTP causing his acute medical conditions and was started on plasmapheresis and corticosteroid therapy, stabilized and transferred to an LTAC. He was further started on hemodialysis three times per week for his ARF, and plasmapheresis twice weekly for suspicion of TTP while at the LTAC. He presented to our institution because his CBC showed down-trending platelets without any active bleeding and because his TTP workup was incomplete. Upon admission to our institution, the patient was hemodynamically stable, blood pressure was 140's systolic. Labs were significant for a BUN of 68 and Creatinine of 8.8. Other electrolytes were within normal limits. t was agreed that further workup would be needed to determine the cause of his ARF.

Nephrology and hematology were consulted on the case and a renal biopsy was agreed upon as the next step in management after labs including LDH, ANCA, Anti-GBM, Complements C3/C4, ANA, ADAMTS-13, hepatitis panel and HIV were negative. On admission day 2, the patient underwent ultrasound guided biopsy of the left kidney, and on admission day 3, he began having severe left lower quadrant abdominal and suprapubic pain, with an appreciable drop in hemoglobin from 8.9 to 5.4 within a 24-hour period. His blood pressure acutely elevated with from167/91 to 213/116, HR 104.CT abdomen/pelvis revealed a large complex left retroperitoneal hematoma extending along the left para-colic gutter and into the pelvis (**Figure 1**). An ultrasound of the kidneys again revealed the mass without any focal changes in the kidneys themselves.

Surgical consultants recommended conservative management and the patient was controlled with PRN transfusions to maintain adequate hemoglobin and the patient was subsequently admitted to the MICU service on day 4 and started on nicardipine drip for management of accelerated hypertension refractory to oral antihypertensive medical management until further interval resolution of the hematoma occurred and hypertensive management was able to be de-escalated.

Renal biopsy revealed severe interstitial fibrosis and tubular atrophy involving the entire cortex, severe arterial sclerosis and arteriolar hyalinosis consistent with hypertension and NSAID use which the patient admitted he had been taking for his migraine headaches. The patient's medication was adjusted and his blood pressure was refractory requiring high doses of clonidine, nifedipine, coreg, hydralazine, minoxidil, and furosemide. The patient came to our institution with a known history of hypertension, however his acute refractory surge in blood pressure after development of a renal hematoma, enabled a diagnosis of Page Kidney as a complication of the renal biopsy and then was confirmed by CT imaging. The expected outcome for this patient was favorable and outpatient follow-up was established which has further allowed for further de-escalation of antihypertensive medication and now he is controlled on only two oral antihypertensives.

3. Discussion

Renal hematoma can be managed either surgically or medically. Acute onset of flank/abdominal pain, tenderness, as well as an acute drop in hemoglobin and hematocrit after a potential injury should all raise concern for retroperitoneal bleed [4]. Many cases of Page Kidney can be successfully managed by controlling the associated hypertensive disorder [5]. A CT scan without contrast should be ordered immediately followed by prompt surgical evaluation. In the Page phenomenon the rapid acute rise in blood pressure can be very dangerous—resulting

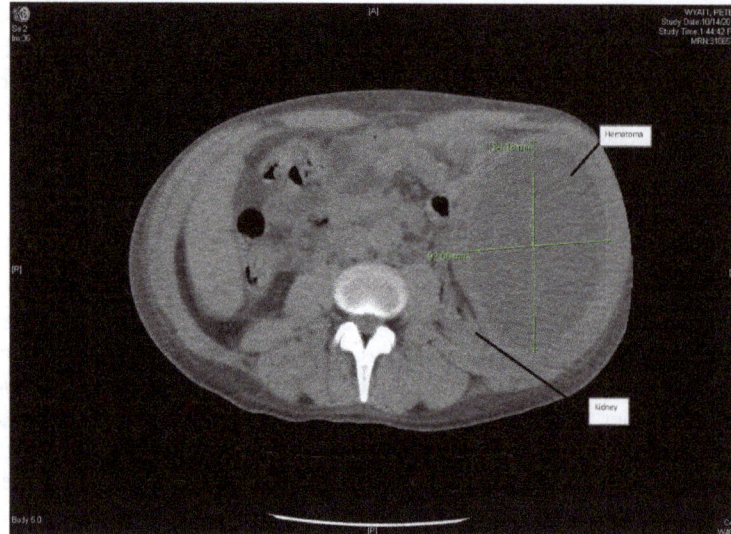

Figure 1. Retroperitoneal hematoma post left renal biopsy.

in stroke, MI, or worsening of the bleed itself [6]. In this case, we advocate the importance of rapid blood pressure control with intravenous anti-hypertensive medication to prevent the size of the hematoma from progressing, thereby worsening the Page phenomenon [7]. Oral medications can be unpredictable in this scenario and often times may not be tolerated by the patient due to the severe abdominal pain [8]. The calcium channel blocker nicardipine, was successful in this case and may be considered a good choice as it can be administered intravenously in an ICU setting with close monitoring, and can be titrated quickly to maintain a systolic blood pressure less than 140. After 24 - 48 hours of strict control, the patient should be reassessed clinically to determine resolution of symptoms. A repeat CT scan should then be ordered to reassess the size of the bleed. If stable, the patient can then be safely transitioned to oral medications. As the hematoma resolves, the hypertension and ARF will also resolve [9].

4. Conclusion

In conclusion, we have reported a case of Page Kidney that has been successfully treated with medical management. There have been studies showing the use of anti-hypertensive medications to manage subcapsular hematomas, in our case of an extracapsular bleed the same medical management was used to resolve the hematoma [10]. The patient's clinical course was favorable with complete resolution of symptoms and stabilization on oral medications. The patient currently comes to the clinic for follow-up of his hypertension and kidney disease.

References

[1]   Smyth, A., Collins, C., Thorsteinsdottir, B., Madsen, B., Oliveira, G., Kane, G. and Garovic, V. (2012) Page Kidney: Etiology, Renal Function Outcomes and Risk for Future. *The Journal of Clinical Hypertension*, **14**, 216-221. http://dx.doi.org/10.1111/j.1751-7176.2012.00601.x

[2]   Kim, M., Parks, K. and Miller, E. (2013) Page Kidney: Hypertension Secondary to Extra-Renal Compression. *Journal of Diagnostic Medical Sonography*, **29**, 26-29. http://dx.doi.org/10.1177/8756479312457593

[3]   Dopson, S., Jayakumar, S. and Velez, J. (2009) Page Kidney as a Rare Cause of Hypertension: Case Report and Review of the Literature. *American Journal of Kidney Diseases*, **25**, 334-339. http://dx.doi.org/10.1053/j.ajkd.2008.11.014

[4]   Mathew, A., Brahmbhatt, B., Rajesh, R., Kurian, G. and Unni, V.N. (2009) Page Kidney. *Indian Journal of Nephrology*, **19**, 170-171. http://dx.doi.org/10.4103/0971-4065.59342

[5]   Brotfain, E., Koyfman, L., Frenkel, A., Smolikov, A., Zlotnik, A. and Klein, M. (2013) Traumatic Page Kidney Induced Hypertension in Critical Care: Immediately Resolved or Long-Term Resistant Problem. *Case Reports in Critical Care*, **2013**, Article ID: 201424. http://dx.doi.org/10.1155/2013/201424

[6]   Chung, J., Caumartin, Y., Warren, J. and Luke, P. (2008) Acute Page Kidney Following Renal Allograft Biopsy: A

Complication Requiring Early Recognition and Treatment. *American Journal of Transplantation*, **8**, 1323-1328. http://dx.doi.org/10.1111/j.1600-6143.2008.02215.x

[7]   Nakano, S., Kigoshi, T., Uchita, K., Morimoto, S., Tsugawa, R. and Matsunou, H. (2008) Hypertension and Unilateral Renal Ischemia (Page Kidney) Due to Compression of a Retroperitoneal Paraganglioma. *American Journal of Nephrology*, **16**, 91-94. http://dx.doi.org/10.1159/000168976

[8]   Myrianthefs, P., Aravosita, P., Tokta, R., Louizou, L., Boutzouka, E. and Baltopoulos, G. (2007) Resolution of Page Kidney-Related Hypertension with Medical Therapy: A Case Report. *Heart & Lung*: *The Journal of Acute and Critical Care*, **36**, 377-379. http://dx.doi.org/10.1016/j.hrtlng.2006.10.009

[9]   Kapil, S., Ashish, S., Viswaroop, S., Arul, M. and Gopalakrishnan, G. (2011) Page Kidney—Rare but Correctable Cause of Hypertension. *UroToday International Journal*, **4**, art54. http://dx.doi.org/10.3834/uij.1944-5784.2011.10.10

[10] Patel, T.V. and Goes, N. (2007) Page Kidney. *Kidney International*, **72**, 1562. http://dx.doi.org/10.1038/sj.ki.5002580

22

Higher Endogenous Erythropoietin Levels in Hemodialysis Patients with Hepatitis C Virus Infection and Effect on Anemia

Karima Boubaker[1], Madiha Mahfoudhi[1*], Amel Gaieb Battikh[1], Azza Bounemra[2], Chokri Maktouf[3], Adel Kheder[1]

[1]Department of Internal Medicine A, Charles Nicolle Hospital, Tunis, Tunisia
[2]Cellular Immunology, Blood Transfusion Center, Tunis, Tunisia
[3]Nuclear Medicine and Clinical Research Department, Pasteur institute, Tunis, Tunisia
Email: *madiha_mahfoudhi@yahoo.fr

Abstract

Study for influence of chronic Hepatitis C (HCV) on endogenous erythropoietin production and on anemia in dialysis patients remains inconclusive. We hypothesize that chronic hemodialysis patients with co-existing Hepatitis C infection will have higher hemoglobin levels than chronic hemodialysis patients without hepatitis C infection. Secondly, we hypothesize that the higher hemoglobin levels will be associated with higher erythropoietin levels. Therefore we conducted a cross-sectional study of chronic hemodialysis patients with and without hepatitis C infection and evaluated associations with hemoglobin and erythropoietin levels. Our primary outcome was level of hemoglobin. Secondary outcome included association of hemoglobin and erythropoietin levels. 57 chronic hemodialysis patients (33 male, 24 female, mean age 46.05 ± 12.7 years) were included. The mean time spent on hemodialysis was 7.16 ± 6.2 years. None of the patients received any recombinant EPO therapy. Biochemical analyses include ALT, AST, Albumin, C-Reactive Protein, cholesterol levels and complete blood counts. Iron status of patients (transferrin saturation and serum ferritin levels) and parathyroid hormone were measured. Endogenous EPO serum levels were measured by a standardized enzyme-linked immunoassay. 23 of the hemodialysed patients (38.5%) were HCV (+). There was no difference in age, sex, distribution of primary renal diseases, iron status, albumin, C-Reactive-Protein and parathyroid hormone levels between HCV (+) and (−) patients. Mean duration time on dialysis was higher in HCV (+) than HCV (−) patients. Hemoglobin levels were similar between study groups. However serum endogenous erythropoietin levels were significantly higher in HCV (+) patients than HCV (−) patients (19.6 ± 10 mUI/ml vs 7.8 ± 7.7 mUI/ml, p = 0.03). No correlation has been found between the severity of anemia and HCV infection. However, HCV (+) hemodialysed patients had higher serum endogenous erythropoietin levels

*Corresponding author.

as compared to HCV (−) patients. Further studies are needed to clarify why high endogenous erythropoietin level does not improve anemia in HCV infected hemodialysis patients.

Keywords

Anemia, Hepatitis C, Hemodialysis, Erythropoietin

1. Introduction

Hepatitis C virus (HCV) was cloned and identified as the major cause of parenterally transmitted non-A and non-B hepatitis in 1989 [1]. In hemodialysis patients, HCV infection is the most common cause of acute and chronic hepatitis and it increases risk for death. In this population, HCV infection is mainly handily transmitted since transmission by blood product transfusion is virtually eliminated with the screening of blood products for anti-HCV [2] [3]. The prevalence of anti-HCV using standardized enzyme-linked immunoassay among dialysis patients is variable in different countries. Study for influence of chronic HCV on anemia in dialysis patients remains inconclusive. Lessened anemia was observed in chronic HCV positive hemodialysis patients, which demanded less erythropoietin (EPO) dose than in HCV negative hemodialysis patients [4]-[8]. On the other hand, increased endogenous EPO production was reported in hemodialysis patients with hepatitis virus infections [6] [9] [10].

In this study, we hypothesize that chronic hemodialysis patients with co-existing Hepatitis C infection will have higher hemoglobin levels than chronic hemodialysis patients without hepatitis C infection. Secondly, we hypothesize that the higher hemoglobin levels will be associated with higher erythropoietin levels. Therefore we conducted a cross-sectional study in our department of chronic hemodialysis patients with and without hepatitis C infection and evaluated associations with hemoglobin and erythropoietin levels. Our primary outcome was level of hemoglobin. Secondary outcomes included association of hemoglobin and erythropoietin levels.

2. Material and Methods

One hundred thirty two chronic hemodialysis patients were followed-up in our hemodialysis unit in 2006. Demographic data were collected including age and sex. Duration of hemodialysis, Anti-HCV antibody, Hepatitis B surface antigen and antibody were investigated in all patients. Laboratory parameters are done retrospectively before patients identified and investigated complete blood count, iron status (transferrin saturation (TSAT) and serum ferritin levels) and parathyroid hormone (PTH) levels. As a marker of inflammation, serum C-reactive protein (CRP) was measured. Functional iron deficiency (defined on the basis of TSAT <20% and serum ferritin <100 ng/ml) was treated by intravenous iron saccharate treatment. None of the patients received any recombinant EPO therapy because this treatment is not present in our country for economical reasons.

Inclusion criteria were a stable clinical state, hemodialysis duration 12 hours since at least 12 weeks, TSAT between 20% and 50% and serum ferritin between 100 and 800 ng/ml.

Exclusion criteria were blood transfusion, major surgery and massive blood loss with worsening anemia in the preceding 3 months, treatment with angiotensin II receptor blocker or any drug containing aluminum.

Fifty seven chronic hemodialysis patients (33 male, 24 female, mean age 46.05 ± 12.7 years) were enrolled in the cross-sectional study. Primary renal diseases were primary glomerular disease in 20 cases, diabetic nephropathy in 3 cases, secondary amyloidosis in 1 case, lupus nephritis in 2 cases, hypertensive nephropathy in 6 cases, interstitial nephritis in 10 cas, polycystic kidney disease in 3 cases and unknown nephropathy in 12 cases. The mean time spent on hemodialysis was 7.16 ± 6.2 years (1 - 33 ans).

Dialyses were performed for 4 hours, three times a week with carbonate-containing dialysate bath using a double-needle technique with native arteriovenous fistulas. Blood flow rate was 250 - 300 ml/min with a dialysate flow of 500 ml/min. All patients were dialyzed with polysulfone membranes which were discarded after dialysis session. All patients were taking folic acid, vitamins and calcium carbonate, and some of them were treated with antihypertensive drugs.

Regarding coexisting infectious, autoimmune or neoplastic diseases, 2 patients had systemic lupus erythematosus, 1 patient had Tuberous sclerosis and 1 patient had Epidermolysis Bullosa Simplex. One patient with secondary amyloidosis had a history of pleural tuberculosis. These diseases were clinically inactive and not requiring therapy while on dialysis. None of the patients with HCV infection undergo treatment for hepatitis C.

Complete blood counts and blood chemistries were performed on an auto analyzer using routine laboratory methods. TSAT was calculated by expressing serum iron as a percentage of plasma total iron-binding capacity.

$$TSAT(\%) = (iron/total\ iron\ binding\ capacity) \times 100.$$

Endogenous EPO serum levels were measured by a standardized enzyme-linked immunoassay.

Biochemical analyses including ALT, AST, Albumin and cholesterol levels were measured.

Only one study visit was made.

Statistical analysis was performed using Statview logician. Data were presented as mean ± standard deviation. Two groups were compared for numerical variables by using unpaired Student's test. For non-numerical data, Chi2-tests were used for the comparison of the two groups. The criterion of statistical significance was p<0,05.

3. Results

Demographic features and the results of biochemical analysis, hemogram and parameters related to iron status are shown in **Table 1** and **Table 2**. There was no difference in age, sex, distribution of primary renal diseases,

Table 1. Epidemiologic and clinical data of patients.

	Anti-HCV (+) (n = 23)	Anti-HCV (−) (n = 34)	Statistics (p)
Gender (Males/Females)	14/9	19/15	0.916
Age (years)	46.4 ± 11.8	45.8 ± 13.4	0.8676
Time on hemodialysis (years)	10.6 ± 7.7	4.5 ± 3	0.0022
Primary renal disease	17	28	0.1055
Primary glomerular disease	8	12	
Diabetic nephropathy	0	3	
Secondary amyloidosis	1	0	
Lupus nephritis	2	0	
Interstitial nephritis	4	6	
Polycystic kidney disease	2	1	
Hypertensive nephropathy	0	6	
Unknown	6	6	
Vasoactive drug	10	17	0.6291
Calcium channel antagonist	7	10	0.057
β-blocker	0	3	0.297

Values are given as mean ± standard deviation.

Table 2. Biological and viral data of patients.

Viral hepatitis B seropositive	1	4	0.615
Albumin (g/l)	39.7 ± 4.1	40.7 ± 3.9	3.926
C-Reactive-Protein (mg/l)	4.07 ± 2.7	5.25 ± 4.6	0.3349
AZT (IU/l)	22.2 ± 11.4	18.6 ± 19	0.528
ALT (IU/l)	23.6 ± 21.7	20.1 ± 29.7	0.7
Ferritin (g/dl)	261.5 ± 146.9	352.2 ± 214.1	1.894
TSAT (%)	32.7 ± 10.5	28.4 ± 10.7	0.3353
Cholesterol (mmol/l)	3.7 ± 0.97	3.7 ± 0.89	0.7562
PTH (pg/ml)	217.54 ± 150	186.8 ± 129.8	0.5827

Values are given as mean ± standard deviation.

albumin, PTH, AST, ALT serum, ferritin levels, TSAT and CRP levels between HCV (+) and HCV (−) hemodialysis patients. Mean duration time on dialysis was higher in HCV (+) than HCV (−) patients.

Hemoglobin levels were similar between study groups. However serum endogenous erythropoietin levels were significantly higher in HCV (+) patients than HCV (−) patients (19.6 ± 10 mUI/ml vs 7.8 ± 7.7 mUI/ml, p = 0.03) (**Table 3**).

4. Discussion

In this study, no correlation has been found between the severity of anemia and HCV infection. However, endogenous EPO levels were significantly higher in anti-HCV positive hemodialysis patients than in HCV-negative patients.

Patients in maintenance hemodialysis are at increased risk of acquiring HCV infection and consequently have a higher prevalence than general population [11], but large variations in HCV infection occur among dialysis units in different geographic areas. For example, the prevalence of HCV infection among dialysis patients in different European and Mediterranean countries varied between 2% and 63% [3]. In Tunisia, prevalence of HCV infection was 20.4% among dialysis patients in 2006 and 11.7% in 2008 according to immunology laboratory research of Tunisia. In our department, prevalence was 19 % in 2006.

In literature was reported that the time on hemodialysis dialysis was significantly longer among HCV-positive patients than HCV-negative patients [12]. The risk of acquiring HCV infection on hemodialysis has been estimated at 10% per year [13] [14]; so that the time on hemodialysis is an independent risk factor for acquiring HCV infection [15]. Our data were concordant with literature data.

In this study, we did not report any significantly difference in hemoglobin level between HCV-positive and -negative hemodialysis patients. None of the patients with HCV infection undergo treatment for hepatitis C as some of the drugs can cause anemia. Our result was consistent with some reports [6]. However, in other reports hemoglobin was significantly higher in HCV-positive or after hepatitis B virus infection in hemodialysis patients [10] [16]-[19].

Endogenous EPO is mainly produced by kidneys [20]. Ability of the EPO production is well preserved in end-stage-renal disease patients [21]. In fact, serum EPO level despite severe anemia or hypoxia, is similar in end-stage-renal disease patients and in normal subjects (respectively 37.4 ± 15.3 mU/ml and 24 - 42 mU/ml) [21] [22]. In dialysis patients, anemia is ascribed mainly to reduced sensitivity of bone marrow to EPO, probably as a result of retention of uremic toxins and inhibitors of erythropoiesis.

In our study, patients did not received exogenous EPO and than endogenous EPO levels measurement was possible.

We demonstrated that HCV-positive hemodialysis patients had higher endogenous EPO levels compared to HCV-negative patients. There are few data on serum endogenous EPO in hemodialysis patients with chronic viral infection with HCV or hepatitis B virus [5] [6]. Since 1980, some authors reported in hemodialysis or normal subjects, an increase in the hepatic synthesis of EPO by regenerating hepatocytes after viral and toxic cytolysis or hepatocellular carcinoma [10] [18] [23]. Hepatic production of EPO is maximal in experimental animals, during liver regeneration or anemia and is the main source for production of endogenous EPO in the fetal stage [5] [16] [18] [24] [25]. High endogenous EPO level in infected HCV patients may be explained by hepatic synthesis.

In our study, high endogenous EPO level does not improve anemia in HCV-positive patients perhaps because the level of EPO in these patients was very low to improve anemia. On the other hand, some authors reported suppression of EPO by humeral factors, possibly cytokines or growth factors [26] [27].

Table 3. Comparison of the anti-HCV-negative and -positive patients levels of hemoglobin and endogenous erythropoietin.

	Anti-HCV (−) (n = 23)	Anti-HCV (+) (n = 34)	Statistics
Hemoglobin (g/dl)	9.7 ± 3.01	9.3 ± 2.56	0.583
Mean corpuscular volume	86.9	86.9	0.972
Erythropoïetin level (mU.I./ml)	19.6 ± 10	7.8 ± 7.7	0.0347

Values are given as mean ± standard deviation.

Among the limitations of this study, we cite the reduced number of the sample. The initial values of the endogenous EPO before HCV infestation was also missing in our study. This has prevented us from performing a comparison before and after the occurrence of hepatitis C. The findings of this study can't be formally considered. Only a prospective study on more extended sample could draw objective and interesting conclusions.

5. Conclusion

In our hemodialysis patients no correlation has been found between the severity of anemia and HCV infection. However, higher endogenous EPO levels were observed in these patients explained probably by hepatic synthesis. Further studies are needed to clarify other causes of higher endogenous EPO levels and to define etiologies of EPO resistance in HCV-pstositive hemodialysis patients.

Conflicts of Interest

The authors declare no conflict of interest.

References

[1]   Kuo, G., Choo, K.L., Alter, H.J., Gitnick, G.L., Redeker, A.G., Purcell, R.H., et al. (1989) An Assay for Circulating Antibodies to a Major Etiologic Virus of Human Non-A, Non-B Hepatitis. Science, 244, 362-364. http://dx.doi.org/10.1126/science.2496467

[2]   Pereira, B.J. (1999) Hepatitis C Virus Infection in Dialysis: A Continuing Problem. Artificial Organs, 23, 51-60. http://dx.doi.org/10.1046/j.1525-1594.1999.06274.x

[3]   Akpolat, T., Turkish Multicentre CAPD Study Group (TULIP) (2001) CAPD: A Control Strategy to Prevent Spread of HCV Infection and End Stage Renal Disease (Short Reports). Peritoneal Dialysis International, 21, 77-79.

[4]   Di Bisceglie, A.M., Axiotis, C.A., Hoofnagle, J.H. and Bacon, B.R. (1992) Measurement of Iron Status in Patients with Chronic Hepatitis. Gastroenterology, 102, 2108-2113.

[5]   Radovic, M., Jelkmann, W., Djukanovic, L. and Ostric, V. (1999) Serum Erythropoietin and Interleukin-6 Levels in Hemodialysis Patients with Hepatitis Virus Infection. Journal of Interferon & Cytokine Research, 19, 69-73. http://dx.doi.org/10.1089/107999099314072

[6]   Altintepe, L., Kurtoglu, E., Tonbul, Z., Yeksan, M., Yildiz, A. and Türk, S. (2004) Lower Erythropoietin and Iron Supplementation Are Required in Haemodialysis Patients with Hepatitis C Virus Infection. Clinical Nephrology, 61, 347-351. http://dx.doi.org/10.5414/CNP61347

[7]   Lin, Y.L., Lin, C.W., Lee, C.H., Lai, I.C., Chen, H.H. and Chen, T.W. (2008) Chronic Hepatitis Ameliorates Anemia in Haemodialysis Patients. Nephrology, 13, 289-293. http://dx.doi.org/10.1111/j.1440-1797.2008.00937.x

[8]   Khurana, A., Nickel, A.E., Narayanan, M. and Foulks, C.J. (2008) Effect of Hepatitis C Infection on Hemodialysis Patients. Hemodialysis International, 12, 94-99. http://dx.doi.org/10.1111/j.1542-4758.2008.00248.x

[9]   Brown, S., Caro, J., Erslev, A.J. and Murray, T.G. (1980) Spontaneous Increase in Erytropoietin and Hematocrit Value Associated with Transient Liver Enzyme Abnormalities in an Anephric Patient Undergoing Hemodialysis. The American Journal of Medicine, 68, 280-284. http://dx.doi.org/10.1016/0002-9343(80)90367-8

[10] Brown, S., Caro, J., Erslev, A.J. and Murray, T.G. (1999) Impact of Hepatitis B and C Virus on Kidney Transplantation Outcome. Hepatology, 29, 257-263. http://dx.doi.org/10.1002/hep.510290123

[11] Natov, S.N. and Pereira, B.J.G. (1994) Hepatitis C Infection in Patients on Dialysis. Seminars in Dialysis, 7, 360-368. http://dx.doi.org/10.1111/j.1525-139X.1994.tb00855.x

[12] Weiner, A.J., Kuo, G., Bradley, D.W., Bonino, F., Saracco, G., Lee, C., et al. (1990) Detection of Hepatitis C Viral Sequences in Non A, Non-B Hepatitis. The Lancet, 335, 1-3. http://dx.doi.org/10.1016/0140-6736(90)90134-Q

[13] Hardy, N.M., Sandroni, S., Danielson, S. and Wilson, W.J. (1992) Antibody to Hepatitis C Virus Increases with the Time on Dialysis. Clinical Nephrology, 38, 44-48.

[14] Medici, G., Depetri, G.C. and Mileti, M. (1992) Anti-Hepatitis C Virus Positivity and Clinical Correlations in Hemodialyzed Patients. Nephron, 61, 363-364. http://dx.doi.org/10.1159/000186945

[15] Pereira, B.J. and Levey, A.S. (1999) Hepatitis C Virus Infection in Dialysis and Renal Transplantation. Kidney International, 51, 981-999. http://dx.doi.org/10.1038/ki.1997.139

[16] Chan, N., Barton, C.H., Mirahmadi, M.S., Gordon, S. and Vaziri, N.D. (1984) Erythropoiesis Associated with Viral Hepatitis in End-Stage Renal Disease. The American Journal of the Medical Sciences, 287, 56-57. http://dx.doi.org/10.1097/00000441-198401000-00017

[17] Pololi-Anagnostou, A., Westenfelder, C. and Anagnostou, A. (1981) Marked Improvement of Erythropoiesis in an Anephric Patient. *Nephron*, **29**, 277-279. http://dx.doi.org/10.1159/000182389

[18] Simon, P., Meyrier, A., Tanquerel, T. and Ang, K.S. (1980) Improvement of Anaemia in Haemodialyzed Patients after Viral or Toxic Hepatic Cytolysis. *British Medical Journal*, **280**, 892-894. http://dx.doi.org/10.1136/bmj.280.6218.892

[19] Sahin, I., Arabaci, F. and Sahin, H.A. (2003) Does Hepatitis C Virus Infection Increase Hematocrit and Haemoglobin Levels in Hemodialyzed Patients? *Clinical Nephrology*, **60**, 401-404. http://dx.doi.org/10.5414/CNP60401

[20] Jelkmann, W. (1992) Erythropoietin: Structure, Control of Production and Function. *Physiological Reviews*, **72**, 449-489.

[21] Zadrazil, J., Bachleda, P. and Zahálková, J. (1997) Endogenous Erythropoietin in Patients on Regular Dialysis Therapy. *Vnitřní Lékařství*, **43**, 649-654.

[22] Kato, A., Hishida, A., Kumagai, H., Furuya, R., Nakajima, T. and Honda, N. (1994) Erythropoietin Production in Patients with Chronic Renal Failure. *Renal Failure*, **16**, 645-651. http://dx.doi.org/10.3109/08860229409044892

[23] Kew, M.C. and Fisher, J.W. (1986) Serum Erythropoietin Concentrations in Patients with Hepatocellular Carcinoma. *Cancer*, **58**, 2485-2488.
http://dx.doi.org/10.1002/1097-0142(19861201)58:11<2485::AID-CNCR2820581122>3.0.CO;2-N

[24] Brox, A.G., Zhang, F., Guyda, H. and Gagnon, R.F. (1996) Subtherapeutic Erythropoietin and Insulin-Like Growth Factor-1 Correct the Anemia of Chronic Renal Failure in the Mouse. *Kidney International*, **50**, 937-943.
http://dx.doi.org/10.1038/ki.1996.394

[25] Bondurant, M.C. and Koury, M.J. (1985) Anemia Induces Accumulation of Erythropoietin mRNA in the Kidney and Liver. *Molecular and Cellular Biology*, **6**, 2731-2733.

[26] Birgegård G. (1989) Erythropoiesis and Inflammation. *Contrib Nephrol*, **76**, 330-339; discussion 339-341.

[27] Mecans, R.T. and Krantz, S.B. (1992) Progress in Understanding the Pathogenesis of the Anemia of Chronic Disease. *Blood*, **80**, 1639-1647.

List of Abbreviations

HCV: Hepatitis C virus
EPO: Erythropoietin
TSAT: Transferrin saturation
PTH: Parathyroid hormone
CRP: C-reactive protein
ALT: Alanine aminotransferase
AST: Aspartate aminotransferase

23

Quality of Life of Chronic Haemodialytic Patients at Cotonou Teaching Hospital (BENIN)

Elhadji Fary Ka[1], Jacques Vigan[2*], Ahmed Tall Lemrabott[1], Noriace Excelle Zohoun[2], Mohamedou Moustapha Cissé[1], Séraphin Ahoui[2], Maria Faye[1], Younoussa Keita[1], Khodia Fall[1], Bruno Léopold Agboton[2], Abdou Niang[1], Boucar Diouf[1]

[1]Nephrology Department, Aristide Le Dantec Hospital, Dakar, Senegal
[2]Nephrology and Hemodialysis Clinic, Hubert Koutoukou Maga Teaching Hospital, Cotonou, Benin
Email: *viques2@yahoo.fr

Abstract

Introduction: The objectives of this work were to assess haemodialytic patients' quality of life (QoL) and to identify factors affecting this QoL. **Patients and Methods:** It was a three (03) month monocentric and transversal study (from October 24, 2011 to January 27, 2012) conducted in the haemodialysis unit at Hubert Koutoukou Maga Teaching Hospital (CNHU-HKM) in Cotonou. Patients included were residents of Benin, aged 18 years and above, chronic haemodialysis in this unit for over 3 months, and willfully gave their consent. Quality of life was evaluated using questionnaire on Kidney Disease Quality of Life Short-Form French version 1.2 (KDQoL-SF 36). Epidemiological data, nephropathy etiologies and purification parametres were recorded in patients files. Data statistical analysis was performed using SPSS software 11.5. **Results:** In total 131 patients were involved in the study. The average age was 50.27 ± 12.17 years with a sex ratio of 1.69. Nephroangiosclerosis was the 1st cause. Most patients 128 (97.71 %) received two haemodialysis sessions on weekly basis. The Average Overall Score (AOS) based respectively on SF 36 and KDQoL was 48.55 and 58.55. The average of both SF 36 and KDQoL AOS was 53.55. Factors affecting hemodialytic patients quality of life were vitality, limitations related to mental health and physical condition, burden of kidney disease, effect of the disease on daily life and occupational status. The study revealed that: Patients education level was correlated with vitality ($p < 0.017$); The number of haemodialyses sessions was correlated with the consequences of kidney disease on daily life ($p < 0.025$). **Conclusion:** It is necessary to strengthen the staff by providing a psychologist and a dietician and also build new haemodialysis centres.

Keywords

Quality of Life, Haemodialysis Patients, Chronic Kidney Disease, Benin

---

*Corresponding author.

1. Introduction

Chronic kidney disease is the consequence of gradual and definite loss of kidneys functions. It is secondary to irreversible lesion of the kidney parenchyma [1]. At the terminal phase, the treatment uses kidney substitution techniques such as haemodialysis, peritoneal dialysis, in the absence of kidney transplant. Haemodialysis implies patient's short and long term constraints, despite countless progress made in recent years.

For the past few years, in the field of health, quality of life assessment has become widespread. This is one of the reasons the Kidney Disease and Quality of Life—Short Form (KDQoL-SF) has been proposed as an instrument for the assessment of haemodialytic patients' quality of life [2]. It is intended to measure both the impact of kidney disease and its treatment on the daily life of patients and their level of satisfaction [3]. The concept of "quality of life" is a very important topic in the sense that, from a subjective point of view its study helps to know the impact of diseases on patients' life [4].

In developed countries, haemodialysis care is well codified and abides by the recommendations set by learned societies. In Africa, it is not the case in all countries, because of the poorly equipped technical facilities. If haemodialytic patients' quality of life has thoroughly been studied in some African countries particularly in South and North African Countries, it is the contrast in sub-Saharan Africa where dialysis is not yet accessible to all patients and is therefore scarcely appreciated.

In West Africa, particularly in Senegal, a study has been made in Dakar on this theme in 2008 [5]. In Benin, it is the daily conventional haemodialysis that is practiced. Conventional haemodialysis corrects the renal failing and the hydroelectrolytics disorders; but it's little tolerated, and is not bound to a reduction of mortality. It's freely provided by the Government, but no study has been made so far on chronic haemodialytic patient's quality of life. Factors that are affecting their quality of life are unknown. That is why this study having the objectives below has been initiated:

General Objective:

Assessing haemodialytic patients' quality of life at CNHU-HKM of Cotonou and their determinants.

Specific Objectives:

- Assessing haemodialytic patients' quality of life in CNHU-HKM;
- Identifying factors that affect haemodialytic patients' quality of life;
- Determining the correlation between quality of life domains and epidemioclinical characteristics.

2. Patients and Methods

This work has been conducted in the haemodialysis unit at Hubert Koutoukou Maga Teaching Hospital (CNHU-HKM) in Cotonou, within the Nephrology-Haemodialysis University Hospital. It was a three (03) month monocentric and transversal study from October 24, 2011 to January 27, 2012 using self completed questionnaire for patients. Patients included in the study were residents of Benin, aged 18 years and above, chronic haemodialysis in the unit for over 3 months, and willfully gave their consent.

Quality of life was evaluated using Kidney Disease Quality of Life Short-Form French version 1.2 (KDQoL-SF) [2]. It was a self completed questionnaire comprising 79 items and made up of 2 modules.

A generic module: Short-Form (SF-36) made-up of 36 questions grouped into eight domains namely:
- General health (D1);
- Physical activity (D2);
- Limitations due to physical conditions (D3);
- Limitations due to mental state (D4);
- Life and relationships with others (D5);
- Physical pain (D6);
- Vitality (D7);
- Mental health (D8).

These eight domains were also divided into 2 dimensions:
- Physical health dimension was in correlation with "general health", "physical activities", "limitations due to physical activity", "physical pain", and "vitality";
- Mental health dimension was in correlation with "limitations due to mental activity", "life and relationship with others" and "mental health".

A specific module adapted to kidney pathology, comprising 43 items and divided into 11 domains:

- Burden of kidney disease (D9);
- Quality of the immediate circle (D10);
- Cognitive functions (D11);
- Symptoms and problems (D12);
- Effects of the disease on daily life (D13);
- Quality of sexual activity (D14);
- Sleep (D15);
- Family and friendly relationship (D16);
- Occupational status (D17);
- Patient's satisfaction (D18);
- Encouragement from dialysis team (D19).

These 19 domains were also divided into 04 dimensions:

- A physical health dimension in correlation with "general health", "physical functioning", "limitations due to physical activity", "physical pain", "vitality" and "occupational status";
- A mental health dimension in correlation with "limitations due to mental activity", "life and relationship with others" "mental health", "quality of the immediate circle", "burden of kidney disease";
- A dialysis specific dimension in correlation with "cognitive functions", "symptoms and problems", "effects of the disease on daily life", "quality of sexual activity" and "sleep";
- A dimension related to patient's care satisfaction along with a question concerning "patient satisfaction" as well as "encouragement from dialysis team".

Scoring of answers was based on a 0 to 100 scale, whereby 0 represented the worst quality of life and 100 the best. An average score was calculated for each domain (DAS) to help identify most affected domains, based on the following formula $[(100/S-s) * (Y-s)]$.

"S" being the maximum score that an individual might have in the field, "s" the minimum score and Y is the patient score in the domain.

Furthermore, an average score was calculated for each SF-36 and KDQoL dimension. The overall average score (OAS) was obtained through the calculation of the quotations average; the higher the score, the better the quality of life.

The interpretation of our results was made on the basis of 50 as average for the DAS.

Patients had to fill out the questionnaire by themselves, though sometimes they are assisted by the only one doctor available to either help patients check their chosen answers or translate in local dialect for uneducated patients. The assistance offered by this doctor complied with the recommendations of KDQoL. The formulations in the local dialect have been selected and validated by the research team so as to minimize biases. Epidemiological characteristics (age, sex, level of education, occupational status, marital status, standard of living), etiologies of nephropathy, and dialysis related parametres (number of haemodialyses sessions on weekly basis, vascular access) were filled out by the doctor through each patient's medical record. The standard of living was evaluated on the basis of housing stress, education challenges, lack of financial resources, and poor access to health care. With regard to chronic kidney disease patients, the lack of one of these elements taken separately was regarded as a sign of underprivileged life conditions (UNDP, 2006). On that basis, high, average and low standards of living were clearly defined.

Data were recorded and analyzed using SPSS software 11.5. Univariate and bivariate analyzes were conducted, and 0.05 was the adopted threshold of significance.

3. Results

In total, 133 patients met our inclusion criteria. Out of that figure, there was 1 refusal and 1withdrawal during our investigation, so this brings the figure to 131 patients who effectively took part in the study.

3.1. Characteristics of the Population

3.1.1. Socio-Economic Characteristics of the Study Population

The average age of patients was 50.27 ± 12.17 with 18 and 76 years as extremes. It is worth noting that males were predominant, with a sex ratio of 1.69. Uneducated patients accounted for 12.50%. The other socio-economic characteristics were found in **Table 1**.

3.1.2. Etiologies of Kidney Disease

Nephroangiosclerosis and diabetic nephropathy were respectively the first and second cause of chronic kidney disease, with respectively 25.58% and 15.19%. Other etiologies are found on **Figure 1**.

Table 1. Socio-economic characteristics of the population.

	Effective N = 131	Percentage
Age		
18 - 38	23	18
38 - 58	69	52.4
58 - 76	39	29.6
Sex		
Male	82	62.88
Female	49	37.12
Level of education		
Out-of-school	16	12.50
Primary	24	18.75
Secondary	46	35.94
Tertiary	42	32.81
Occupational status		
With a profession	47	40.87
Pensioners	42	36.52
Without a profession	26	22.61
Marital status		
Married	95	72.73
Unmarried	36	27.27
Benefit from a PEC*		
Yes	131	100
Standard of living		
High	38	06.82
Average	84	64.39
Low	09	28.79

*Benefit from free haemodialysis provided by the Government of Benin.

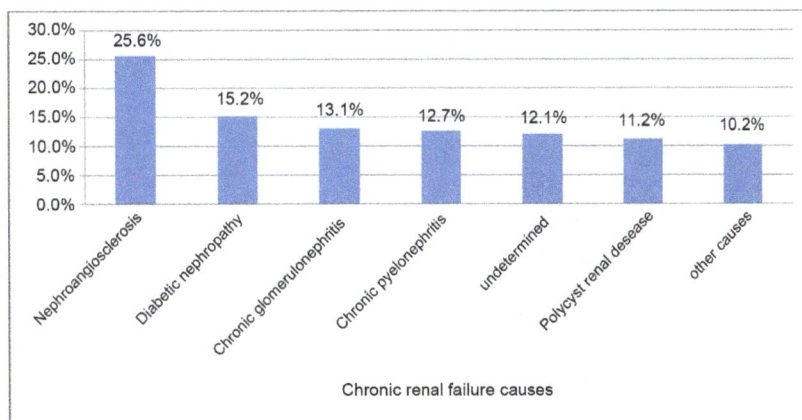

Figure 1. Patients classification per different kidney disease etiologies.

3.1.3. Required Haemodialysis Parametres

Only 3 patients received 3 haemodialysis sessions on weekly basis. And all our patients had an arteriovenous fistula as shown in **Table 2**.

3.1.4. Complications of the Patients

Frequents complications were dominated by anaemia (72.51%) and infection (35.51%). **Table 3** showed the frequent complications of our patients.

3.2. Overall Assessment of Hemodialytic Patients Quality of Life

The average of SF 36 and AOS of KDQoL Overall Average Score (AOS) was 53.55. The different domains average scores ranged from 27.46 to 80.44 as shown in **Table 4**.

3.3. Factors Affecting Quality of Life

According to the generic module, vitality, limitations due to mental health and physical condition were factors that affect hemodialytic patients' quality of life of in CNHU-HKM of Cotonou (**Figure 2**).

Depending on the specific module, occupational status, burden of the disease and consequences of kidney disease on daily life together with those found in the generic module, constituted factors which adversely affect the quality of life of hemodialytic patients in CNHU HKM-Cotonou (**Figure 3**).

3.4. Correlations between Different Domains and Epidemioclinical Data

- Patients education level was significantly correlated with vitality ($p < 0.017$);
- Patients number of haemodialyses sessions was significantly correlated with the effects of kidney disease on daily life ($p < 0.025$);
- Patients' living standard was significantly correlated with physical functioning ($p < 0.020$);
- Patients occupational status was significantly correlated with cognitive functions ($p < 0.001$);

Table 2. Patients classification per required haemodialysis parameters.

	Effective N = 131	Percentage
Number of weekly sessions		
- 2	128	97.71
- 3	3	2.29
Type of vascular access		
- Arteriovenous fistula	131	100

Table 3. Frequent complications of the patients.

	Effective N = 131	Percentage
Anemia	95	72.51
Infection (lung, urinary, otolaryngology)	46	35.11
Carpal chennal syndrom	35	26.71
Hepatitis C	31	23.66
Hyperkaliemia	28	21.37
Undernutrition	23	17.55
Malaria	12	09.16
Unchecked high blood pression	12	09.16
Hepatitis B	08	06.10
Dysfonction of vascular access	04	03.05

Table 4. Average scores for different domains and dimensions.

KDQoL and SF 36 domains	Average score	Standard deviation
• **SF 36**		
General Health (D1)	52.84	±19.69
Physical activities (D2)	50.39	±23.51
Limitations due to physical conditions (D3)	27.46	±35.34
Limitations due to mental state (D4)	31.57	±39.85
Life and relationship with others (D5)	62.45	±23.05
Mental pain (D6)	55.47	±24.44
Vitality (D7)	46.70	±16.33
Mental health (D8)	50.09	±19.32
Physical Health Dimension (PHD)	**46.54**	**±25.75**
Mental Health Dimension (MHD)	**47.70**	**±24.64**
AOS of SF36	**48.55**	**±16.85**
• **KDQoL**		
Burden of illness (D9)	38.07	±25.11
Quality of immediate circle (D10)	62.10	±14.89
Cognitive functions (D11)	70.18	±18.29
Symptoms/problems (D12)	66.98	±18.26
Effects of the disease on daily life (D13)	47.43	±22.19
Quality of sexual activity (D14)	55.21	±33.64
Sleep (D15)	56.66	±15.60
Family and friendly relationship (D16)	62.75	±28.12
Occupational status (D17)	45.45	±29.16
Patient's satisfaction (D18)	58.79	±16.65
Encouragement from dialysis team (D19)	80.44	±21.07
Physical Health Dimension (PHD)	**46.54**	**±17.55**
Mental Health Dimension (MHD)	**50.56**	**±17.74**
Specific Dialysis Dimension (SDD)	**56.79**	**±15.30**
Patient Satisfaction Dimension (PSD)	**69.09**	**±15.35**
AOS of KDQoL	**58.55**	**±22.09**

- Patients sex was respectively significantly correlated with vitality and symptoms/problems ($p < 0.043$ and $p < 0.008$);
- Patients marital status was significantly correlated with vitality and support from healthcare team ($p < 0.008$ and $p < 0.009$).

Patients age was respectively significantly correlated with physical functioning, physical pain, perceived health and sexual function ($p < 0.005$, $p < 0.047$, $p < 0.019$ and $p < 0.000$) (see **Table 4**).

Table 5 shows domains which were statistically significant correlated with epidemioclinical variables.

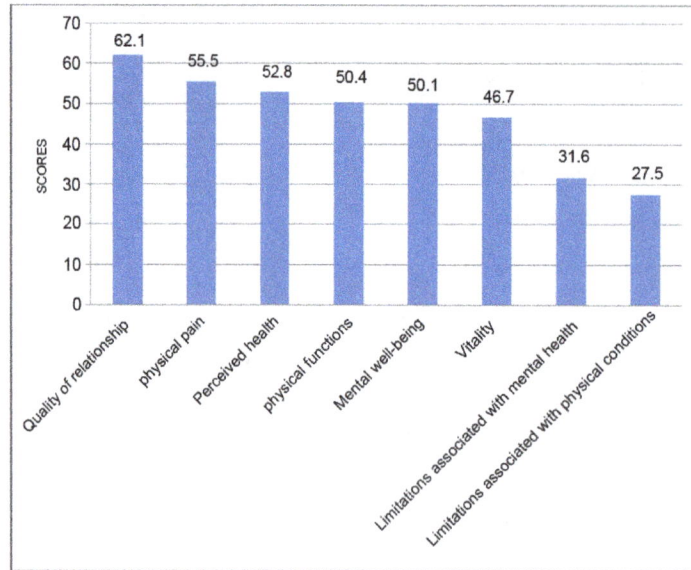

Figure 2. Average Scores for haemodialytic patients SF-36 domains.

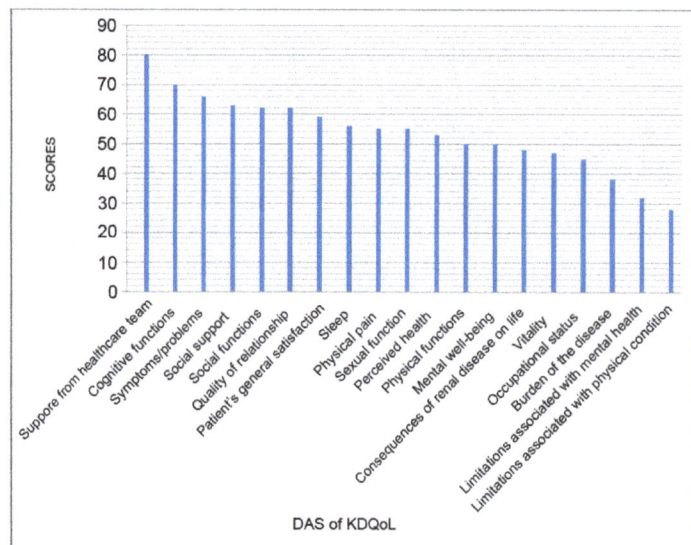

Figure 3. Average scores of haemodialytic patients KDQoL domains.

Table 5. Correlation between epidemioclinical characteristics and KDQoL domains.

	D1	D2	D6	D7	D11	D12	D13	D14	D19
Level of education				0.017*					
Age	0.019*	0.005**	0.047*					0.000**	
Sex				0.043*		0.008**			
Number of sessions							0.025*		
Marital status				0.008**					0.009**
Occupational status					0.001**				
Standard of living		0.020*							

** Correlation is significant at 0.01 level; * Correlation is significant at 0.05 level.

4. Discussion

Nowadays, Quality of Life (QoL) assessment is very interesting in haemodialysis therapeutic programmes. All surveys were mainly facing problems of non homogeneity of study populations, and the choice of the evaluation tool to use. It is the French version of the questionnaire that was used because it has been used repeatedly for studies on quality of life in the African context.

The choice of KDQoL is linked not only to its use in many studies [3] [6]-[9], but also to its specific dimension to dialysis which helps to separate levels of perceived health of dialytic patients from the duration of its execution requiring only 20 to 30 minutes. Its acceptability was good since we only recorded one refusal in our study and also only one missing answer (0.8%). Bioni *et al.* [10] in France and Mohamed Nasr *et al.* [11] in Tunisia respectively found 5.5% and 32% missing answers.

4.1. Overall Quality of Life

The overall quality of life of haemodialytic patients at CNHU-HKM of Cotonou during the period of our study is average. We found the same result as Ouattara in Senegal in 2008 who found an average overall quality of life evaluated at 50.50 of haemodialytic patients [5]. This could be explained by an average treatment of haemodialytic patients. In France in 2008, Boini found an average quality of life. Furthermore, the author showed that quality of life for haemodialytic patients during the study impaired very much in relation to the general population [10].

4.2. Factors Affecting Quality of Life of Haemodialytic Patients

4.2.1. Per SF 36

Out of the 08 domains, only 03: namely vitality, limitations related to physical activity and mental activity impaired. Water and food restrictions as well as complexity of treatment could explain severe impairment of the domain "limitations due to physical condition". **Figure 4** shows the results of several studies compared to those of this study [11]-[14].

The low Domain Average Score (DAS) of limitations associated with physical conditions, which was observed by most authors, tallies effectively with our results [5] [12]-[14]. Mohamed, N., Jose, A. and Peter, B. observed like this study a low DAS for vitality [11]-[13]. This could be explained by the complexity of the treatment. Moreover, DAS of limitations related to mental health is average in most studies, while it is low in our study [11]-[14]. This could be explained by anxiety for dialysis and insufficient psychological support probably due to the absence of a psychologist in our team. With regard to the physical health dimension of our study, our patients' quality of life was higher when compared to that of Jose, A. and Peter, B. who found 35.2 and 33.3 respectively, while mental health dimension was like those of Jose, A. and Peter, B. respectively 47.9 and 47.5 [12] [13].

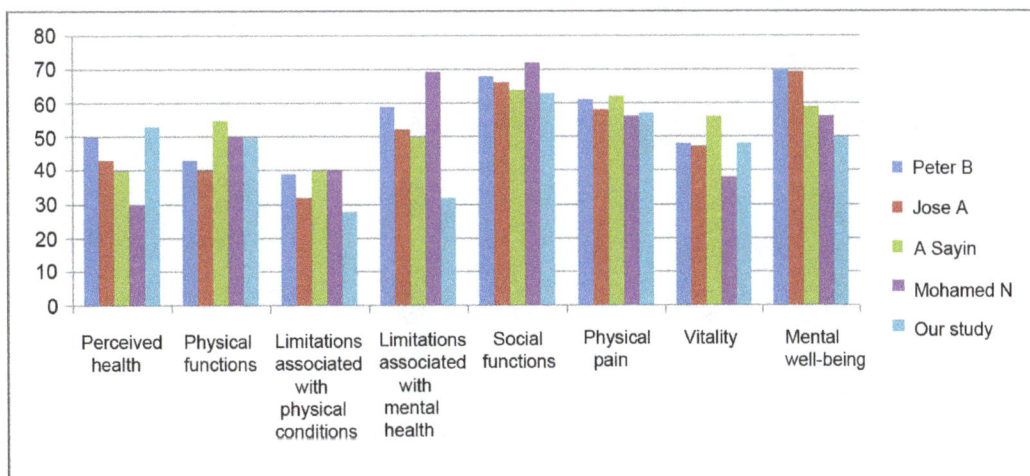

Figure 4. Study histograms comparing quality of life per SF-36.

The two SF-36 dimensions impaired but physical dimension was a bit more impaired than the mental dimension. This observation was made by several authors [5] [15]. These results could be explained by the following factors: Physical inactivity, damage of the musculoskeletal system, low dose of dialysis, anaemia.

Globally, our haemodialytic patients DAS of KDQoL were comparable to those in the study of Boini Stephanie and Mohamed Nasr [10] [11] except for domains namely "limitations due to mental state", "limitations due to physical activity" and "quality of sexual activity" (**Figure 5**).

Indeed, it appears that our patients had better sex quality than those of Mohamed and Boini; however, they were more limited physically and mentally compared to Stephanie Boini and Mohamed Nasr's patients [10] [11]. Anaemia associated with dialysis could explain these results.

4.2.2. Per KDQoL

The analysis of KDQoL scores dimensions showed similar results to those found by Boini Stephanie and Mohamed Nasr [10] [11], except that mental health dimension (MHD) score is higher in the Tunisian study, and patient satisfaction dimension (PSD) score is higher in the French study (**Figure 6**).

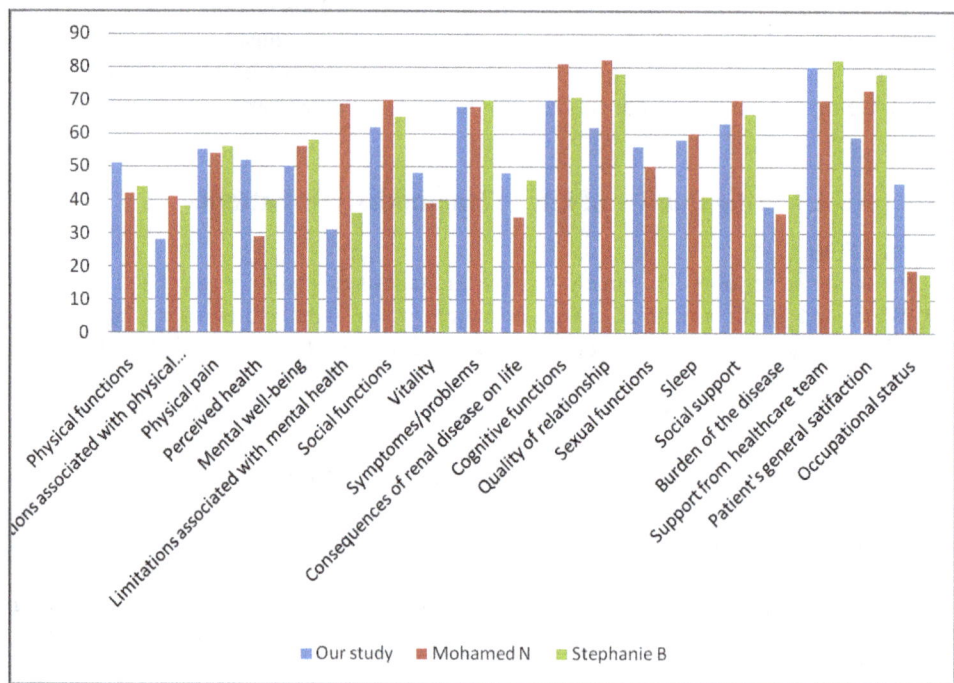

Figure 5. Study histogram comparing quality of life per KDQoL.

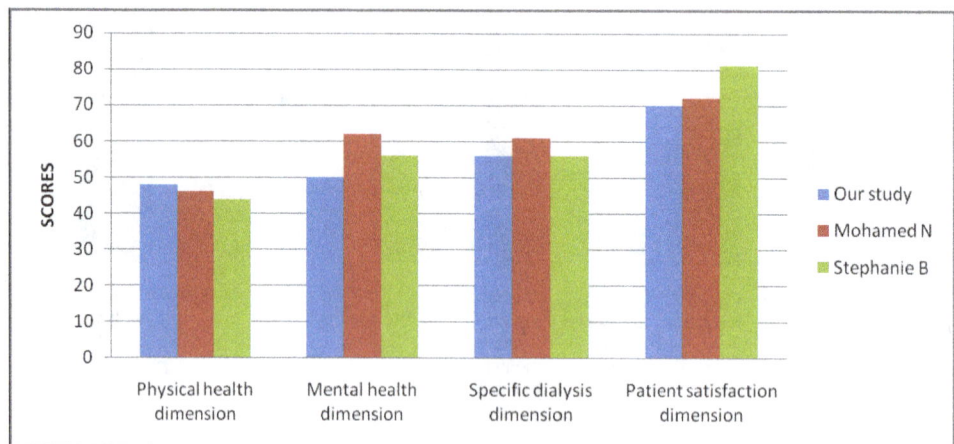

Figure 6. Study histograms comparing different KDQoL dimensions.

4.3. Correlation between Quality of Life and Patients Epidemioclinical Characteristics

Age was correlated with physical functioning, physical pain, perceived health and sexual functions. Literature reports that a higher age is correlated with these domains. This could be explained by a deterioration of physical health and a decline in general adaptive capacity with growing age [11] [14] [15].

Patients education level was correlated with vitality. Low education levels associated with impairment of quality of life (QoL) were found by Mohamed Nasr and Valderrabano who highlighted that a high level of education protects against impairment of QoL [11] [16].

With regard to marital status, Neto observed that married haemodialytic patients had better QoL [17]. Indeed, the presence of the spouse helps the patient to overcome difficulties associated with renal disease [11]. In our study, patients marital status is correlated with vitality and also with support from healthcare team. This could be explained by the fact that haemodialytic patients recognize the support provided to them by healthcare team.

With regard to sex, Sayin, A. found in his study that women had high scores compared to men [14]. Other authors on the contrary, reported that female sex was associated with QoL impairment [11] [15] [16].

To some extent, QoL is influenced by inadequate number of dialyses sessions. We believed that the inadequate number of generators could explain this result. It is therefore logical that patients with inadequate dialysis dose had a slightly impaired QoL than others.

5. Conclusions

The overall assessment of chronic haemodialysis patients' quality of life at CNHU-HKM of Cotonou is broadly average (53.55). Factors impairing the quality of life of haemodialysis patients are according to SF36: vitality and limitations related to mental health and physical condition; and according to KDQoL: burden of kidney disease, effect of the disease on daily life and occupational status.

Age was correlated with physical functioning, physical pain, perceived health and sexual functions. Patients education level was correlated with vitality. Patients number of haemodialyses sessions was correlated with the effects of kidney disease on daily life. Patients occupational status was correlated with cognitive functions.

The recourse to the haemodiafiltration online and the increase of the number of the sessions will contribute to improve the quality of life of these patients. It has the advantage to offer a better tolerance. It's associated with a reduction of the carpal channel and of the mortality.

In the same way, it is necessary to increase staff by providing a psychologist and a dietician, and to build new haemodialysis centres in the city.

Disclosure of Conflict of Interest

None.

References

[1] MerkusM.P.,Jager, K.J., Dekker, F., Boeschoten, E.W., Stevens, P. and Krediet, R.T. (1997) Quality of Life in Patients on Chronic Dialysis: Self-Assessment 3 Months after the Start of Treatment. *American Journal of Kidney Dis- eases*, **29**, 584-592. http://dx.doi.org/10.1016/S0272-6386(97)90342-5

[2] Boini, S., Leplege, A., Loos, C., Français, P., Ecosse, E. and Briançon, S. (2007) Mesure de la qualité de vie dans l'insuffisance rénale chronique terminale. Adaptation transculturelle et validation du questionnaire spécifique kidney disease quality of life. *Néphrologie et Thérapeutique*, **3**, 372-383. http://dx.doi.org/10.1016/j.nephro.2007.05.005

[3] Hays, R.D., Kallich, J.D., Mapes, D.L., Coons, S.J., Amin, N. and Carter, W.B. (1994) Development of the Kidney Disease Quality of Life (KDQOL) Instrument. *Quality of Life Research*, **3**, 329-338. http://dx.doi.org/10.1007/BF00451725

[4] Martin, P. and Ferreri, M. (1997) Le concept de qualité de vie. *Ardix Medical*, **45**, 345-375.

[5] Ouattara, F. (2008) Qualité de vie des hémodialysés à dakar. Thèse Med, Dakar, No. 120.

[6] Korevaar, J.C., Jansen, M., Merkus, M.P., Dekker, F.W. and Boeschoten, E.W. (2000) Quality of Life in Predialysis End-Stage Disease Patients at the Initiation of Dialysis Therapy. *Peritoneal Dialysis International*, **20**, 69-75.

[7] Gentile, S., Delarozière, J.-Ch., Fernandez, C., Tardieu, S., Devictor, B., Dussol, B., Daurès, J.-P., Berland, Y. and Sambuc, R. (2003) Qualité de vie et insuffisance rénale chronique terminale: Le point sur les différents questionnaires existants. *Néphrologie*, **24**, 291-299.

[8]   Rebollo, P., Ortega, F. and Baltar, J.M. (2001) Is the Loss of Health-Related Quality of Life during Renal Replacement Therapy Lower in Elderly Patients than in Younger Patients? *Nephrology Dialysis Transplantation*, **16**, 1675-1680. http://dx.doi.org/10.1093/ndt/16.8.1675

[9]   Wu, A.W., Fink, N.E., Cagney, K.A., Bass, E.B. and Rubin, H.R. (2001) Developing a Health-Related Quality-of-Life Measure for End Stage Renal Disease: The Choice Health Experience Questionnaire. *The American Journal of Kidney Diseases*, **37**, 11-21.

[10] Boini, S., Bloch, J. and Briançon, S. (2011) Surveillance de la qualité de vie des sujets atteints d'insuffisance rénale chronique terminale. *Néphrologie et Thérapeutique*, **7**, S215-S300. http://dx.doi.org/10.1016/S1769-7255(11)70021-9

[11] Mohamed, N., Mohamed, H.A., Sami, K., Dhia, N.B. and Anouar, G. (2008) L'hémodialyse et son impact sur la qualité de vie. *Néphrologie et Thérapeutique*, **4**, 21-27. http://dx.doi.org/10.1016/j.nephro.2007.07.008

[12] Jose, A.D.B., Edmund, G.L. and Nancy, L.L. (2000) Quality-of-Life Evaluation Using Short Form 36: Comparison in Hemodialysis and Peritoneal Dialysis Patients. *American Journal of Kidney Diseases*, **35**, 293-300.

[13] Peter, B.D. (1997) Hemodialysis Patient-Assessed Functional Health Status Predicts Continued Survival, Hospitalization, and Dialysis-Attendance Compliance. *American Journal of Kidney Diseases*, **30**, 204-212. http://dx.doi.org/10.1016/S0272-6386(97)90053-6

[14] Sayin, A., Mutluay, R. and Sindel, S. (2007) Quality of Life in Hemodialysis, Peritoneal Dialysis, and Transplantation Patients. *Transplantation Proceedings*, **39**, 3047-3053. http://dx.doi.org/10.1016/j.transproceed.2007.09.030

[15] Anca, S., Liviu, S. and Constantin, V. (2008) Factors Affecting the Quality of Life of Haemodialysis Patients from Romania: A Multicentric Study. *Nephrology Dialysis Transplantation*, **1**, 1-4.

[16] Valderrabano, F. (2000) Quality of Life Benefits of Early Anemia Treatment. *Nephrology Dialysis Transplantation*, **15**, 23-28. http://dx.doi.org/10.1093/oxfordjournals.ndt.a027972

[17] Neto, J.F., Ferraz, M.B. and Cendoroglo, M. (2000) Quality of Life at the Initiation of Maintenance Dialysis Treatment—A Comparison between the SF-36 and the KDQ Questionnaires. *Quality of Life Research*, **9**, 101-107. http://dx.doi.org/10.1023/A:1008918609281

24

Correction of Severe Anemia in a Patient with End Stage Renal Disease and Myelodysplastic Syndrome

Ankita Patel, Suchita Mehta*, Ahmad Waseef, Subodh Saggi

Department of Nephrology, SUNY Downstate Medical Center, New York, USA
Email: *mehtasuchita@gmail.com

Abstract

Background: Anemia is a common complication of end-stage renal disease (ESRD) and is effectively managed by Erythropoietin Stimulating Agents (ESAs) and intravenous iron therapy. Management of anemia in ESRD patients with myelodysplastic syndrome (MDS) poses a unique challenge. ESAs even at extremely high doses do not result in a desired response, especially if the patients are iron-overloaded. Case: A 72-year-old man with history of ESRD and MDS on hemodialysis since September 2009 was severely anemic requiring massive doses of ESA in excess of 90,000 units/week. Iron saturation was consistently >60%; ferritin was >2500. Desferrioxamine (DFO) 125 mg IV/week was begun in November 2010. His PRBC transfusion and ESA requirements declined after the initiation of this therapy. He had 33 ER visits for PRBC transfusions (1 - 3 transfusions/visit) from September 2009 to November 2010 (average: 2.35/month), which decreased to 18 visits in 20 months (average: 0.9/month) after getting DFO. Conclusion: We report a case of MDS with ESRD on hemodialysis where anemia was managed with Desferrioxamine therapy along with ESA, after which it was noted that there was a significant reduction in the number of PRBC transfusions that the patient received along with a decrease in ESA requirements and a decrease in number of hospitalizations, which in the long term could be cost effective.

Keywords

Anemia, Desferrioxamine, ESRD

1. Background

Myelodysplastic Syndrome (MDS) comprises a heterogeneous group of malignant stem cell disorders characte-

---

*Corresponding author.

rized by dysplastic and ineffective blood cell production from ineffective iron incorporation. Most of these patients require multiple packed red blood cell transfusions. Anemia is a common complication of end-stage renal disease (ESRD) and is effectively managed by Erythropoietin Stimulating Agents (ESAs) and intravenous iron therapy. Management of anemia in ESRD patients with MDS poses a unique challenge. ESAs, even at extremely high doses do not result in a desired response, especially if the patients are iron-overloaded [1]. Patients become dependent on frequent packed red blood cell (PRBC) transfusions, which result in many adverse effects, one of which includes iron overload and its toxicity. We report a case of MDS with ESRD on hemodialysis whose anemia was managed with Desferrioxamine therapy along with EPO, after which it was noted that there was a significant reduction in the dose of ESA as well as the number of PRBC transfusions that the patient received. Further, this patient benefited from a decrease in number of hospitalizations, which in the long term could be cost effective.

2. Case Presentation

A 72-year-old African American man with history of Diabetes Mellitus Type II and Hypertension for 15 years was diagnosed with MDS in 2008. He developed End stage renal disease (ESRD) due to Diabetic nephropathy and was started on hemodialysis three times a week in September 2009. He was profoundly anemic requiring massive doses of Erythropoietin (EPO) in excess of 90,000. Despite such high doses of ESA requirement, patient's response was suboptimal and he required multiple hospitalizations for PRBC transfusions, averaging 1 - 2 per week. His iron saturations' were persistently above 60% and his ferritin's were always greater than 2500 ng/ml, on occasions even above 10,000 ng/ml, in part related to the excess blood transfusions. In an effort to control his excess iron overload, patient was started on Desferrioxamine (DFO) therapy in November 2010. He was prescribed 125 mg intravenously once a week as a maintenance therapy on an ongoing basis.

After initiation of DFO, his requirements of blood transfusion and multiple hospitalizations were greatly decreased. Overall he had 33 emergency room visits requiring 1 to 3 PRBC transfusions during each visit from September 2009 to November 2010 (an average of 2.35 admissions per month). Remarkably after initiation of DFO he had 18 emergency room visits for transfusions in 20 months (an average of 0.9 admissions per month). Average EPO requirements declined simultaneously over this time period. His hemoglobin, and iron indices are shown in **Figure 1**.

3. Discussion

Anemia is one of the most common presenting features of MDS, apart from disturbances of platelets, white cells and coagulation. Most of the patients with MDS become transfusion dependent. Secondary iron overload from frequent red blood cell transfusions and poor iron incorporation into red blood cells (RBCs) is associated with poor survival in these patients [2]-[4]. Transfusion requirement has been recently recognized as an independent prognostic factor for survival in MDS patients [5]. Benefits of iron chelation therapy have been described in MDS patients who did not have any kidney injury or ESRD [6]-[8]. Such treatments resulted in a reduction of transfusions in such patients in association with a reduction in their iron overload. Iron chelation therapy has also been shown to reduce iron overload in ESRD patients but an effect on their anemia has not been reported before. Here we report a case of a patient who had both ESRD and MDS with profoundly high iron load who benefited from chelation therapy. To our knowledge this is the first case with both ESRD and MDS, where we show his anemia improved and his ESA requirements reduced. We present a hypothesis by which we believe iron chelation might be working under these circumstances where the kidneys and bone marrow are not functioning optimally.

The expression of erythropoietin (EPO) mRNA and protein is regulated primarily at the transcriptional level. Hypoxia is the most physiologically important stimulus for EPO production. It results in the activation of hypoxia inducible factor (HIF), a $\alpha\beta$ heterodimer transcription factor that contains an oxygen-labile α subunit and a constitutively expressed β subunit. At normal oxygen tension the α-subunit of HIF undergoes post-translational modification by proline hydroxylation and ubiquitylation, causing it to be rapidly degraded. At low oxygen tension, HIF-1α is not hydroxylated and therefore escapes degradation and it thus translocates into the nucleus, and heterodimerizes with β subunit to form the HIF complex [9] [10]. HIF-1α can be activated in oxygenated cells by inhibitors of prolyl hydroxylase (PH). Desferrioxamine (DFO) has been shown to activate HIF-1α *in vitro*, with kinetics similar to those associated with hypoxia, and to increase expression of HIF-1α target genes, including EPO [11]. We believe this happens via inhibition of prolyl hydroxylase by DFO (see **Figure 2**).

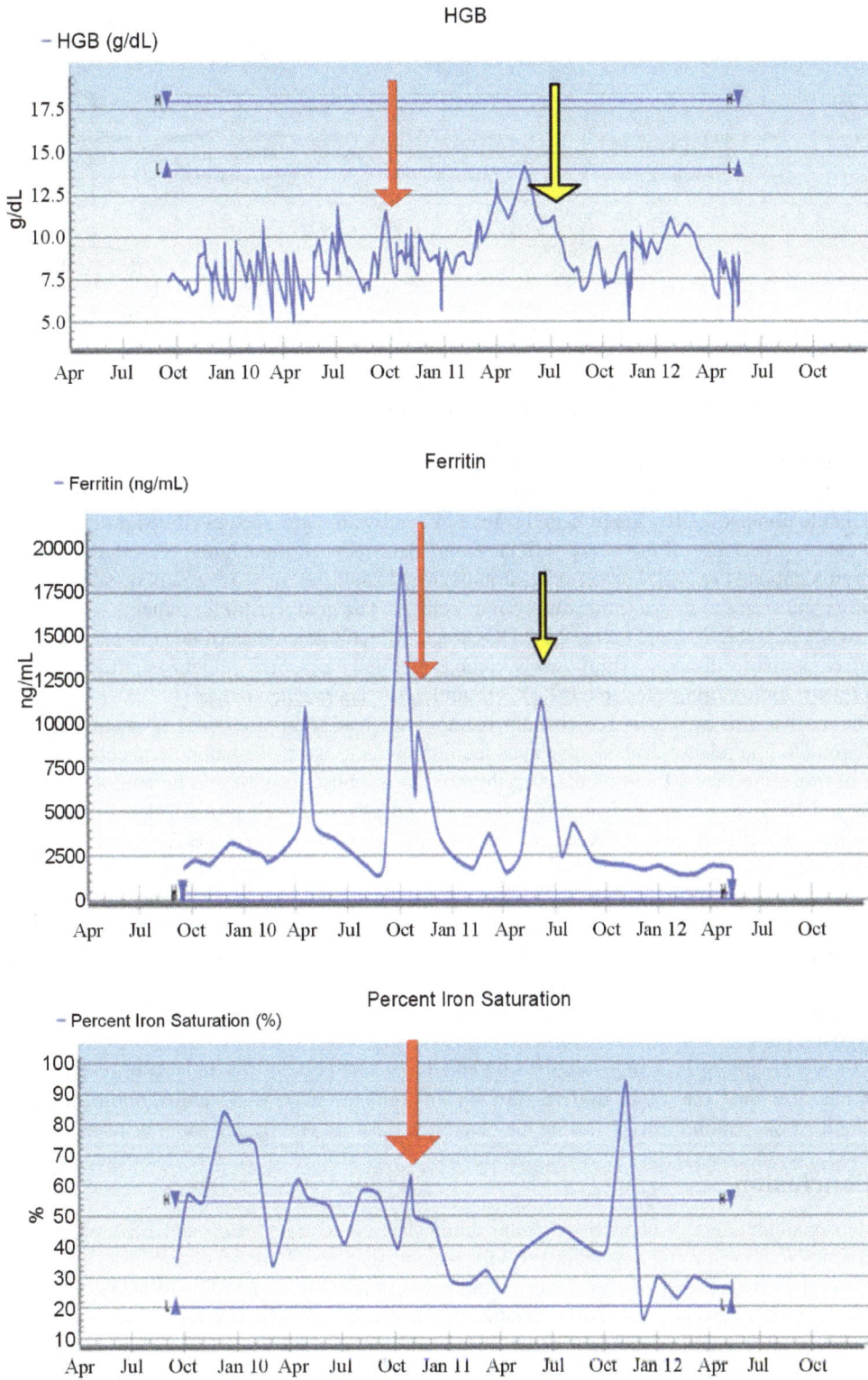

Figure 1. The red arrow represents initiation of DFO therapy. The yellow arrow depicts a rise in ferritin and subsequent decrease in hemoglobin when DFO therapy was held temporarily.

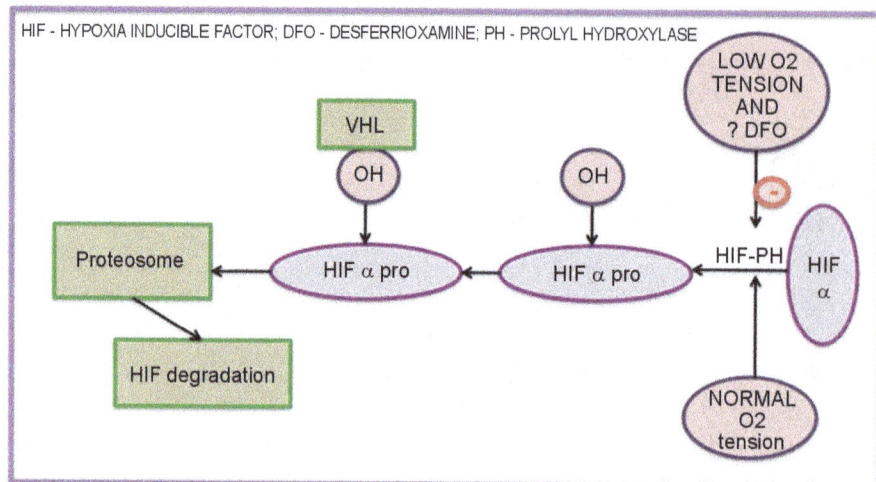

Figure 2. Degradation of hif-α under normal oxygen tension by prolyl hydroxylase. Inhibition of hydroxylation under hypoxic conditions and also possibly by desferrioxamine.

Iron excess is also associated with increased oxidative stress: the accumulation of non-transferrin-bound iron caused by chronic blood transfusions which results in excess extracellular labile plasma iron (LPI) and intracellular labile iron pool (LIP), the principal source of reactive oxygen species (ROS) production. Iron accumulation also causes a decrease of the major cellular antioxidant reduced glutathione (GSH) and increases membrane lipid peroxidation [12] [13]. Furthermore, iron overload itself has an *in vitro* suppressive effect on erythroid progenitors and seems to increase transfusion requirement. The goal ferritin for patients with chronic kidney disease is now set at 500ug/l, based up on the KDOQI and KDIGO guidelines of anemia management in patients with chronic kidney disease. (http://www.kdigo.org/clinical_practice_guidelines/pdf/KDIGO-Anemia_GL.pdf; http://www.kidney.org/professionals/KDOQI/guidelines_anemia/ped32.htm)

The mechanisms by which iron chelator therapy may lead to improvement in anemia are unclear. Iron chelators promote iron release from storage sites facilitating its usage by hematopoietic cells. Furthermore, the reduction of iron store seems to up regulate erythropoietin response, resulting in hemoglobin increase [14]. Perhaps, DFO and EPO have a synergistic effect on erythroid precursor cell proliferation [15]. In MDS patients, iron chelation significantly reduces ROS, membrane lipid peroxidation and the LIPs, and concomitantly increases GSH in RBC [16].

Now, with reimbursement rates by Center for Medicare and Medicaid Services (CMS) being dependent on average dose of ESA requirement in a month and also with a possible further cut by 9.4% in the bundling system for the dialysis centers as proposed by CMS in 2014; cost effective measures to reduce ESA requirements would be beneficial to the patient as well as to a dialysis facility. (http://www.cms.gov/Outreach-and-Education/Medicare-Learning-Network-MLN/MLNMattersArticles/downloads/se0406.pdf; http://www.renalbusiness.com/news/2013/07/cms-proposes--pay-cut-for-dialysis-providers.aspx)

In our case, once the use of desferrioxamine was initiated there was stabilization of his hemoglobin thus reducing his ESA requirements, reducing his blood transfusions, emergency room visits and hospitalizations.

4. Conclusion

Desferrioxamine therapy improves anemia, diminishes blood transfusion and ESA requirements, and reduces emergency room visits and hospitalizations for patients that have both MDS and ESRD. Larger studies would be hard to do as the number of cases with combined co-morbidity of ESRD and MDS are too few. However, if measurements of endogenous and exogenous erythropoietin levels and assessment of intracellular signaling pathways were available, we might better understand the mechanisms of chelation therapy and its role in iron incorporation into RBC. In our patient, we think there must have been a reservoir of endogenous EPO production (possibly cystic kidneys), which was being modulated by chelation therapy with its likely effect on prolyl hydroxylases.

Disclosures

None.

Conflicts of Interest

None.

Funding

None.

References

[1] El-Reshaid, K., *et al.* (1994) Erythropoietin Treatment in Haemodialysis Patients with Iron Overload. *Acta Haematologica*, **91**, 130-135. http://dx.doi.org/10.1159/000204318

[2] Malcovati, L., *et al.* (2005) Prognostic Factors and Life Expectancy in Myelodysplastic Syndromes Classified According to WHO Criteria: A Basis for Clinical Decision Making. *Journal of Clinical Oncology*, **23**, 7594-7603. http://dx.doi.org/10.1200/JCO.2005.01.7038

[3] Jabbour, E., *et al.* (2008) Red Blood Cell Transfusions and Iron Overload in the Treatment of Patients with Myelodysplastic Syndromes. *Cancer*, **112**, 1089-1095. http://dx.doi.org/10.1002/cncr.23280

[4] Alessandrino, E.P., *et al.* (2010) Prognostic Impact of Pre-Transplantation Transfusion History and Secondary Iron Overload in Patients with Myelodysplastic Syndrome Undergoing Allogeneic Stem Cell Transplantation: A GITMO Study. *Haematologica*, **95**, 476-484. http://dx.doi.org/10.3324/haematol.2009.011429

[5] Malcovati, L., *et al.* (2007) Time-Dependent Prognostic Scoring System for Predicting Survival and Leukemic Evolution in Myelodysplastic Syndromes. *Journal of Clinical Oncology*, **25**, 3503-3510. http://dx.doi.org/10.1200/JCO.2006.08.5696

[6] Badawi, M.A., *et al.* (2010) Red Blood Cell Transfusion Independence Following the Initiation of Iron Chelation Therapy in Myelodysplastic Syndrome. *Advances in Hematology*, **2010**, 164045.

[7] Jensen, P.D., Jensen, I.M. and Ellegaard, J. (1992) Desferrioxamine Treatment Reduces Blood Transfusion Requirements in Patients with Myelodysplastic Syndrome. *British Journal of Haematology*, **80**, 121-124. http://dx.doi.org/10.1111/j.1365-2141.1992.tb06411.x

[8] Praga, M., *et al.* (1987) Improvement of Anaemia with Desferrioxamine in Haemodialysis Patients. *Nephrology Dialysis Transplantation*, **2**, 243-247.

[9] Semenza, G.L. (1998) Hypoxia-Inducible Factor 1: Master Regulator of O2 Homeostasis. *Current Opinion in Genetics & Development*, **8**, 588-594. http://dx.doi.org/10.1016/S0959-437X(98)80016-6

[10] Wenger, R.H. (2000) Mammalian Oxygen Sensing, Signalling and Gene Regulation. *The Journal of Experimental Biology*, **203**, 1253-1263.

[11] Wang, G.L. and Semenza, G.L. (1993) Desferrioxamine Induces Erythropoietin Gene Expression and Hypoxia-Inducible Factor 1 DNA-Binding Activity: Implications for Models of Hypoxia Signal Transduction. *Blood*, **82**, 3610-3615.

[12] Schmid, M. (2009) Iron Chelation Therapy in MDS: What Have We Learnt Recently? *Blood Reviews*, **23**, S21-S25. http://dx.doi.org/10.1016/S0268-960X(09)70006-2

[13] Prus, E. and Fibach, E. (2008) Flow Cytometry Measurement of the Labile Iron Pool in Human Hematopoietic Cells. *Cytometry Part A*, **73**, 22-27. http://dx.doi.org/10.1002/cyto.a.20491

[14] Vreugdenhil, G., *et al.* (1993) Iron Chelators May Enhance Erythropoiesis by Increasing Iron Delivery to Haematopoietic Tissue and Erythropoietin Response in Iron-Loading Anaemia. *Acta Haematologica*, **89**, 57-60. http://dx.doi.org/10.1159/000204488

[15] Aucella, F., *et al.* (1999) Synergistic Effect of Desferrioxamine and Recombinant Erythropoietin on Erythroid Precursor Proliferation in Chronic Renal Failure. *Nephrology Dialysis Transplantation*, **14**, 1171-1175. http://dx.doi.org/10.1093/ndt/14.5.1171

[16] Ghoti, H., *et al.* (2010) Changes in Parameters of Oxidative Stress and Free Iron Biomarkers during Treatment with Deferasirox in Iron-Overloaded Patients with Myelodysplastic Syndromes. *Haematologica*, **95**, 1433-1434. http://dx.doi.org/10.3324/haematol.2010.024992

25

Renal Replacement Therapy in Patients over 65 Years Old

Imen Gorsane, Madiha Mahfoudhi*, Mondher Ounissi, Fathi Younsi, Imed Helal, Taieb Ben Abdallah

Internal Medicine A Department, Charles Nicolle Hospital, Tunis, Tunisia
Email: *madiha_mahfoudhi@yahoo.fr

Abstract

Age at onset of renal replacement therapy (RRT) is increasing in all countries. Two substitution methods of renal function remain available: hemodialysis (HD) and peritoneal dialysis (PD). It was a retrospective study carried out on January 2015 and it included patients older than 65 years, monitored for HD and PD. We studied their epidemiological and clinical profile, their evolution, and the elements of prognosis. Two groups of 42 patients were included. The first was about 30 HD patients representing 25% of all patients on HD with an average age of 71 ± 4.5 years. The second was concerning 12 patients on PD having a mean age of 69.8 ± 3.5 years and representing 11.7% of all patients on PD. Functional and vital prognosis of a patient with end stage renal disease (ESRD) depends, in the elderly, on psychological, cognitive functions, and the degree of autonomy.

Keywords

Renal Replacement Therapy, Elderly, Hemodialysis, Peritoneal Dialysis

1. Introduction

The aging of the current population and future is recognized by all demographic studies. The health professional currently holds the age of 75 to define an old person.

The incidence of end stage renal disease and age at onset of renal replacement therapy (RRT) is increasing in all countries. The number of older patients requiring dialysis therapy is rising, reflecting the ageing of the general population [1]. Kidney transplantation is not generally given to this category of the population, two substitution methods of renal function remain available: HD and PD.

We report our experience of care in RRT of the elderly population.

---

*Corresponding author.

2. Material and Methods

It was a single-center retrospective study carried out in our department of nephrology, in January 2015 and included patients older than 65 years in RRT: HD and PD.

Exclusion criteria: Patients on hemodialysis for less than 3 months and patients with acute infection, or active neoplasia.

We studied their epidemiological and clinical profile, the different complications during RRT and the elements of the prognosis.

Clinical, biological and radiological parameters were identified from medical records. Patient's records were point data of patients at the time of the study in January 2015.

The ethics committee had no objections against this study since it reflects our clinical work habits and did not include supplementary measures (other biological or radiological examinations).

We performed a comparative study of these parameters between patients on HD and those in PD.

Baseline characteristics were described as means and standard deviations for continuous variables, and frequencies and proportions for categorical variables.

A study of the correlation was made between the various parameters by the statistical test CHI2. P value $\leq$ 0.05 was regarded as significant.

3. Results

Two groups of patients were included.

For the first group, there were 30 chronic HD patients, 13 women and 17 men representing 25% of all patients on HD. The average age was 71 ± 4.5 years. The initial nephropathy was vascular nephropathy in 7 cases, diabetic nephropathy in 11 cases, indeterminate nephropathy in 5 cases, chronic interstitial nephritis in 5 cases and nephropathy secondary to polycystic kidney disease in 2 cases. The age of initiation of hemodialysis was 69 ± 3.5 years.

Vascular access was an arteriovenous fistula (AVF) in 16 cases, an AV graft (AVG) in 2 cases and a tunneled catheter in 2 cases. Seven patients were anuric, 14 patients were oliguric and 9 patients had residual diuresis.

The number of sessions per week was 3 times in 8 cases, 2 times in 11 cases and only one session per week in 11 cases.

Several patients had comorbidities with myocardial infarction in 4 cases, heart rhythm disorder in 3 cases, sleep apnea syndrome in 2 cases, and dementia in 2 cases.

Fifteen patients were not autonomous. The impossibility of walking was observed in 3 cases, a limitation of walking in 7 cases, bilateral blindness in one case, and decreased auditory acuity in 4 cases.

The average hemoglobin (Hb) was 8.28 ± 1.9 g/dl, the mean serum cholesterol was 3.98 ± 1.01 mmol/l, the mean triglyceride level was 1.29 ± 0.9 mmol/l, the mean serum calcium was 2.1 ± 0.4 mmol/l, the mean serum phosphorus was 1.46 mmol /l ± 0.5, the mean parathyroid hormone (PTH) was 848.07 ± 490 pg/ml, the mean serum albumin was 31 ± 4.2 g/l.

Hemodynamic tolerance of hemodialysis was good in 14 cases only. Two deaths occurred following a cardiovascular complication.

The second group was concerning 12 patients on PD: 7 men and 5 women, having a mean age of 69.8 ± 3.5 years and representing 11.7% of all patients on PD. Seven were on automatic peritoneal dialysis and 5 on continuous ambulatory peritoneal dialysis. Kidney diseases were diabetes nephropathy in 58.3% of cases and vascular nephropathy in 41.6% of cases. Patients were not autonomous, they were helped by their children in 62.5% of cases and their partners in 38.5% of cases. Comorbidity was important: hypertension 91.6% of cases; Diabetes 66.6% of cases and heart disease 33.3% of cases.

Peritonitis was present in 5 cases, recurrent in 1 case. Staphylococcus was the causative organism in 3 cases.

The average biological values were: Hb: 9.6 ± 0.9 g/dl, Albumin: 27 ± 2.6 g/l, cholesterol: 4.1 ± 1 mmol/l, triglyceride: 1.09 ± 1.2 mmol/l, Serum Calcium: 2.21 ± 0.28 mmol/l, phosphorus: 1.79 ± 0.15 mmol/l and PTH: 524 ± 378 pg/ml.

One death occurred after a bronchopulmonary infection.

The differences on Socio-demographic characteristics, comorbidities and biological data between the 2 groups are presented in **Table 1**.

They were not statistically significant except for albumin level.

Table 1. Clinical and biological parameters.

	HD (N = 30)	PD (N = 12)	P
Age (Years)	71 ± 4.5	69.8 ± 3.5	0.1
Sex (M/F)	17/13	7/5	0.15
Diabetes (%)	11 (36.66%)	8 (66.66%)	0.09
HTA (%)	7 (23.33%)	11 (91.66%)	0.8
Heart Disease (%)	7 (23.33%)	4 (33.33%)	0.5
Dementia (%)	2 (0.06%)	0	0.9
No autonomy (%)	15 (0.5%)	8 (66.66%)	0.1
Death (%)	2 (6.66%)	1 (8.33%)	0.9
Hemoglobin (g/dl)	8.28 ± 1.9	9.6 ± 0.9	0.75
Albumin (g/l)	31 ± 4.2	27 ± 2.6	**0.05**
Calcium (mmol/l)	2.1 ± 0.4	2.21 ± 0.28	0.8
Phosphorus (mmol/l)	1.46 ± 0.5	1.79± 0.15	0.5
PTH (pg/ml)	848.07 ± 490	524 ± 378	0.07
Cholesterol (mmol/l)	3.98 ± 1.01	4.1 ± 1	0.1
Triglyceride (mmol/l)	1.29 ± 0.9	1.09 ± 1.2	0.5

4. Discussion

Reduced mortality and morbidity, prolongation of the patient's life, and better clinical outcomes of RRT allowed having older patients regularly monitored in dialysis units.

The age of patients with end-stage renal disease is increasing in all countries. The dialysis population is old with a median age mostly in the 60s and even over 70 years in some European regions [2]. In France, patients older than 75 years represent 40% of the patients who start RTT [3]. In Belgium, patients above 75 years comprise 41% of dialysis patients, as compared to 20% in the United Kingdom and 17% in Japan [4].

Older dialysis patients have a tendency to present later for dialysis, have a higher number of comorbid conditions, are at higher risk of cognitive dysfunction, impaired physical function, falls, poor nutrition and have increased levels of frailty [5] [6].

Old patients with terminal chronic renal failure can be offered conservative medical treatment or active renal replacement therapy. Advanced dementia and severe neurological sequels of stroke were shown as the conditions underlying the nephrologists' decision making not to provide dialysis in elderly patients [7].

The demographic, psychological, and health-related factors create a net of interdependences. Elderly patients with complex medical problems are a challenge to the health care team, clearly requiring the cooperation of physician, nurse, dialysis technician, social worker, dietician, physical medicine specialist, and a host of other subspecialists [8].

Many older patients do not have the opportunity for transplantation, so quality of life (QOL) in RRT is particularly important. The choice of dialysis modality has a major impact on many aspects of an individual's life [9].

A prospective study of incident and prevalent patients starting on dialysis over the age of 70 years, is the only study to have focused on older patients showed that outcomes, survival and QOL were not different for patients on HD and PD [10] [11].

The perception that older patients are more likely to have barriers to PD related to physical problems, social circumstances and cognitive dysfunction can result in the healthcare team believing that PD at home is not feasible in this patient group [12].

No difference in the course of functional status was observed between patients treated with PD or HD [13].

PD confers a substantial advantage in reducing rates of hospitalization for sepsis as compared with HD with central venous catheters among many older patients [14].

Risks and benefits of vascular access strategies in patients with differing life expectancies are controversial. AVF do not result in a lower lifetime risk of bacteremia compared with AVG in older patients without a permanent access at onset of ESRD, and that only those with longer life expectancy will benefit from pre-emptive AVF placement [14].

In our study, the differences on socio-demographic characteristics, comorbidities and biological data between the 2 groups of patients (HD and PD) were not statistically significant except for albumin level. This is probably due to the fact that there is a loss of albumin greater on DP compared to HD which adds to the poor nutrition on the elderly. However retrospective nature of our analysis and the small number of patients precludes any meaningful conclusion.

Recent studies suggested that dialysis provided a survival advantage compared to conservative management for most of stages 4 - 5 of chronic kidney disease patients over the age of 75. However, this advantage was lost for patients with multiple co-morbidities and ischemic heart disease [15] [16].

Regardless of the treatment choice, a multidisciplinary and multidimensional approach in the care of these patients is strongly needed [17].

5. Conclusions

Nephrologists are increasingly confronted with an elderly population of patients who have a large number of comorbid conditions requiring ongoing care.

Older patients on dialysis have unique needs and characteristics, and their outcomes vary from that of their younger counterparts.

RRT decision in the elderly requires consideration of functional and cognitive impairment and cardiovascular disease.

Both life expectancy and life quality should be taken into account.

Our results cannot be generalized because of the small size of our series.

Conflict of Interest

There are no conflicts of interest.

References

[1] Berger, J.R. and Hedayati, S.S. (2012) Renal Replacement Therapy in the Elderly Population. *Clinical Journal of the American Society of Nephrology*, **7**, 1039-1046. http://dx.doi.org/10.2215/CJN.10411011

[2] ERA-EDTA (2009) 2007 ERA-EDTA Annual Report. Ann Rep, 21 September 2009.

[3] Moranne, O., Couchoud, C. and Vigneau, C. (2012) Characteristics and Treatment Course of Patients Older than 75 Years, Reaching End-Stage Renal Failure in France. The PSPA Study. *The Journals of Gerontology: Series A*, **67**, 1394-1399. http://dx.doi.org/10.1093/gerona/gls162

[4] Canaud, B., Long, T., Tentori, F., Akiba, T., Karaboyas, A., Gillespie, B., *et al.* (2011) Clinical Practices and Outcomes in Elderly Hemodialysis Patients: Results from the Dialysis Outcomes and Practice Patterns Study (DOPPS). *Clinical Journal of the American Society of Nephrology*, **6**, 1651-1662. http://dx.doi.org/10.2215/CJN.03530410

[5] Kimmel, P.L., Cohen, S.D. and Weisbord, S.D. (2008) Quality of Life in Patients with End-Stage Renal Disease Treated with Hemodialysis: Survival Is Not Enough! *Journal of Nephrology*, **21**, S54-S58.

[6] Anand, S., Kurella Tamura, M. and Chertow, G.M. (2010) The Elderly Patients on Hemodialysis. *Minerva Urologica e Nefrologica*, **62**, 87-101.

[7] Clement, R., Chevalet, P., Rodat, O., Ould-Aoudia, V. and Berger, M. (2005) Withholding or Withdrawing Dialysis in the Elderly: The Perspective of a Western Region of France. *Nephrology Dialysis Transplantation*, **20**, 2446-2452. http://dx.doi.org/10.1093/ndt/gfi012

[8] Stel, V.S., Kramer, A., Zoccali, C. and Jager, K.J. (2009) The 2006 ERA-EDTA Registry Annual Report: A Precis. *Journal of Nephrology*, **22**, 1-12.

[9] Tamura, M.K., Tan, J.C. and O'Hare, A.M. (2012) Optimizing Renal Replacement Therapy in Older Adults: A Framework for Making Individualized Decisions. *Kidney International*, **82**, 261-269. http://dx.doi.org/10.1038/ki.2011.384

[10] Harris, S.A., Lamping, D.L., Brown, E.A. and Constantinovici, N., North Thames Dialysis Study (NTDS) Group. (2002) Clinical Outcomes and Quality of Life in Elderly Patients on Peritoneal Dialysis versus Hemodialysis. *Peritoneal Dialysis International*, **22**, 463-470.

[11] Lamping, D.L., Constantinovici, N., Roderick, P., Normand, C., Henderson, L., Harris, S., *et al.* (2000) Clinical Outcomes, Quality of Life, and Costs in the North Thames Dialysis Study of Elderly People on Dialysis: A Prospective Cohort Study. *The Lancet*, **356**, 1543-1550. http://dx.doi.org/10.1016/S0140-6736(00)03123-8

[12] Finkelstein, F.O., Afolalu, B., Wuerth, D. and Finkelstein, S.H. (2008) The Elderly Patient on CAPD: Helping Patients Cope with Peritoneal Dialysis. *Peritoneal Dialysis International*, **28**, 449-451.

[13] Jassal, S.V., Chiu, E. and Hladunewich, M. (2009) Loss of Independence in Patients Starting Dialysis at 80 Years of Age or Older. *The New England Journal of Medicine*, **361**, 1612-1613. http://dx.doi.org/10.1056/NEJMc0905289

[14] Tamura, M.K., Tan, J.C. and O'Hare, A.M. (2012) Optimizing Renal Replacement Therapy in Older Adults: A Framework for Making Individualized Decisions. *Kidney International*, **82**, 261-269. http://dx.doi.org/10.1038/ki.2011.384

[15] Murtagh, F.E., Marsh, J.E., Donohoe, P., Ekbal, N.J., Sheerin, N.S. and Harris, F.E. (2007) Dialysis or Not? A Comparative Survival Study of Patients over 75 Years with Chronic Kidney Disease Stage 5. *Nephrology Dialysis Transplantation*, **22**, 1955-1962. http://dx.doi.org/10.1093/ndt/gfm153

[16] Demoulin, N., Beguin, C., Labriola, L. and Jadoul, M. (2011) Preparing Renal Replacement Therapy in Stage 4 CKD Patients Referred to Nephrologists: A Difficult Balance between Futility and Insufficiency. A Cohort Study of 386 Patients Followed in Brussels. *Nephrology Dialysis Transplantation*, **26**, 220-226. http://dx.doi.org/10.1093/ndt/gfq372

[17] Kooman, J.P., Cornelis, T., van der Sande, F.M. and Leunissen, K.M. (2012) Renal Replacement Therapy in Geriatric End-Stage Renal Disease Patients: A Clinical Approach. *Blood Purification*, **33**, 171-176. http://dx.doi.org/10.1159/000334153

Abbreviations

Arteriovenous fistula: AVF
Arteriovenous graft: AVG
End stage renal disease: ESRD
Hemodialysis: HD
Hemoglobin: (Hb)
Peritoneal dialysis: PD
Parathyroid hormone: PTH
Quality of life: QOL
Renal replacement therapy: RRT

26

Why Did Sudanese End Stage Renal Failure Patients Refuse Renal Transplantation?

Amin S. Banaga[1*], Elaf B. Mohammed[2], Rania M. Siddig[2], Diana E. Salama[2],
Sara B. Elbashir[2], Mohamed O. Khojali[2], Rasha A. Babiker[3], Khalifa Elmusharaf[4],
Mamoun M. Homeida[5]

[1]Department of Medicine & Nephrology, University of Medical Sciences and Technology, Academy Charity Teaching Hospital, Khartoum, Sudan
[2]Clinical Research Assistants, Department of Nephrology, Academy Charity Teaching Hospital, Khartoum, Sudan
[3]Department of Basic Sciences, Faculty of Medicine, University of Medical Sciences & Technology, Khartoum, Sudan
[4]Department of Epidemiology & Public Health Medicine, Royal College of Surgeon in Ireland (RCSI), Dublin, Ireland
[5]Department of Medicine, Faculty of Medicine, University of Medical Sciences & Technology, Khartoum, Sudan
Email: [*]amin.banaga@gmail.com

Abstract

Renal transplantation remains the most effective treatment of End Stage Renal Failure (ESRF). In this cross sectional study we explore the reasons behind refusal of renal transplantation among adults' Sudanese haemodialysis patients. The subjects of the study are ESRF adults' patients on regular haemodialysis treatment in 15 haemdoialysis centres in Khartoum/Sudan. All patients who are on regular haemodialysis were interviewed by questionnaire to explore the reasons of refusal of renal transplantation. A total of 1583 ESRF adults' patients on regular haemodialysis have been participated in the study, 381 (24.1%) patients refused kidney transplantation. The mean age of patients refusing kidney transplantation was (58.5 + 15.1 years); 77.4% of them were ≥50 years old, 59.2% were males and 88.1% were unemployed, patients older than 50 years old and unemployed are tend to refuse renal transplantation (P < 0.001). The main reason of refusal was that the patients refuse to accept kidney from living donors (34.8%). 17.6% of patients decline kidney transplantation because of financial reason, 18.1% of patients refused to do transplantation because of fear of transplant surgery, 15.7% of patients believe that kidney transplantation is against their religious values, 11.9% of patients refused transplantation because they don't have enough knowledge on renal transplantation, only 0.5% of patients refuse transplantation because of side effect of immunosuppressive drugs. In conclusion, in this study we found that elderly and unemployed ESRF patients tend to refuse renal transplantation, the most important

---

[*]Corresponding author.

reason behind refusal of renal transplantation is refusal of accepting kidney donation from living related donors. This reflects the need for development of cadaveric donors program in the Sudan. ESRF patients need education and counseling on renal transplantation.

Keywords

Sudan, ESRF, Transplantation, Refusal

1. Introduction

Renal transplantation remains the most effective treatment of End Stage Renal Failure (ESRF). Only seven countries in Sub Saharan Africa (SSA) including Sudan have renal transplantation program [1]. Renal transplantation in Sudan is from living donors and no cadaveric donation program is available. The first patient transplanted from a living donor in Sudan was in 1974. Renal transplantation constitutes 28.4% of total Renal Replacement Therapy (RRT) in Sudan [2] [3].

Known the fact that renal transplantation improves the quality of life of ESRF patients, still some patients refuse renal transplantation. A previous study conducted in Sudan explored the barriers to kidney transplantation among 462 ESRF patients who are on maintenance haemodialysis [4]. In this study, we focused on ESRF patients who refused renal transplantation exploring in depth the main reasons behind their refusal and the determinants of their decision.

2. Materials and Methods

This study is a cross sectional hospital based descriptive study. All patients on regular haemodialysis in 15 hemodialysis centers in Khartoum-Sudan were approached to participate in the study in the period from 1/11/2014 to 1/12/2014. Out of 1602 patients a total of 1583 ESRF adults' patients on regular haemodialysis participated in the study with response rate of 98.8%. A questionnaire was used to collect the personal data (age, gender, occupation, duration of dialysis), and for those who refuse renal transplantation we explored the reasons for non acceptance of transplantation. We excluded haemodialysis patients who are less than 18 years old and haemodialysis unit where located in rural area of Khartoum State. Statistical analysis was performed using SPSS 21 software package (SPSS Inc, Chicago, IL, USA); results were presented in number, percent, mean and standard deviation. Chi-square and student t tests have been used to test the statistical significance and P values < 0.05 were considered significant. Ethical clearance was obtained from the ethics and research committees of the ministry of health/Sudan. Permission for the study was obtained from directors of the dialysis units. An informed consent was obtained from each patient participated in the study.

3. Results

A total of 1583 ESRF adults' patients on regular haemodialysis participated in the study, 381 (24.1%) patients refused kidney transplantation. The mean age ± (SD) of patients refusing kidney transplantation was 58.5 ± 15.1 years , 77.4% of them were ≥50 years old, 59.2% were males and 88.1% were unemployed (**Table 1**). In this study we found that patients who are older than 50 years old and unemployed tend to refuse renal transplantation (P < 0.0001) (**Table 1**).

The reasons of refusal of kidney transplantation are shown on **Table 2**. The main reason was that patients do not want to accept kidney from life related donors (34.8%). Other mentioned reasons were financial reason (17.6%), fear of transplant surgery (18.1%), believes that kidney transplantation is against their religious values (15.7%), they do not have enough knowledge on renal transplantation (13.4%), fear of the side effects of immunosuppressive drugs (0.5%).

4. Discussion

In this study, we found that elderly patients (≥50 years) tend to refuse renal transplantation more than young

Table 1. Characteristic of patients refuse kidney transplantation.

	Accept Transplantation	Refuse transplantation	P value
Age[1]	46.18 ±15.13 years	58.5±15.1 years	<0.0001
≥50 years old[2] <50 years old	530 (44.1%) 672 (55.9%)	295 (77.4%) 86 (22.6%)	<0.0001
Occupation[2]	Employed 331(27.5%) Unemployed 871 (72.5%)	Employed 44 (11.5%) Unemployed 337 (88.5%)	<0.0001
Gender[2]	Male 775 (64.5%) Female 427 (35.5%)	Male 229 (60.1%) Female 152 (39.9%)	0.12
Duration of dialysis[1]	4.37 ± 3.9 years	4.41 ± 4.96 years	0.89

[1]Mean ± SD. [2]Number (percentage).

Table 2. Reasons behind refusal of renal transplantation.

Reasons behind refusal of renal transplantation	Frequency (%)
Financial	67 (17.6%)
Fear of renal transplant surgery	69 (18.1%)
Refuse to accept kidney from living donors	132 (34.8%)
Religious	60 (15.7%)
Lack of knowledge about renal transplantation	51 (13.4%)
Immunosuppressive treatments side effects	2 (0.5%)

patients. As has been shown before in previous study, age was a factor in refusal of renal transplantation [5]. Patients who are employed tend to accept renal transplantation. This might reflect that frequent visits to hospital to receive hemodialysis affect the working life of our patients. However, we found no significant difference regarding gender or duration of dialysis.

Almost one in four ESRF patients refused to perform renal transplantation. Several studies pointed out that renal transplantation is associated with better quality of life when it compare with dialysis [6]-[8]. However, there were many studies reported increase number of patients who are refusing renal transplantation. In Morocco a study reported that 37.4% of ESRF patients were wouldn't like to go for renal transplantation [9]. In Slovenia, 13.7% of ESRF patients refused renal transplantation [10].

One in three patients who refused to go for renal transplantation stated that they do not want to accept kidney from living related donor. This raises the importance of establishing a cadaveric donor program in Sudan. In SSA, only South Africa has a cadaveric donor program [1]. Published data clearly reported that living kidney donation from healthy persons is associated with minimal perioperative risk [11]. A review of medical literature on living kidney donation found that unilateral nephrectomy is not harmful to healthy persons [12]. Increase awareness of ESRF patients and potential kidney donors about the living kidney donation is essential to increase the number of transplanted patients.

Financial constrains was one of the causes for refusal of renal transplantation despite that renal transplantation surgery in Sudan is free and the immunosuppressive treatments are distributed free for patients. However, patients and donors still need to pay for the necessary investigations and work-up pre transplant. On the other hand, some patients wish to do renal transplantation outside Sudan. The reason for that is the long waiting list. In previous study conducted in Sudan about attitude of patients toward renal transplantation reported that 24.2% of ESRF patients could not proceed to renal transplantation because of financial problems [4]. The same results were obtained from developed countries where reported that low socioeconomic status and lack of medical insurance was associated with failure of or delay of renal transplantation [13].

One in five of patients who refused renal transplantation were due to fear from the transplant surgery. There is a need to raise awareness about the risk of transplant surgeries. Transplanted patients have long term lower mortality risk in comparison with dialysis patients [14]. The survival rate after one year of transplantation is about 95% and around 90% on five years' post transplantation [15]. The quality of life is markedly improved with transplantation [16].

Among those who refused renal transplantation, 15.7% of patients reject transplantation because of religious reasons believing that Islam is against renal transplantation. Islam does not prohibit transplantation. In 1988, the Islamic Jurisprudence Assembly Council in Saudi Arabia approved cadaveric and live kidney donations [17]. The same decision about kidney donation has been approved in Iran and Egypt [18]. Despite that, some patients still refuse transplantation based on religious values in Muslims countries. One third of ESRF patient in Morocco refused transplantation on the belief that Islam is against it [9]. In a study conducted in Saudi Arabia, 26.2% believes that Islam is against renal transplantation [19]. So an increasing awareness is needed from Muslims' scholars and Islamic institutions to promote renal transplantation.

In the current study, 13.4% of those who refused transplantation stated that they have no enough information about renal transplantation. This reflects the poor counseling on renal transplantation, which should be carried out by physicians and following nephrologists. Several studies pointed out the attitude of health worker toward renal transplantation. In one study, 49% of physicians they did not agree with live kidney donation and 53% of them didn't have enough information on renal transplantation [20]. Other study, conducted in Tunisia, reported that 41% of physicians refused organ transplantation [21]. In previous study in Sudan among haemodialysis patients, 31.6% of patient reported that they haven't been counseled for renal transplantation [4]. Education of health workers about renal transplantation might play an important role in increasing the acceptance rate of kidney transplant among ESRF patients.

In the current study, we reported that a minority of patient (<1%) refused transplantation because they fear the side effect of immunosuppressive medications. In contrast, other study reported that side effects of immunosuppressive medications are a major reason behind refusal of renal transplantation among ESRF patients [5].

There was limitation in our study, we focused only in patients who refuse renal transplantation however more researches are needed to explore the barriers toward renal transplantation among patients who accept but couldn't perform renal transplantation, in other hand a decision of refusal of renal transplantation may be affected by the cause of the original kidney disease and definitely more researches are needed to explore such association.

5. Conclusion

In conclusion, in this study, we found that elderly and unemployed ESRF patients tend to refuse renal transplantation. The most important reason behind refusal of renal transplantation is refusal of accepting kidney donation from living related donors. This reflects the need to develop cadaveric donors program in Sudan. ESRF patients need education and counseling on renal transplantation.

References

[1]   Naicker, S. (2013) End-Stage Renal Disease in Sub-Saharan Africa. *Kidney International Supplements*, **3**, 161-163.

[2]   Suliman, S.M., Beliela, M.H. and Hamza, H. (1995) Dialysis and Transplantation in Sudan. *Saudi Journal of Kidney Diseases and Transplantation: An Official Publication of the Saudi Center for Organ Transplantation, Saudi Arabia*, **6**, 312-314.

[3]   Elamin, S., Obeid, W. and Abu-Aisha, H. (2010) Renal Replacement Therapy in Sudan, 2009. *Arab Journal of Nephrology and Transplantation*, **3**, 31-36. http://dx.doi.org/10.4314/ajnt.v3i2.58903

[4]   Abdelwahab, H.H., Shigidi, M.M.T., Ibrahim, L.S. and El-Tohami, A. (2013) Barriers to Kidney Transplantation among Adult Sudanese Patients on Maintenance Hemodialysis in Dialysis Units in Khartoum State. *Saudi Journal of Kidney Diseases and Transplantation*, **24**, 1044-1049. http://dx.doi.org/10.4103/1319-2442.118093

[5]   Nizič-Kos, T., Ponikvar, A. and Buturović-Ponikvar, J. (2013) Reasons for Refusing Kidney Transplantation among Chronic Dialysis Patients. *Therapeutic Apheresis and Dialysis*, **17**, 419-424. http://dx.doi.org/10.1111/1744-9987.12090

[6]   Maglakelidze, N., Pantsulaia, T., Tchokhonelidze, I., Managadze, L. and Chkhotua, A. (2011) Assessment of Health-Related Quality of Life in Renal Transplant Recipients and Dialysis Patients. *Transplantation Proceedings*, **43**, 376-379. http://dx.doi.org/10.1016/j.transproceed.2010.12.015

[7]   Chkhotua, A., Pantsulaia, T. and Managadze, L. (2011) The Quality of Life Analysis in Renal Transplant Recipients and Dialysis Patients. *Georgian Medical News*, **11**, 10-17.

[8]   Balaska, A., Moustafellos, P., Gourgiotis, S., Pistolas, D., Hadjiyannakis, E., Vougas, V. and Drakopoulos, S. (2006) Changes in Health-Related Quality of Life in Greek Adult Patients 1 Year after Successful Renal Transplantation. *Experimental and Clinical Transplantation: Official Journal of the Middle East Society for Organ Transplantation*, **4**, 521-524.

[9]   Kabbali, N., Mikou, S., El Bardai, G., Tazi, N., Ezziani, M., Batta, F., Arrayhani, M. and Houssaini, T. (2014) Attitude of Hemodialysis Patients toward Renal Transplantation: A Moroccan Interregional Survey. *Transplantation Proceedings*, **46**, 1328-1331. http://dx.doi.org/10.1016/j.transproceed.2014.03.008

[10]   Buturović-Ponikvar, J., Gubenšek, J., Arnol, M., Bren, A., Kandus, A. and Ponikvar, R. (2011) Dialysis Patients Refusing Kidney Transplantation: Data from the Slovenian Renal Replacement Therapy Registry. *Therapeutic Apheresis and Dialysis*, **15**, 245-249. http://dx.doi.org/10.1111/j.1744-9987.2011.00945.x

[11]   Weitz, J., Koch, M., Mehrabi, A., Schemmer, P., Zeier, M., Beimler, J., Büchler, M. and Schmidt, J. (2006) Living-Donor Kidney Transplantation: Risks of the Donor—Benefits of the Recipient. *Clinical Transplantation*, **20**, 13-16. http://dx.doi.org/10.1111/j.1399-0012.2006.00595.x

[12]   Tarantino, A. (2000) Why Should We Implement Living Donation in Renal Transplantation? *Clinical Nephrology*, **53**, 55-63.

[13]   Schold, J.D., Gregg, J.A., Harman, J.S., Hall, A.G., Patton, P.R. and Meier-Kriesche, H.-U. (2011) Barriers to Evaluation and Wait Listing for Kidney Transplantation. *Clinical Journal of the American Society of Nephrology*, **6**, 1760-1767. http://dx.doi.org/10.2215/CJN.08620910

[14]   Wolfe, R.A., Ashby, V.B., Milford, E.L., Ojo, A.O., Ettenger, R.E., Agodoa, L.Y., Held, P.J. and Port, F.K. (1999) Comparison of Mortality in All Patients on Dialysis, Patients on Dialysis Awaiting Transplantation, and Recipients of a First Cadaveric Transplant. *New England Journal of Medicine*, **341**, 1725-1730. http://dx.doi.org/10.1056/NEJM199912023412303

[15]   Briggs, J.D. (2001) Causes of Death after Renal Transplantation. *Nephrology Dialysis Transplantation*, **16**, 1545-1549. http://dx.doi.org/10.1093/ndt/16.8.1545

[16]   Evans, R.W., Manninen, D.L., Garrison Jr., L.P., Hart, L.G., Blagg, C.R., Gutman, R.A., Hull, A.R. and Lowrie, E.G. (1985) The Quality of Life of Patients with End-Stage Renal Disease. *New England Journal of Medicine*, **312**, 553-559. http://dx.doi.org/10.1056/NEJM198502283120905

[17]   Golmakani, M.M., Niknam, M.H. and Hedayat, K.M. (2005) Transplantation Ethics from the Islamic Point of View. *Medical Science Monitor*, **11**, RA105-RA109.

[18]   Einollahi, B. (2008) Cadaveric Kidney Transplantation in Iran: Behind the Middle Eastern Countries? *Iranian Journal of Kidney Diseases*, **2**, 55-56.

[19]   Mohamed, E. and Guella, A. (2013) Public Awareness Survey about Organ Donation and Transplantation. *Transplantation Proceedings*, **45**, 3469-3471. http://dx.doi.org/10.1016/j.transproceed.2013.08.095

[20]   Nadoushan, M.S., Heshmati, B.N., Pirsaraee, A.S., Nodoushan, I.S., Nadoushan, R.J. and Yazdi, F. (2014) Knowledge and Attitude of Iranian Physicians towards Organ and Tissue Donation. *International Journal of Organ Transplantation Medicine*, **5**, 66-70.

[21]   Tebourski, F., Jaouadi, N., Ben, A.D., Benamar-Elgaaied, A. and Ayed, M. (2003) Attitude of Health Personnel to Organ Donation and Transplantation. *La Tunisie Medicale*, **81**, 482-487.

27

Unusual Case of Idiopathic Membranous Later Developing Non-Hodgkin's Lymphoma

Rubina Naqvi

Department of Nephrology, Sindh Institute of Urology and Transplantation (SIUT), Karachi, Pakistan
Email: rubinanaqvi@gmail.com

Abstract

A 30-year-old male presented to nephrology services as a case of nephrotic syndrome and membranous nephropathy was found on renal biopsy. He was treated for this pathology with steroid and cytotoxic drugs and remained in remission for 3 years and then presented with non Hodgkin's lymphoma.

Keywords

Nephrotic Syndrome, Idiopathic Membranous Nephropathy, Non-Hodgkin's Lymphoma

1. Introduction

Membranous nephropathy is among the most common causes of the nephrotic syndrome in adults, accounting for up to one-third of biopsy diagnoses. Most common form in adults is idiopathic (approximately 75 percent of cases) while secondary could be due to a variety of drugs, infections, and underlying diseases. These include gold, penicillamine, systemic lupus erythematosus, malignancy, and hepatitis B and C virus infection [1]-[3].

We aim to present here an unusual case of a young male who initially came as idiopathic membranous nephropathy, treated, got remission for 3 years and then presented with non Hodgkin's lymphoma.

2. Case

A 30-year-old male was referred to nephrology clinic of Sindh Institute of Urology and Transplantation, which is a tertiary care center for nephro-urological disorders. He was a farmer by profession, in rural area of province of Sindh, living at a distance of 350 Km from this hospital, non-smoker, having history of asthma and atopic allergies for last at least 15 years, he only took salbutamol and steroid inhaler off and on for his asthma during this period and there was no history of herbal or homeopathic drug ingestion in past. Beside that he had history of acquiring pulmonary tuberculosis a year earlier, for which he received Rifampicin, Isoniazid, Ethambutol and

Pyrazinamide based antituberculous regimen for 8 months, he did required in addition indwelling catheter in pleural cavity for drainage of pleural effusion, which remained in for 4 - 5 days. He was father of 3 and there was no positive history of any medical condition in his siblings, parents or children.

At the time of presentation to this hospital, which was July 2004, he had generalized body swelling, passage of frothy urine and malaise of 2 months duration. There was no noticeable weight loss during this period. He was started on Prednisolone in dose of 0.65 mg/kg/day and on diuretics 10 days prior to referring to this hospital.

On examination at initial presentation he was afebrile with blood pressure of 120/80, heart rate of 80 beats per minute and weight of 57 Kg. He had bilateral pedal edema to the knees, periorbital swelling, no rash, no lymphadenopathy and normal jugular venous pressure. Abdomen was soft with ascitis and no organomegaly. Lungs auscultation revealed occasional fine basal crackles. Heart examination revealed regular rate and rhythm with no murmurs. Loco motor and nervous system examination was unremarkable.

Initial laboratory tests revealed Hemoglobin of 11.5, hematocrit 34, TLC 8, platelet 234, ESR 15 mm 1st hour, urea 18 mg/dl, creatinine 0.8 mg/dl, K 4.2, Na 139, Ca 7.0 mg/dl, albumin 1.4 g/dl, random blood sugar 121 mg/dl, liver enzymes and bilirubin were in normal limits, urinalysis revealed specific gravity of 1025, albumin 3+, no red cells, white cells, casts or crystal. 24 hours urinary protein excretion was 3.1 Gm. Abdominal sonography revealed normal size non hydronephrotic both kidneys, normal spleen and pancreas, thick walled gall bladder, mild hepatomegaly and minimal ascitis. Renal veins were patent bilaterally. Chest roentgenogram was unremarkable except for blunt right cardio phrenic angle. Echocardiography showed normal chambers and valves with mild pericardial effusion. Serological tests revealed within normal range immunoglobulins (IgA, IgG, and IgM) and complement levels (C3 and C4) and negative HbsAg, AntiHCV, ANA, AntiDNA, ASOT, RA factor and ANCA. Renal biopsy was initially postponed as he went in remission on steroids he was started before coming to us, which were tapered to stop at 4 months duration. He came in relapse in May 2005 and this time renal biopsy was done which showed membranous thickening and spikes (**Figure 1**).

After routine laboratory and radiological tests, diagnosis of idiopathic membranous nephropathy was made and he was started on diuretic, ARB, Prednisolone from 0.5 mg/kg/day and cyclophosphamide 2 mg/kg/day (cumulative dose of 160 mg/Kg). Steroid tapered to stop over 4 months. Edema disappeared at 4 weeks and proteinuria disappeared completely by 7 weeks of start of treatment.

This man remained in remission while examined in outpatient clinic in Jan. 2006, then June 2006. In Mar. 2007 he came to us with fever and productive cough of 10 days duration, was afebrile when examined, had no enlarged lymph-nodes, bilateral lower zone crackles over auscultation of lungs. He was still in remission, sputum was unremarkable. Chest roentgenogram reported as having opacifications in both lower lung fields suggestive of pulmonary infection. He was assessed by pulmonologist and given Levofloxacin and Klarithromycin for 10 days.

He returned in June 2007 with history of intermittent fever of 3 weeks duration, found afebrile in clinic, on chest auscultation right lower zone coarse crackles, and again treated with Levofloxacin.

His clinic follow up in May 2008 was unremarkable with no protein in urine and no active complaint. In Dec. 2008, he came with swelling of right eye with decrease in vision in this eye, fever with productive cough and significant weight loss over 2 - 3 weeks.

On examination found afebrile with blood pressure of 110/80, heart rate of 95 BPM had palpable cervical and preauricular lymph nodes on right side, which were mobile and non-tender. His right eye was bulged out, had mobility in all directions, conjunctiva was congested and pupils were non reactive. Intra ocular pressure was normal but visual acuity was reduced to 6/60. Left eye was normal.

Systemic examination revealed hepato-spleenomegaly, bilateral coarse crackles over lungs, no cardiac murmur, intact higher mental function and motor and sensory, except for local abnormality in right eye described earlier.

Routine laboratory tests were Hemoglobin 12, HCT 38, TLC 10 (N = 15%, L = 80%), Anisocytosis, normochromic, ESR 5 mm 1st hour, urea 19 mg/dl, creatinine 1 mg/dl, K 4.2, Na 140, Ca 7.8 mg/dl Alb 2.4 liver enzymes normal, Alk. phos. 75, LDH 176 IU/L (ref. range 90 - 180). Urinalysis specific gravity of 1020, no albumin, red blood cells, white blood cells, or casts. Cultures from urine blood and sputum found negative. Sputum also looked for acid fast bacilli on 3 occasions found negative.

On radiological work up chest roentgenogram showed wide mediastinum, CT chest showed mediastinal lymphadenopathy and patchy consolidation in basal segments of lower lobes, differential included lymphoma and

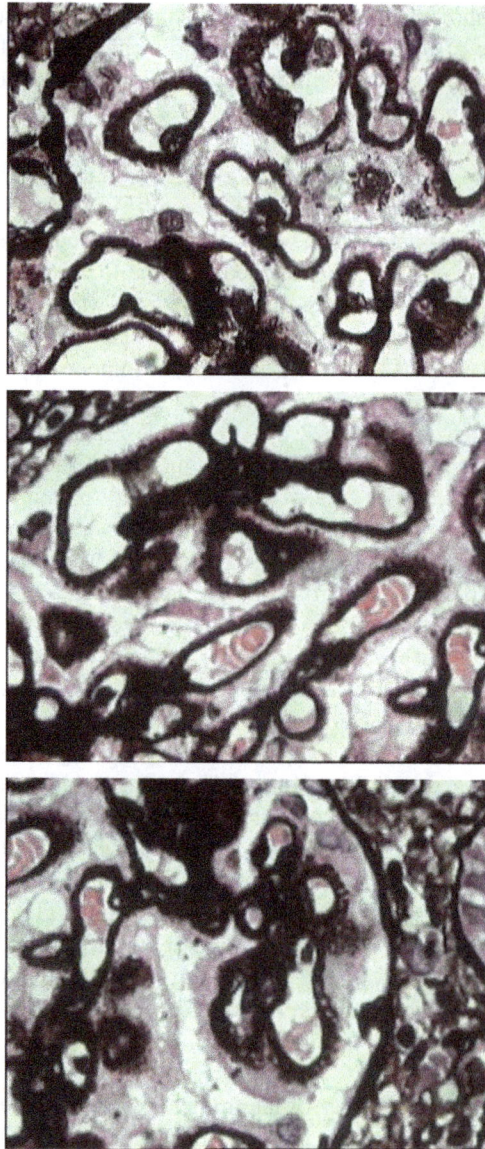

Figure 1. Renal biopsy low and medium power view of silver stain.

Wegener's (**Figure 2**). Abdominal CT revealed hypo dense area in upper pole of right kidney and multiple mesenteric, Para-aortic and inguinal lymph nodes of variable size (**Figure 3**). MRI head revealed soft tissue mass in right orbit (**Figure 4**).

Fluorescent Angiography revealed retinal detachment and area of hyper florescence with a small area of hypo-florescence in it (**Figure 5**).

Lymph node biopsy was performed which revealed diffuse sheets of small and medium size lymphoid cells (**Figure 6**). Tumor markers showed positivity of CD20 and scattered background cells were also positive for CD3 and CD138.

Bone Marrow biopsy performed which revealed hyper active marrow.

Patient received 4 cycles of CHOP (Jan., Feb., Mar., Apr. 2009), he tolerated cycles acceptably well except for transient decrease in cell line and derangement in renal function. He was last discharged from hospital on 16th Apr. 2009, with Hemoglobin of 11.3, TLC 10.1, Platelet 501 and serum creatinine 0.78. He was advised to come back for 5th cycle of chemotherapy scheduled for 5th May 2009, which he never did. When contacted on his cell number some relative informed that he died in quite after 2 weeks of leaving from hospital.

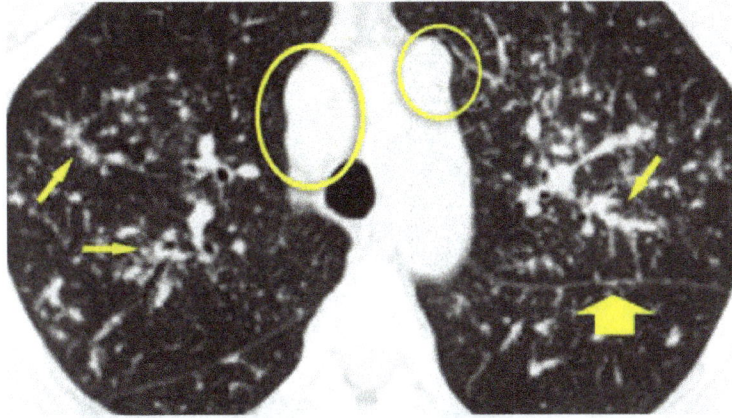

Figure 2. CT chest showing mediastinal enlarged lymph nodes and bilateral nodular infiltrates.

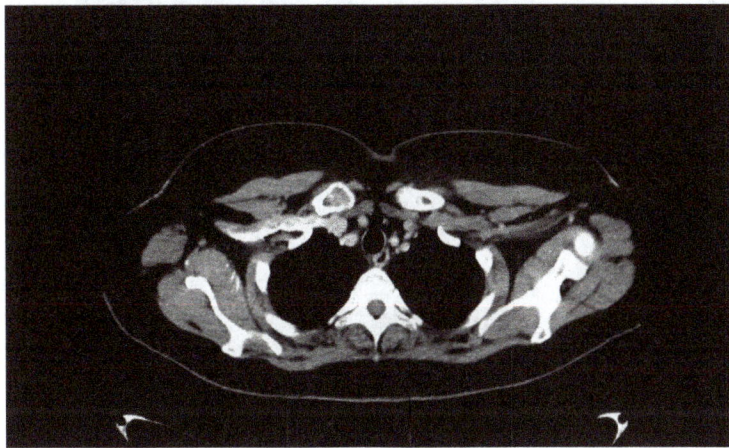

Figure 3. CT abdomen multiple enlarged lymph nodes.

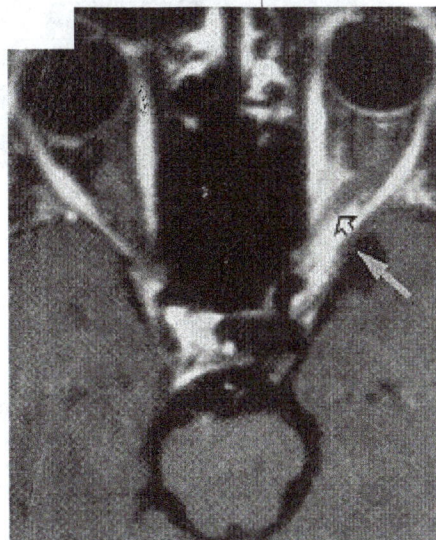

Figure 4. MRI brain after gadolinium enhancement reveals mass at the apex of the orbit (white arrow), causing displacement of optic nerve sheath (plain arrow).

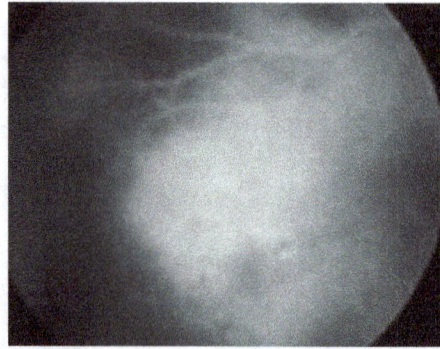

Florescent angiogram venous phase

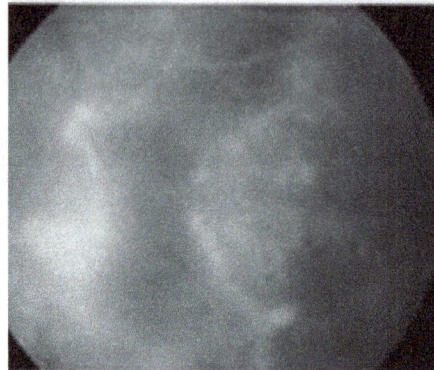

Florescent angiogram recirculation phase

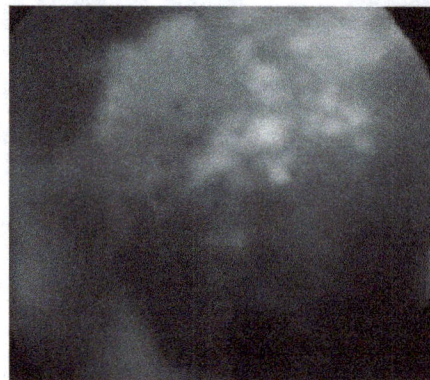

Florescent angiogram late phase

Figure 5. Lymphomatous sub retinal infiltrate.

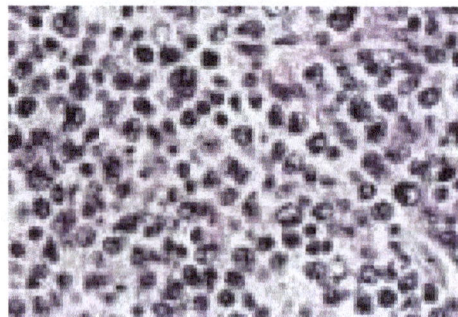

Figure 6. Lymph node biopsy diffuse lymphocytic infiltrates.

3. Discussion

Over 50 years ago David Jones identified the pathologic features of membranous nephropathy (MN); distinguishing it from other causes of nephrotic syndrome [4]. MN is characterized by uniform thickening of glomerular capillary wall which is caused by sub-epithelial deposits of immune complexes. In about two third of cases the etiology of MN is unknown and disease is called as idiopathic MN(IMN) [1]. IMN remains the most common cause of nephrotic syndrome in adults [2] [3]. Management of MN remained a topic of debate since early 1970s and consensus regarding therapy remains a question. Remuzzi *et al.* have published a review on immunosuppressive (IS) therapy for IMN, they included all randomized controlled trials (RCTs) on IS searching literature according to Cochrane Collaboration guidelines [5]. Their searches on 18 RCTs (1025 patients) proved no difference between IS therapy and placebo or no treatment group. Groups included here were steroid alone, alkylating agent alone or in combination with steroid, calcineurin inhibitor alone or in combination with steroid and anti-proliferative agent alone [5]. Whereas, a study from region (RCT) has proven favorable long term results of use of combination of steroid and cytotoxic in IMN [6]. As IMN is diagnosis of exclusion, a search for secondary causes of MN is a routine. History of NSAIDs, Solvents, Gold salts, Serological examination for HBV, HCV, SLE and radiological screening to evaluate any cancer are usual in any nephrology setting.

Published reports cite membranous nephropathy as the most common malignancy-associated glomerulopathy, occurring with many carcinomas and occasionally with leukemia and lymphoma [7].

Non-Hodgkin's lymphomas are a heterogeneous group of neoplasm arising from the lymphopoietic system including a wide range of subtypes of either B-cells or T-cells lymphomas. The few established risk factors for the development of these neoplasms include viral infections and immunological abnormalities, but their etiology remains largely unknown.

The immunomodulators can exhaust cytotoxic T lymphocytes and induce an imbalance in the control of EBV infection thus giving EBV associated B Cell lymphoma [8] [9]. We have not assessed EBV status in our patient, though our 90% general population is IgM positive for EBV (unpublished data).

Renal involvement as part of systemic lymphoma is quite frequent and most common presentation is with acute renal failure, glomerulonephritis has also rarely been reported in association with lymphoma [10].

A case of diffuse large B cell lymphoma been reported recently after treatment for aplastic anemia which was consisted of anti-thymocyte globulin and cyclosporine [11].

Our patient was a unique presentation; he initially had only IMN received cytotoxic and steroid combination therapy and after 3 years came with B cell non-Hodgkin's lymphoma. During this period he was coming up regularly and never raised any suspicion of lymphoproliferative disease. His interim presentation with respiratory symptoms could be any viral infection, which is all hypothetical. Reported prognosis of lymphoma with CHOP therapy is reasonably good but this patient was unfortunate enough of not having medical facilities available at his near distance.

4. Conclusion

More than one pathology can always exist, or one occurring after it should be kept in mind. Poor health care facilities in developing world continue to result in loss of young lives.

References

[1]   Pontecelli, C. (2007) Membranous Nephropathy. *Journal of Nephrology*, **20**, 268-287.

[2]   Cattarn, D.C. (2002) Membranous Nephropathy: Quo Vadis? *Kidney International*, **61**, 349-350. http://dx.doi.org/10.1046/j.1523-1755.2002.00125.x

[3]   Fervenza, F.C., Sethi, S. and Specks, U. (2008) Idiopathic Memranous Nephropathy: Diagnosis and Treatment. *Clinical Journal of the American Society of Nephrology*, **3**, 905-919. http://dx.doi.org/10.2215/CJN.04321007

[4]   Jones, D.B. (1957) Nephrotic Glomerulonephritis. *American Journal of Pathology*, **33**, 313-329.

[5]   Perna, A., Schieppati, A., Zamora, J., Giuliano, G.A., Braun, N. and Remuzzi, G. (2004) Immunnosuppressive Therapy for Idiopathic Memranous Nephropathy: A Systemic Review. *American Journal of Kidney Diseases*, **44**, 385-401. http://dx.doi.org/10.1053/j.ajkd.2004.05.020

[6]   Jha, V., Gangoli, A., Saha, T.K., Sud, K., Gupta, K.L., Joshi, K. and Sakhuja, V. (2007) A Randomized, Controlled Trial of Steroid and Cyclophosphamide in Adults with Nephrotic Syndrome Caused by Idiopathic Memranous Nephropathy. *Journal of the American Society of Nephrology*, **18**, 1899-1904. http://dx.doi.org/10.1681/ASN.2007020166

[7]   Gupta, K., Nada, R., Das, A. and Kumar, M.S. (2008) Membranoproliferative Glomerulonephritis in a Carcinoma with Unknown Primary: An Autopsy Study. *Indian Journal of Pathology and Microbiology*, **51**, 230-233. http://dx.doi.org/10.4103/0377-4929.41665

[8]   Richendollar, B.G., His, E.D. and Cook, J.R. (2009) Extramedullary Plasmacytoma like Posttransplantation Lympho-proliferative Disorders: Clinical and Pathological Features. *American Journal of Clinical Pathology*, **132**, 581-588. http://dx.doi.org/10.1309/AJCPX70TIHETNBRL

[9]   Hasserjian, R.P., Chen, S., Perkin, S.L., del Leval, L., Kinney, M.C., Barry, T.S., Said, J., Lim, M.S., Finn, W.G., Me-deiros, L.J., Harris, N.L. and O'Malley, D.P. (2009) Immunomodulator Agent Related Lymphoproliferative Disorders. *Modern Pathology*, **22**, 1532-1540.

[10] Da'as, N., Polliak, A., Cohen, Y., Amir, G., Darmon, D., Kleinman, Y., Goldfarb, A.W. and Ben-Yahuda, D. (2001) Kidney Involvement and Renal Manifestation in Non-Hodgkin's Lymphoma and Lymphocytic Leukemia: A Retros-pective Study in 700 Patients. *European Journal of Haematology*, **67**, 158-164. http://dx.doi.org/10.1034/j.1600-0609.2001.5790493.x

[11] Suzuki, Y., Niitsu, N., Hayama, M., Katayama, T., Ishii, R., Osaka, M., Miyazaki, K., Danbara, M., Horie, R., Yoshida, T., Nakamura, N. and Higashihara, M. (2009) Lymphoproliferative Disorders after Immunosuppressive Therapy for Aplastic Anemia: A Case Report and Literature Review. *Acta Haematologica*, **121**, 21-26. http://dx.doi.org/10.1159/000209225

28

Renal Cortical Necrosis:
An Unusual Complication of
Plasmodium malariae Malaria

Ahmed Tall Lemrabott[1*], Mouhamadou Moustapha Cissé[1], Sidy Mohamed Seck[2], Elhadji Fary Ka[1], Maria Faye[1], Aliou Ndongo[1], Cherif Dial[3], Younoussa Keita[1], Khodia Fall[1], Abdou Niang[1], Boucar Diouf[1]

[1]Department of Nephrology, Aristide Le Dantec University Hospital, Dakar, Senegal
[2]Faculty of Medicine, Gaston Berger University, Saint-Louis, Senegal
[3]Anatomo-Pathology Laboratory, Grand-Yoff General Hospital, Dakar, Senegal
Email: *ahmedtall35@hotmail.com

Abstract

Renal cortical necrosis (RCN) is anecdotal in malaria. To our knowledge, RCN secondary to *Plasmodium malariae* has not yet been published. We report a case of severe malaria complicated by RCN. A 29 year old Senegalese patient was transferred to our department for anuria in a context of severe malaria. The diagnosis was RCN secondary to a severe *Plasmodium malariae* malaria. Physical examination showed anuria, anaemic syndrome, haemorrhagic syndrome and a generally impaired condition. There was a normocytic normochromic anaemia aplastic, thrombocytopenia leukocytosis of 11.580/mm^3, serum creatinine of 12.45 mg/dl and blood urea of 252 mg/dl. The *Plasmodium malariae* had been shown to thick blood film with high parasite density. The molecular study was able to confirm the infestation of this parasite. Treatment consisted of four haemodialysis sessions and antimalarial molecules. Initial evolution was favourable with a recovery through diuresis and a partial improvement in renal function. Given the persistence of impaired renal function, a renal biopsy was performed. This confirmed the RCN. At last consultation, he had no symptoms and his last glomerular filtration rate (GFR) was 30 mL/min/1.73 m^2.

Keywords

Renal Cortical Necrosis, *Plasmodium malariae*, Acute Kidney Injury, Malaria

---

*Corresponding author.

1. Introduction

Malaria is a major public health problem with significant morbidity and mortality in sub-Saharan Africa [1]. Life-threatening malaria is mainly determined by visceral effects including kidney damage [1]. These lesions are varied, including renal cortical necrosis (RCN), although this remains anecdotal. Several cases of RCN secondary to infestation by *Plasmodium falciparum* and *Plasmodium vivax* have been published. To our knowledge, RCN secondary to *Plasmodium malariae* (*PM*) has not been published. We propose to present the case of a patient who presents severe malaria with *PM* complicated by kidney failure as RCN.

2. Case Report

Mr. D.S., a 29 year old Senegalese patient, was transferred on 09/11/2012 to the Department of Nephrology at Aristide Le Dantec University Hospital in Dakar, for the management of persistent anuria in a context of severe malaria.

He suddenly complained on November 2nd, 2012 of intense and permanent headaches and profuse bilious vomit. This was followed a few hours later by polyarthralgia and intense myalgia. He felt worse on the night of 06 to 07/11/2012 with the appearance of high fever and profuse sweating. He had been prescribed an oral anti-malarial treatment (based on an Artemisinin derivative) at a local health clinic. Generalised tonic-clonic seizures and persistent fever had caused his transfer to the Department of Infectious Diseases at Fann University Hospital Centre where he stayed three days. A gradual break in his diuresis appeared, progressing to persistent anuria which led to a transfer to the Department of Nephrology at the Aristide Le Dantec University Hospital.

At admission, the patient was conscious. He was afebrile. He had a pulse rate of 102/min, respiratory rate of 19/min and his blood pressure was 130/90 mm Hg. Physical examination revealed a total lack of diuresis, bilateral and symmetrical oedema of the lower limbs, anaemic syndrome, haemorrhagic syndrome with bilateral epistaxis and gingival bleeding, and ascites of moderate abundance.

Biological investigations at admission revealed: anaemia normochromic normocytic hypoplastic with haemoglobin at 7.8 g/dl, thrombocytopenia 72,000/mm^3, leukocytosis 11,580/mm^3, creatinine 12.45 mg/dl, blood urea 252 mg/dl, serum calcium 8.2 mg/dl and hyperphosphatemia 9.67 mg/dl. In blood electrolytes, sodium was 127 mmol/l, potassium 4.5 mmol/l. Transaminases were normal with SGOT 21.6 IU/l, and SGPT 26.9 UI/l. blood sugar was 90 g/dl. CRP was 9.6 mg/dl (**Table 1**).

On the third day after his admission, investigation of urine revealed that 24 h urine volume was 400 ml, urine protein 0.04 g/day, leukocytes 5208/min and erythrocytes 3472/min.

Table 1. Showing laboratory values.

Laboratory parameter	Laboratory result	Normal range
Hemoglobin (g/dl)	7.8	12 - 16
Total leucocytes count (/mm^3)	11,580	4000 - 10,000
Platelet count (/mm^3)	72,000	150 - 350,000
Blood urea (mg/dl)	252	15 - 45
Serum creatinine (mg/dl)	12.45	0.6 - 1.2
Serum sodium (mmol/l)	127	135 - 145
Serum potassium (mmol/l)	4.5	3.5 - 5.5
SGPT* (U/l)	26.9	5 - 35
SGOT* (U/l)	21.6	5 - 40
Blood sugar (g/dl)	90	70 - 110
Serum calcium (mg/dl)	8.5	8.5 - 10.5
Serum phosphorus (mg/dl)	9.67	2.5 - 4.5
Parasitemia load (trophozoites/μl)	18,402	0

*SGOT: serum glutamic-oxaloacetic transaminase; *SGPT: serum glutamic-pyruvic transaminase.

The *Plasmodium malariae* was highlighted in the thick coloured drop by 10% of Giemsa. This led to the identification of the trophozoites, schizonts and gametocytes of *P. malariae* (**Figure 1**). Molecular diagnostics, based on the amplification of ribosomal gene 18S, had identified a band at 144 bases pair confirming infection with *P. malariae* (**Figure 2**). The parasitemia load was 18,402 trophozoites/μl.

An abdominal ultrasound showed normal sized kidneys with poor cortico-medullary differentiation.

Treatment consisted of: parenteral quinine salt at 250 mg three times daily for five days followed by a relay with oral association Artemether-Lumefantrine, furosemide at a dose of 250 mg/day on Day 1 and 500 mg/day on Day 2 and 3 to stimulate diuresis and fluid restriction.

A worsening of renal impairment (serum creatinine at 16.62 mg/dl, blood urea to 313 mg/dl and hyperkalemia 6.4 mmol/l) occurred on the fourth day of hospitalization. Renal replacement therapy was therefore indicated. In total, the patient received four sessions of haemodialysis. Secondarily, evolution during hospitalisation was favourable with a recovery of diuresis to 2 litres per day, a partial improvement of renal function (creatinine decreased from 12.7 mg/dl on 20/11/2012 at 3.45 mg/dl on 02/12/2013) and a normalisation of the platelets count. Normocytic normochromic anaemia persisted to 9.9 g/dl, however.

Given the persistence of impaired renal function, renal biopsy was realised and showed an abundant and mutilating band of interstitial fibrosis encompassing destroyed glomeruli (**Figure 3**). This fibrosis band around areas of parenchyma preserved tubular atrophy (**Figure 4**) and 80% of nephron reduction, a secondary segmental

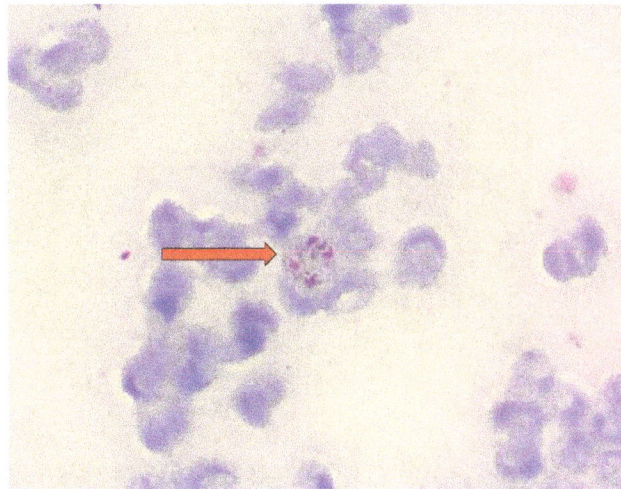

Figure 1. Giemsa-stained thin smear of patient'speripheral blood: Trophozoites of *Plasmodium malariae* "Basket-form"(arrow) × 1000.

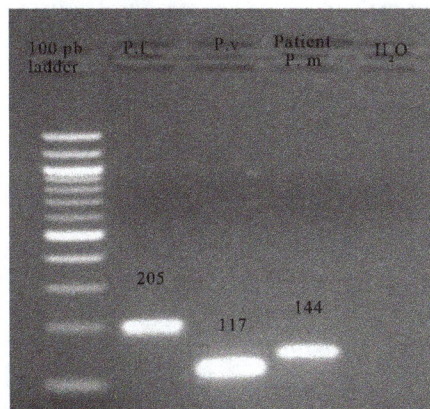

Figure 2. Confirmation of *Plasmodium malariae* by molecular biology. *P.v*: *Plasmodium vivax*, *P.f*: *Plasmodium falciparum*, *P.m*: *Plasmodium malariae*.

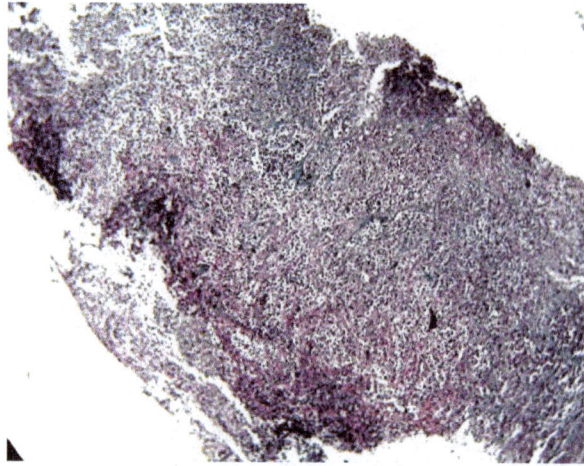

Figure 3. Zone of total necrosis of the renal parenchyma. Masson Trichrome × 200.

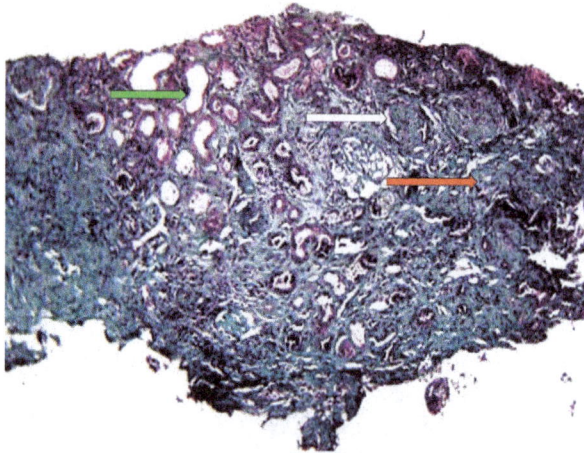

Figure 4. Area of diffuse inter stitial fibrosis (red arrow) tubularatrophy (green arrow) and glomerulosclerosis (white arrow). Masson Trichrome × 200.

lesions glomerulosclerosis according to 30% of residual glomeruli. This element was in favour of subtotal cortical necrosis. The patient is currently monitored as a nephrology outpatient. At his last check up, he had a good general condition and his GFR was 30 mL/min/1.73 m^2.

3. Discussion

Post-malaria renal failure occurs in the context of severe malaria [2]. In developing countries, the incidence of acute kidney injury (AKI) in malaria is not known, but in hospital studies, it ranges from 6% to 30.4% of cases [3] [4].

Acute tubulointerstitial nephropathy is the most common complication [5], however, cortical necrosis is exceptional and prognosis is especially bad in its complete form [3] [5]-[7]. To our knowledge, this clinical case remains the first RCN post-malaria *Plasmodium malariae* reported in sub-Saharan Africa and the world.

RCN is a rare clinicopathological AKI form. It consists of a bilateral ischemic necrosis, symmetrical, "patchy" diffuse to renal cortex, sparing the renal medulla and a thin strip of subscapular cortex [8]. The prognosis of RCN is often pejorative, requiring the use of chronic haemodialysis, apart from cases where segmental renal cortical necrosis and delayed partial recovery can be observed.

RCN post-malaria remains unusual. To our knowledge, four cases have been reported [3] [6] [7] [9]. The first two cases involved the RCN post *Plasmodium falciparum* [3] [7]. The third and fourth cases, published in 2012 and 2014, dealt with *Plasmodium vivax* RCN [6] [9].

RCN in malaria can be explained by four main phenomena: massive intravascular haemolysis causing haemoglobinuria; dehydration and hypovolemia secondary to fever, with profuse sweating, a lack of water intake and digestive disorders resulting in renal hypoperfusion, also cytoadherence and erythrocyte sequestration with intravascular coagulation, head of hypoperfusion, and monocyte activation with release of free radicals. The first two mechanisms were excluded in our patient because there was no clinicobiological evidence for a massive intravascular haemolysis or severe hypovolemia. In our case, the RCN could have been due to cytoadherence and erythrocyte sequestration with intravascular and/or coagulation monocyte activation with the release of free radicals [2].

Clinically, the patient had persistent anuria. In RCN, the main symptom for Chugh and Kleinknecht [10] [11] was anuria that was almost constant. The patient had clinical anaemia on admission. On CBC (count blood cells), this anaemia was normochromic normocytic hypoplastic (reticulocyte count in 5680/mm^3) with 7.8 g/dl of haemoglobin. The aplastic anaemia could be explained by dyserythropoiesis. The increase in inflammatory cytokines TH1 has effects on bone marrow, inducing cell hyperplasia and dyserythropoiesis, resulting in a slowing in production of reticulocytes, and anaemia. Some authors believe that the effect of cytokines alone cannot explain the significant morphological changes observed in the spinal cord and suggest that this is a direct effect of haemozoin [12]. Haemorrhagic disease in our patient could be explained by the DIC (disseminated intravascular coagulation). This haemorrhagic syndrome may be missing. Indeed, disorders of haemostasis occur, and about half the time, only by a biological syndrome [13].

In the imaging plane, only renal ultrasonography was performed in our patient. It objectified normal size of kidneys with poor cortico-medullary differentiation. The same result was reported in the observation of Baliga and Singhal [3] [7].

The hypothesis of RCN was raised after unfavourable evolution after three weeks of renal function. Confirmation was made by renal biopsy, although this is not necessary for retaining the diagnosis of RCN. Other paraclinical investigations such as renal Doppler, "microbubble" ultrasound or ultrasound contrast, abdomen and pelvis scan or renal MAG3 scintigraphy [14] may be sufficient.

Our patient had the "patchy" form with striped lesions peppered with normal parenchyma. In all four cases published in the literature, the type of RCN has not been clarified [3] [6] [7] [9]. Our patient also had tubulointerstitial lesions as interstitial fibrosis, and tubular atrophy with a case of tubular ghosts. These lesions were also identified in three of the reported cases of RCN post-malaria [3] [6] [7] [9].

In addition to the lesions described above, this patient had an 80% reduction in nephron lesions, with 30% segmental focal glomerulosclerosis in residual glomeruli. This "secondary" SFG is the result of secondary podocytes lesions, demonstrations of functional adaptation and/or structural. RCN is one of its causes.

Plasmodium malariae, which was responsible for RCN in our case, has never been implicated in RCN. Only *Plasmodium falciparum* and *vivax* have been reported so far [3] [6] [7] [9].

Our patient recovered partial renal function. After 18 months of follow-up, he had normal diuresis and stable renal function with a GFR 30 ml/min/1.73 m^2 according to MDRD formula. Of the three cases published on RCN post-malaria, one remained on dialysis [7]; change was not reported for the second case [3], and the third and fourth cases partially recovered and were released from dialysis [6] [9]. Cortical necrosis in our patient was associated with subtotal tubular damage may explain the early anuria, the recovery of diuresis and improvement in renal function.

4. Conclusion

Our case report demonstrates that *Plasmodium malariae* malaria may cause RCN, similar to other forms secondary to *Plasmodium vivax* and *Plasmodium Falciparum*.

Acknowledgements

We would like to thank Dr. Dial Cherif, Anatomo-Pathology Laboratory, Grand-Yoff General Hospital, Dakar, Senegal; and Dr. Badiane Aida, Parasitology Laboratory, Aristide Le Dantec University Hospital.

Conflit of Interest

The authors declare that there is no conflict of interest regarding the publication of this paper.

References

[1]   White, N.J., Pukrittayakamee, S., Hien, T.T., Faiz, M.A., *et al.* (2014) Malaria. *The Lancet*, **383**, 723-735. http://dx.doi.org/10.1016/S0140-6736(13)60024-0

[2]   Mishra, S.K. and Das, B.S. (2008) Malaria and Acute Kidney Injury. *Seminars in Nephrology*, **28**, 395-408. http://dx.doi.org/10.1016/j.semnephrol.2008.04.007

[3]   Baliga, K.V., Narula, A.S., Khanduja, R., Manrai, M., Sharma, P. and Mani, N.S. (2008) Acute Cortical Necrosis in Falciparum Malaria: An Unusual Manifestation. *Renal Failure*, **30**, 461-463. http://dx.doi.org/10.1080/08860220801964293

[4]   Kunuanunua, T.S., Nsibu, C.N., Gini-Ehungu, J.-L., Bodi, J.M., Ekulu, P.M., *et al.* (2013) Acute Renal Failure and Severe Malaria in Congolese Children Living in Kinshasa, Democratic Republic of Congo. *Néphrologie & Thérapeutique*, **9**, 160-165. http://dx.doi.org/10.1016/j.nephro.2013.01.001

[5]   Brocherion, I. and Ferlicot, S. (2008) Glomérulonéphrite et infections parasitaires. In: Noel, L.-H., Ed., *Atlas de Pathologie Rénale*, Flammarion, Paris, 261-283.

[6]   Kute, V.B., Vanikar, A.V., Ghuge, P.P., Patel, M.P., Patel, H.V., *et al.* (2012) Renal Cortical Necrosis and Acute Kidney Injury Associated with *Plasmodium vivax*: A Neglected Human Malaria Parasite. *Parasitology Research*, **111**, 2213-2216. http://dx.doi.org/10.1007/s00436-012-2975-x

[7]   Singhal, M.K., Arora, P., Kher, V., Pandey, R., Gulati, S., *et al.* (1997) Acute Cortical Necrosis in Falciparum Malaria: An Unusual Cause of End-Stagerenal Disease. *Renal Failure*, **19**, 491-494. http://dx.doi.org/10.3109/08860229709047736

[8]   Laurer, D.P. and Schreiner, G.E. (1958) Bilateral Renal Cortical Necrosis. *American Journal of Medicine*, **24**, 519-529. http://dx.doi.org/10.1016/0002-9343(58)90292-4

[9]   Kumar, R., Bansal, N., Jhorawat, R., Kimmatkar, P.D. and Malhotra, V. (2014) Renal Cortical Necrosis: A Rare Complication of *Plasmodium vivax* Malaria. *Indian Journal of Nephrology*, **24**, 390-393. http://dx.doi.org/10.4103/0971-4065.133789

[10]   Hiault, C., Dequiedt, P., Benoit, O., *et al.* (1982) Post Partumrenal Cortical Necrosis. *Journal de Gynécologie Obstétrique et Biologie de la Reproduction*, **11**, 839-848.

[11]   Kleinknecht, D., Grünfeld, J.P., Gomez, P.C., Moreau, J.-F. and Garcia-Torres, R. (1973) Diagnostic Procedures and Long-Term Prognosis in Bilateral Renal Cortical Necrosis. *Kidney International*, **4**, 390-400. http://dx.doi.org/10.1038/ki.1973.135

[12]   Mohandas, N. and An, X. (2012) Malaria and Human Red Blood Cells. *Medical Microbiology and Immunology*, **4**, 593-598. http://dx.doi.org/10.1007/s00430-012-0272-z

[13]   Levi, M. (2009) Guidelines for the Diagnosis and Management of Disseminated Intravascular Coagulation. *British Journal of Haematology*, **145**, 24-33. http://dx.doi.org/10.1111/j.1365-2141.2009.07600.x

[14]   Pruijm, M., Ponte, B., Hofmann, L., *et al.* (2011) New Radiological Techniques to Investigate Patients Suffering from Chronic Kidney Disease. *Revue Médicale Suisse*, **7**, 505-509.

29

Prevalence and the Risk Factors of Renal Insufficiency in the City of Saint Louis in Senegal

Ahmed Tall Lemrabott[1*], Mouhamadou Moustapha Cisse[1], Elhadji Fary Ka[1],
Sidy Mohamed Seck[2], Maria Faye[1], Moussa Sarr[1], Ngoné Diaba Gaye[3], Alassane Mbaye[3],
Abdou Niang[1], Boucar Diouf[1], Abdoul Kane[3]

[1]Department of Nephrology, Aristide Le Dantec University Hospital, Dakar, Senegal
[2]Faculty of Medicine, Gaston Berger University, Saint-Louis, Senegal
[3]Department of Cardiology, Grand-Yoff General Hospital, Dakar, Senegal
Email: [*]ahmedtall35@hotmail.com

Abstract

Background: The true scale of renal insufficiency (RI) in Sub-Saharan Africa remains unknown due to the lack of national registries. The aim of this study is to describe the epidemiological characteristics of renal insufficiency in urban areas in Saint Louis of Senegal. Materials and Methods: It is an observational, cross-sectional and descriptive study. The study was conducted during 27 days starting from 3 to 30 May 2010. All senegalese residents of Saint Louis (older than 15 years at the time of the study) in whom creatinine clearance was performed were included in the study. The sampling method used was a systematic random sampling, stratified cluster. The survey was designed by an expert comitee based on STEPS survey of the World Health Organization. RI was defined as a glomerular filtration rate (GFR) < 60 ml/min/1.73m^2. Results: Among 1424 people initially selected a final selection of 1416 was made. The sex ratio was 0.45. The mean age was 43.4 ± 17.8 years. The overall prevalence of renal insufficiency according to MDRD (Modification of diet in renal disease) formula was 181 cases or 12.7%. The mean age of the people with renal insufficiency was 47.6 ± 17.4 years. Renal insufficiency was correlated to height blood pressure (p = 0.01) and Physical inactivity (p = 0.0001). The prevalence of renal insufficiency was higher in diabetics (71.4%) and obese people (66.6%) than in non-diabetics (64.9%) and non-obese people (56.5%), although the difference was not statistically significant. Dyslipidemia and smoking were not correlated to the risk of occurrence of IR. Conclusions: This study reports the increasing magnitude of RI and its risk factors in the city of Saint Louis in Senegal. It is imperative to establish à national prevention strategies to avoid the dizzying growth of this scourge.

[*]Corresponding author.

Keywords

Renal Insufficiency, Risk Factors, GFR, Saint-Louis, Senegal

1. Introduction

The incidence of renal insufficiency (RI) is growing worldwide in general and in developing countries in particular [1]. In Africa, the real incidence of the disease remains unknown due to the lack of national registries [2]-[4]. In tropical Africa, the impact of environmental and socio-cultural factors on the incidence of RF is more important than the same factors in developed countries. They have changed the epidemiological profile of renal insufficiency in that part of the world. The poor socio-economic conditions and limited access to specialized medical care return the management of CRF more difficult [2].

In Senegal, there is no national registry of kidney failure, and this disease is not listed in reports of the peripheral health structures. The management of the disease poses enormous difficulties because of the serious lack of epidemiological data and the meager means available (few specialist physicians, inadequate number of dialysis centers). Thus, we note a real need to undertake studies to better understand this disease.

The objective of this study is to describe the epidemiological characteristics of renal insufficiency in urban areas in Saint Louis, Senegal.

2. Materials and Methods

An observational, cross-sectional and descriptive study was carried out in Saint Louis located in the north of Senegal [5]. This is the third largest city in Senegal with an estimated population of 271,912 habitants and a surface area of 250 Km^2. The study was conducted during 27 days starting from 3 to 30 May 2010. All senegale seresidents of Saint Louis (older than 15 years at the time of the study) in whom creatinine clearance was performed were included in the study.

Pregnant women, those who refused to participate in the study or whose survey was incomplete or unusable were not included.

The sampling method used was a systematic random sampling, stratified cluster.

Several levels were defined according to the age, with household as sampling unit. The sampling framework was based on Saint Louis' general and housing census. Taking an accuracy of 2%, an expected prevalence of 6.7% and a confidence level of 95%, the calculated sample size was 600 persons. To avoid the cluster effect, the minimum sample size was increased to 1200 persons.

A total of 120 clusters of 10 people were randomly selected to form the study sample. The random selection was made on the basis of proportional probabilities to the size of district.

The more populated was the area the more clusters was selected. In each area, several sociological centers have been identified as centers of clusters. There, directions were randomly selected then interviewers moved forward home by home, recruiting the eligible adults until reaching the number of 10 people in each cluster.

The survey was designed   by an expert comitee based on STEPS survey of the World Health Organization [6]. The form contained 59 questions divided into four sections:
- Social and demographic data;
- Habits and lifestyle: Smoking and physical activity;
- Medical history: Collecting information about hypertension, diabetes, dyslipidemia, healthy lifestyles and family history;
- Clinical parameters and laboratory tests.

Data were collected at the interviewee's home by medical and paramedical personnel. The recruitment was done after signing the consent by the interviewee.

Blood pressure was taken using an electronic sphygmomanometer type OMRON M6. Two values of blood pressures spaced at least of 10 minutes were systematically taken for each subject. Systolic and diastolic blood pressures were taken at rest, on the both arms. The highest numbers were selected.

The weighing was done with a scale placed on a stable and plane surface, the subject was dressed with light clothes and no shoes. The weight unit was kilogram (kg).

A portable measuring rod was used to measure the subject height wearing neither shoes nor hat. The height was assessed in centimeters.

Waist circumference measured by using a new standard tape meter, applied directly to the skin

Kinetic creatinine method was used for the creatinine measurement. Other biological data (Fasting blood sugar, cholesterol, triglyceride and uric acid) were collected from all people included, after a blood test with an automatic controller device, the Reflotron Plus®. A Fasting blood sugar was performed for whom presented a blood sugar >1.26 g/l in first assay.

Operational definitions used in this study were:

Renal insufficiency:

Renal insufficiency (RI) was defined as a glomerular filtration rate (GFR) < 60 ml/min/1.73m². Creatinine clearances were calculated using the MDRD (Modification of diet in renal disease) formula.

Hypertension: All known cases with high blood pressure or anyone with systolic blood pressure ≥ 140 or diastolic blood pressure ≥ 90 mmHg.

Diabetes mellitus: Any known diabetic case or Fasting blood sugar higher than 1.26 g/l, tested two times.

Dyslipidemia: Anyone known with dyslipidemia or with one or more of the following abnormalities:
- Dyslipidemia type I: hypertriglyceridemia (>1.5 g/l).
- Dyslipidemia type II: HypoHDL (<0.4 g/l in women and <0.35 g/l in men).
- Dyslipidemia type III: Total Hypercholesterolemia (>2 g/l).
- Dyslipidemia type IV: A threshold was considered for hyperLDL, one >1 g/l.

BMI: BMI was calculated as the ratio of weight (kg) on the square of height (in m).
- Lean if BMI <18 kg/m².
- Normal if BMI ≥18 and <25 kg/m².
- Over weighted between 25 and 29.9 kg/m² BMI.
- Obese if BMI ≥30 kg/m².

Abdominal obesity: It was defined according to International Diabetes Federation (IDF) [7].

All those with less than 150 minutes physical activity per week were considered as a low physical activity

Metabolic syndrome was defined according to the IDF criteria in 2005 [7].

Ethical aspects:

A writing consent was obtained from all individuals. The data were processed and stored with full privacy considerations. All subject with health issues requiring medical attention were referred to medical centers.

Statistical analysis:

The data collected were entered through an electronic questionnaire elaborated by Epi Info Version 3.5.1.

The analysis plan was as follows:
- The descriptive study of the different variables was carried out by the calculating the proportions for the variables of each category, and the positional and dispersion parameters for quantitative variables;
- The bivariate analysis was made using the chi² test for comparisons of proportions, Student's test for comparison of mean and logistic regression. The difference was considered statistically significant at a p < 0.05.

The risk factor was correlated with RI, if its prevalence was higher in the IR group compared to the group without RI, with a statistically significant difference.

3. Results

3.1. Description of Study Population (Table 1)

Among 1424 people initially selected a final selection of 1416 was made. The sex ratio was 0.45. The mean age was 43.4 ± 17.8 years [range 15 to 96 years]. The most representative occupation was the housekeeping (37%).

The prevalence of obesity and overweight was 22.6% (n = 320) and 22.7% (n = 321) respectively. The weight was normal range in 46.1% of cases (n = 653) and a thinness was found in 8.6% of cases (n = 122). Obesity was more prevalent among female patients (30.9%) than among the males (4.3%) (p < 0.001). The prevalence of abdominal obesity was 48.6% (n = 688). Abdominal obesity was more frequent among female people (65.5%) than among male individuals (11.1%) with a statistically significant difference (p < 0.001). 7.8% (n = 110) subject were smokers. The prevalence of physical inactivity was 64% (n = 907). The prevalence of high blood

Table 1. Clinical characteristics of the study subjects.

Number of participants	1416
Sex-ratio	0.45
Age	43.4 ± 17.8
Obesity	22.6% (n = 320)
Abdominale obesity	48.6% (n = 688)
Smoking	7.8% (n = 110)
Inactivity	64% (n = 907)
Hypertension	45.9% (n = 650)
Diabetes	10.4% (n = 147)
Hypercholesterolaemia	36.4% (n = 515)
Increase LDL-cholesterol	73.9% (n = 1046)
Decrease HDL-cholesterol	21.8% (n = 309)
Increase triglyceride	1.2% (n = 17)
Metabolic syndrome	39% (n = 553)

pressure was 45.9% (n = 650). The prevalence of diabetes was 10.4% (n = 147). The prevalence of dyslipidemia in the overall study population was 77% (n = 1091).

In the overall population, high blood levels of total cholesterol had a prevalence of 36.4% (n = 515), the hyperLDL concerned 73.9% of cases (n = 1046) and 21.8% cases of hypoHDL. Hypertriglyceridemia was less prevalent with a frequency of 1.2% in the population.

The prevalence of metabolic syndrome was 39% (n = 553).

3.2. Epidemiological Profile of Renal Insufficiency in the Population of Saint Louis

Prevalence

Among 1416 person included, the overall prevalence of renal insufficiency according to MDRD was 181 cases or 12.7%. The mean age of the people with renal insufficiency was 47.6 ± 17.4 years with the minimum of 15 and the maximum of 96 years.

The mean value of creatinine clearance was 83.9 ml/min/1, with 73 $m^2 \pm 23.2$ [range from 17.7 to 195 ml/min/1.73m^2]. The modal clearance was 73.4 ml/min/1.73m^2.

The subject with renal insufficiency could be distributed in different proportions according to the stage the disease (**Table 2**).

The prevalence of renal insufficiency increases with age up to 60 years with a peak between 50 and 59 years. It decreased gradually after 60 years (see **Figure 1**).

3.3. Renal Insufficiency and the Population At-Risk

3.3.1. Hypertension

Renal insufficiency was more frequent among people with height blood pressure (74.5%) than among people with normal blood pressure (58%) The difference was statistically significant in these two populations (p = 0.01) (**Table 3**).

3.3.2. Diabetes

The prevalence of renal insufficiency was higher in diabetics (71.4%) than in non-diabetics (64.9%) (**Table 3**). Although the difference was not statistically significant (p = 0.5566).

3.3.3. Obesity

Renal insufficiency was more frequent among obese people (66.6%) than among non obese people (56.5%)

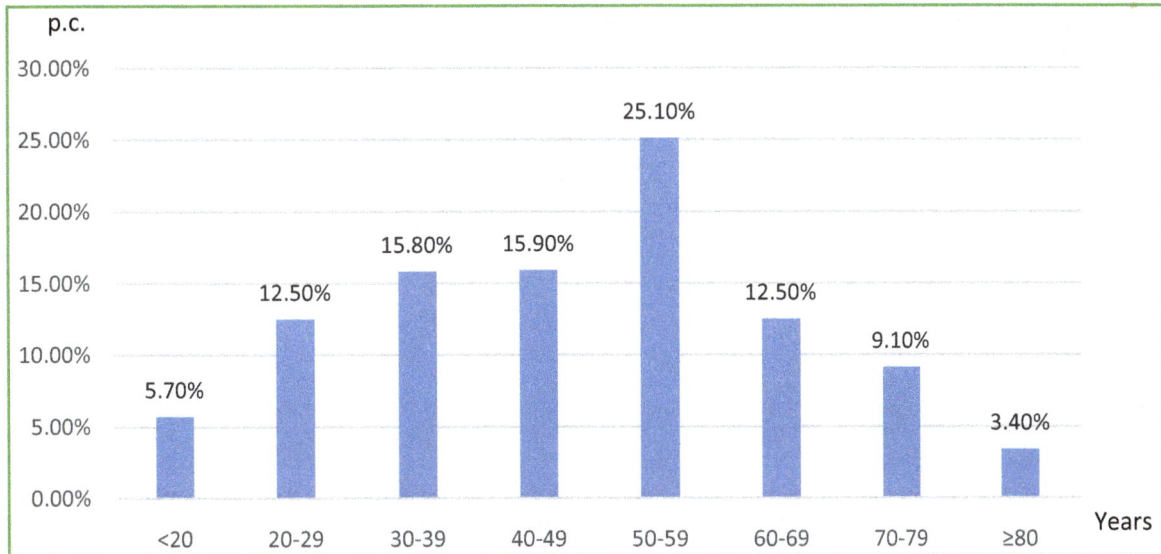

Figure 1. Prevalence of renal insufficiency by age.

Table 2. Prevalence depending on the stage of the CKD.

Stage	GFR ml/min/1.73m^2	Absolute frequency	Prevalence
V	<15	1	0.6%
IV	[15 - 30]	8	
III	[31 - 60]	172	12.1%
II	[61 - 90]	747	52.8%
I	>90	488	34.5%

(**Table 3**). However, the difference was not statistically significant (p = 0. 8655).

3.3.4. Dyslipidemia
Renal insufficiency was less frequent among the subjects with dyslipidemia (56.7%), than among patients who did not have dyslipidemia (96.6%). Dyslipidemia appeared to be a protective factor in renal function (**Table 3**).

3.3.5. Smoking
Among current smokers encountered during the study, renal insufficiency was found in 65.5%. The same frequency was found among nonsmokers.

3.3.6. Physical Inactivity
Among the sedentary subjects, renal insufficiency was found in 74.9% of cases against 48.9% in physically activity subjects. Physical inactivity was strongly associated with the low prevalence of renal insufficiency (p = 0.0001) (**Table 3**).

3.3.7. Association of Two or More Risk Factors
Renal insufficiency was found in 66.6% of people with combined two or more risk factors and 58.3% in patients with more than one risk factor. However, no statistically significant difference was noted (p = 0.4).

   Table 3 shows the prevalence of various risk factors in subjects with renal insufficiency and in people with normal renal function and their correlation with the degree of renal insufficiency.

4. Discussion

Epidemiological profile of renal insufficiency in the general population of Saint Louis:

Table 3. Distribution of various risk factors in patients with renal insufficiency (with RI) and in subjects with normal renal function (without RI).

Risk factors	Absolute frequency		Prevalence		p-value
	With RI (N = 181)	Without RI (N = 1235)	With RI	Without RI	
HTN:					
-Yes	94	420	52.2%	34%	
-No	87	815	47.8%	66%	0.01
Diabetes:					
-Yes	20	106	11.3%	8.6%	
-No	161	1129	88.7%	91.4%	0.5566
Obesity:					
-Yes	42	271	23%	21.9%	
-No	139	964	77%	78.1%	0.8655
Dyslipidemia:					
-Yes	121	1195	66.7%	96.7%	
-No	60	40	33.3%	3.3%	4.107e−08
Smoking					
-Yes	14	96	7.8%	7.8%	
-No	167	1139	92.2%	92.2%	1
Physical inactivity					
-Yes	132	577	73.2%	46.7%	
-No	49	658	26.8%	53.3%	0.0001
Association of two or more risk factors					
-Yes	161	1050	89%	85%	
-No	20	185	11%	15%	0.4

In our series, the prevalence of renal insufficiency was 12.7%. This prevalence was similar to the one found in most countries around the world (between 10% and 20%) [8]-[13]. The high prevalence of renal insufficiency observed in St. Louis could be explained by the higher frequency of hypertension, diabetes and other cardiovascular risk factors in that population. The prevalence of renal insufficiency increased with age up to 60 years with a peak between 50 and 59 years. The glomerular filtration rate gradually decreases with age and this reduction can range from 0.8 to 1.4 ml/min/1, 73 m^2 per year [14]. MRC increases with age independently moreover than physiological decrease of GFR [15].

This high prevalence in the urban environments is to be compared with another study in a rural environment in order to better understand the epidemiology of this disease in Senegal.

Four hundred eighty-eight (488) subject (87.3%) had normal renal function. This prevalence is consistent with the literature data. Indeed, it was respectively 88.8%, 91.9% and 87.7% in the DRC [8], Spain [12] and Japan [9].

Hypertensionis correlated with the risk of of renal insufficiency (p = 0.01) in our study, as in most other series. In Nigeria, renal impairment was associated with elevated systolic blood pressure in 46% of cases and 43.4% in diastolic cases (p < 0.001 in both cases) [10].

The prevalence of renal insufficiency was higher in diabetics (71.4%) than in non-diabetics (64.9%). However diabetes was not correlated with the occurrence of renal insufficiency (p = 0.5566). In France, in 2007, the prevalence of renal insufficiency found in type II diabetes was 62% [16]. Several studies worldwide have shown a strong correlation between renal insufficiency and diabetes mellitus [9] [16]. The unexpected result observed in our study could be explained by the short lasting of diabetes in most of our patients [17].

Obesity was not correlated with RF. This is not consistent with literature data. Indeed, in patients having neither diabetes nor height blood pressure, having a BMI of 25 at the age of 20 increases the risk of CRF 3 times, higher than that provided by a BMI 35 up to adulthood [18].

In long term, the risk of end stage CRF is correlated with BMI, with individual risk of about one case per 1000 patient-years for a BMI ≥ 40 kg/m^2 [19], which shows a relative risk of 7 times more compared to normal weight subjects.

Our study showed that hyperlipidemia does not appear to be risk factor in patients with renal insufficiency. Data on the association dyslipidemia and renal insufficiency appear very controversial in medical literature. In some studies, it was found to be a potent risk factor of renal disease [20] [21], while in others; it confers a benefit rather a paradoxical survival in renal insufficient [22].

The risk of renal insufficiency associated with physical inactivity was statistically significant (p = 0.0001). This result was similar to the one observed in a Palestinian study, where the prevalence of sedentary patients with renal insufficiency was two times higher than in controls (50% vs 25%) [23].

5. Conclusion

This study reports the increasing magnitude of renal insufficiency and its risk factors in the city of Saint Louis, in Senegal. Therefore, strategies for early detection and national preventions should be urgently implemented.

Conflict of Interest

None.

References

[1] Cerda, J., Lameire, N., Eggers, P., *et al.* (2008) Epidemiology of Acute Kidney Injury. *Clinical Journal of the American Society of Nephrology*, **3**, 881-886. http://dx.doi.org/10.2215/CJN.04961107

[2] Lengani, A., Kargougou, D., Fogazzi, G.B., *et al.* (2010) Acute Renal Failure in Burkina Faso. *Nephrology & Therapeutics*, **6**, 28-34.

[3] Sumaili, E.K., Krzesinski, J.-M., Cohen, E.P., *et al.* (2010) Epidemiology of Chronic Kidney Disease in the Democratic Republic of Congo: Review of Cross-Sectional Studies from Kinshasa, the Capital. *Nephrology & Therapeutics*, **6**, 232-239.

[4] Ouattara, B., Kra, O., Yao, H., *et al.* (2011) Characteristics of Chronic Renal Failure in Black Adult Patients Hospitalized in the Internal Medicine Department of Treichville University Hospital. *Nephrology & Therapeutics*, **7**, 531-534.

[5] Economic and Social Situation of the Region of Saint-Louis, Year 2009 (2009) National Agency of Statistics and Demography. http://www.ansd.sn

[6] WHO (2010) The WHO STEPwise Approach to Surveillance (STEPS). http://www.who.int/chp/steps/

[7] Alberti, K.G., Zimmet, P., Shaw, J., *et al.* (2005) IDF Epidemiology Task Force Consensus Group. The Metabolic Syndrome: A New Worldwide Definition. *Lancet*, **366**, 1059-1062. http://dx.doi.org/10.1016/S0140-6736(05)67402-8

[8] Mahon, A. (2008) Epidemiology and Classification of Chronic Kidney Disease and Management of Diabetic Nephropathy. *European Endocrinology*, **2**, 33-36.

[9] Imai, E., Horio, M., Watanabe, T., Iseki, K., *et al.* (2009) Prevalence of Chronic Kidney Disease in the Japanese General Population. *Clinical and Experimental Nephrology*, **13**, 621-630. http://dx.doi.org/10.1007/s10157-009-0199-x

[10] Afolabi, M.O., Adioye-Kuteyi, E.A., Arogundade, F.A. and Bello, I.S. (2009) Prevalence of Chronic Kidney Disease in a Nigerian Family Practice Population. *South African Family Practice*, **51**, 132-137.

[11] Otero, A., de Francisco, A.L.M., Gayosol, P. and Garcia, F. (2010) Prevalence of Chronic Renal Disease in Spain: Results of the EPIRCE Study. *Nefrologia*, **30**, 78-86.

[12] Cirillo, M., Laurenzi, M., Mancini, M., Zanchetti, A., Lombardi, C. and de Santo, N.G. (2006) Low Glomerular Filtration in the Population: Prevalence, Associated Disorders, and Awareness. *Kidney International*, **70**, 800-806. http://dx.doi.org/10.1038/sj.ki.5001641

[13] Zhang, L.X., Zuo, L., Xu, G.B., Wang, F., Wang, M., Wang, S.Y., *et al.* (2007) Community-Based Screening for Chronic Kidney Disease among Populations Older than 40 Years in Beijing. *Nephrology Dialysis Transplantation*, **22**, 1093-1099. http://dx.doi.org/10.1093/ndt/gfl763

[14] Anderson, S., Halter, J.B., Hazzard, W.R., Himmelfarb, J., Horne, F.M., Kaysen, G.A., *et al.* (2009) Prediction, Progression, and Outcomes of Chronic Kidney Disease in Older Adults. *Journal of the American Society of Nephrology*, **20**, 1199-1209. http://dx.doi.org/10.1681/asn.2008080860

[15] Bryson, C.L., Ross, H.J., Boyko, E.J. and Young, B.A. (2006) Racial and Ethnic Variations in Albuminuria in the US Third National Health and Nutrition Examination Survey (NHANES III) Population: Associations with Diabetes and Level of CKD. *American Journal of Kidney Diseases*, **48**, 720-726. http://dx.doi.org/10.1053/j.ajkd.2006.07.023

[16] Villar, E. and Zaoui, P. (2010) Diabetes and Chronic Kidney Disease: Lessons from Renal Epidemiology. *Néphrologie & Thérapeutique*, **6**, 585-590. http://dx.doi.org/10.1016/j.nephro.2010.08.002

[17] Ndaw, M.D. (2010) Epidemiological and Clinical Aspects of Diabetes Mellitus: Results from a Cross-Sectional Study in Saint Louis, Senegal. PhD Thesis, Cheikh Anta Diop University, Dakar.

[18] Hricik, D.E., Chung-Park, M. and Sedor J.R. (1998) Glomerulonephritis. *New England Journal of Medicine*, **339**, 888-899. http://dx.doi.org/10.1056/NEJM199809243391306

[19] Ram, C.V.S. and Silverstein, R.L. (2009) Treatment of Hypertensive Urgencies and Emergencies. *Current Hypertension Reports*, **11**, 307-314. http://dx.doi.org/10.1007/s11906-009-0053-2

[20] Kaba, M.L., Diakite, M., Bah, A.O., Sylla, I.S., Cherif, I., Tolno, A., *et al.* (2010) Lipid Profile of Uremic Patients at Donka National Hospital in Conakry. *Medecine d'Afrique Noire*, **57**, 255-258.

[21] Moorhead, J.F., Chan, M.K., El-Nahas, M. and Varghese, Z. (1982) Lipid Nephrotoxicity in Chronic Progressive Glomerular and Tubulo-Interstitial Disease. *Lancet*, **11**, 1309-1311. http://dx.doi.org/10.1016/S0140-6736(82)91513-6

[22] Chawla, V., Greene, T., Beck, G.J., Kusek, J.W., Collins, A.J., Sarnak, M.J. and Menon, V. (2010) Hyperlipidemia and Long-Term Outcomes in Nondiabetic Chronic Kidney Disease. *Clinical Journal of the American Society of Nephrology*, **5**, 1582-1587. http://dx.doi.org/10.2215/CJN.01450210

[23] Muhaisen, R.M., Sharif, F.A. and Yassin, M.M. (2012) Risk Factors of Cardiovascular Disease among Children with Chronic Kidney Disease in Gaza Strip. *Journal of Cardiovascular Disease Research*, **3**, 91-98. http://dx.doi.org/10.4103/0975-3583.95360

30

A Retrospective Renal Study from a Lupus Vasculitis Clinic

Gaurav Singh[1], Lauren White[2], Patrick Flynn[2], Sajan Thomas[3], Lakshmanan Jeyaseelan[4], Mani Thenmozhi[4], George John[3], Paul Kubler[5], Dwarakanathan Ranganathan[3*]

[1]Department of Internal Medicine, Princess Alexandra Hospital, Brisbane, Australia
[2]Department of Internal Medicine, Royal Brisbane and Women's Hospital, Brisbane, Australia
[3]Department of Nephrology, Royal Brisbane and Women's Hospital, Brisbane, Australia
[4]Department of Biostatistics, Christian Medical College, Vellore, India
[5]Department of Rheumatology, Royal Brisbane and Women's Hospital, Brisbane, Australia
Email: gaurav063@hotmail.com, laurensue.white@gmail.com, patrick.flynn@uqconnect.com.au, docsajan11@gmail.com, ljey@hotmail.com, mani.thenmozhi@gmail.com, george.john@health.qld.gov.au, paul.kubler@health.qld.gov.au, *Dwarakanathan.Ranganathan@health.qld.gov.au

Abstract

Aim: In July 2009, a combined Renal Rheumatology Lupus Vasculitis (RRLV) clinic, the first of its kind for adult patients in Australia, was started at Royal Brisbane & Women's Hospital. This is an audit of progression of renal disease to assess if patients attending this clinic had comparable results to published studies of similar cohorts with lupus Nephritis (LN) and vasculitis. Methods: We conducted a retrospective audit of all the patients who attended this clinic from July 2009 to October 2013. There were 33 patients followed up in the vasculitis group and 36 in the LN group. Patients with other connective tissue disorders were excluded from the analysis as the numbers were insignificant. Results: The mean estimated glomerular filtration rate of vasculitis and LN patients improved from 32.06 to 45.82 ml/min/1.73m^2 and 62.42 to 65.53 ml/min/ 1.73m^2 respectively. The mean urine protein/creatinine ratio of vasculitis and LN patients improved from 420 to 85 and 406 to 70 respectively. No patients died in either group. One vasculitis and two LN patients required maintenance dialysis. Three LN patients underwent renal transplantation. Conclusion: The results show excellent patient and renal survival and support the concept of a combined renal rheumatology clinic in managing renal disease from systemic connective tissue disorders.

Keywords

Vasculitis, Lupus Nephritis, Survival, Estimated Glomerular Filtration Rate, Urinary Protein

---

*Corresponding author.

Creatinine Ratio

1. Introduction

Renal involvement occurs in many autoimmune connective tissue disorders (CTD). Impairment of renal function varies from 50% in Systemic Lupus Erythematosus (SLE) and vasculitis, 5% in Scleroderma, and rarely in Sjogren's syndrome or anti-phospholipid antibody syndrome [1]. The involvement can progress to end stage renal disease (ESRD) [2] [3] reducing life expectancy compared to general population [4] [5].

Patients with CTDs have multi-system involvement and need care from Rheumatology and Renal Medicine. There are a few combined Lupus Vasculitis clinics in UK, USA, and for children, in Australia [6]-[8]. A Renal Rheumatology Lupus Vasculitis Clinic (RRLV) was started at Royal Brisbane and Women's Hospital (RBWH) in July 2009.

The patients in this clinic were managed as per international guidelines (**Tables 1-3**) and detailed records on patient progress were maintained [9]-[18]. Patient survival and progression of kidney disease were measured as key performance indicators.

We conducted a retrospective audit of progression of renal disease in patients attending the combined RRLV clinic to establish whether patients followed up in this clinic had comparable patient and renal survival rates with published reports of cohorts with lupus Nephritis (LN) and vasculitis.

Table 1. Standard therapy used for treatment of renal vasculitis [9] [13]-[15] [18].

Induction therapy		DOSE	Comments
Methylprednisolone then prednisolone	IV PO	MP 500 - 750 mg × 3 consecutive days then prednisone 1 mg/kg/day not exceeding 75 mg; tapered after a few weeks to lowest effective dose	Usually 3 - 6 months
	Plus		
Cyclophosphamide-First Option	IV	Refer **Table 2**, 6 - 12 infusions, 3 - 6 months	
Rituximab-Second Option	IV	375 mg/m^2 × 4 doses	Cannot tolerate or not responding to IV Cyclophosphamide
	Plus		
Plasma Exchange		7 exchanges in 2 weeks	Pulmonary Haemorrhage and or severe renal insufficiency
Maintenance Therapy	**Plus**		
Prednisolone	PO	tapering dose-till 5 - 7 mg/daily	
Azathioprine-*First Option*	PO	1 - 3 mg/kg/day	
MMF Second Option	PO	1 - 1.5 gm twice daily	Usually 18 months since remission
MPS-Second Option	PO	720 - 1080 mg twice daily	

IV, intravenous; PO, per os (oral administration); MP, Methylprednisone; MPS, Mycophenolate Sodium; MMF, MycophenolateMoeftil.

Table 2. Cyclophosphamide dose adjustment according to age and renal function [9] [10].

Age (years)	Cyclophosphamide dose reduction (per pulse, mg/kg) IV Mesna given to minimize toxicity	
	eGFR > 30 ml	eGFR < 30 ml
<60	15	12.5
60 - 70	12.5	10
>70	10	7.5

IV, intravenous.

Table 3. Standard therapy used for treatment of Lupus Nephritis [10]-[12] [17].

Induction therapy		DOSE	Comments
Methylprednisolone then prednisolone	IV PO	MP 500 - 750 mg × 3 days then prednisone 0.5 - 1 mg/kg/day to a maximum of 60 mg tapered after a few weeks to lowest effective dose	Usually 3 - 6 months
	Plus		
MPS-First option	PO	720 - 1080 mg twice daily	Cannot tolerate or not responding to MPS
IV Cyclophosphamide Second option	IV	500 mg IV once in 2 weeks ×6	
Maintenance Therapy	**Plus**		
Prednisolone	PO	slow tapering dose to 5 - 7 mg	
MPS or MMF-First option	PO	MPS-720 mg twice daily/MMF 1 gm bid	
Azathioprine-Second Option	PO	1 - 2 mg/kg/day	Usually 18 months since remission
		Plus	
Hydroxychloroquine	PO	400 mg daily	

IV, intravenous; PO, per os (oral administration); MP, Methylprednisolone; MPS, Mycophenolate Sodium; MMF, Mycophenolate Moeftil.

2. Methods

This is an audit of all patients who attended this clinic from July 2009 to October 2013. They were grouped based on renal involvement with vasculitis or LN and analyzed separately as the reported survival rates are different [2] [3]. Other CTDs were excluded from the analysis as the numbers were small.

We studied trends in estimated glomerular filtration rate (eGFR), urine protein creatinine ratio (uPCR), patient and renal survival.

3. Data

Data collected from medical records included age, gender, cause of renal involvement, renal biopsy, pulmonary involvement and requirement of plasmapheresis and dialysis, were de-identified and recorded on a spread sheet.

Investigations included full blood examination, renal function tests, urine microscopy, uPCR, disease markers of vasculitis *i.e.* perinuclearantineutrophil cytoplasmic antibodies (P-ANCA) and cytoplasmic ANCA(C-ANCA) titres, anti-proteinase3 (PR3), myeloperoxidase (MPO) antibodies and disease markers of LN *i.e.* anti-nuclear antibodies (ANA), anti-double stranded DNA (ds-DNA) antibodies, complement (c) 3 and 4.

Laboratory test results were recorded at six monthly intervals, along with data regarding mortality, renal loss and renal replacement modalities. Duration and details of follow up at renal-rheumatology clinic were collected which included date of first visit, number of clinic visits and total duration of follow up.

4. Statistical Methods

Descriptive statistics and frequency distributions were done for continuous and categorical variables respectively. Associations between eGFR and risk factors were calculated by bi-variate (unadjusted) and multivariate analysis (adjusted). A generalized estimating equations (GEE) model was used to analyze repeated measures on eGFR for the same patient with population-averaged effects of covariates. Exchangeable correlation structure was used. The data were analyzed by using SPSS 16.0 for Windows.

5. Patient Characteristics

There were 31 patients followed up with renal vasculitis and 36 with LN. Fifteen patients with miscellaneous CTD were excluded from the analysis due to small numbers. Among these, there were sixpatients with overlap syndrome, three patients each with Sjogren's syndrome, two patients with Henoch-Schonlein purpura, and one each with scleroderma, polyarteritis nodosa, cryoglobulinemic vasculitis and primary antiphospholipid antibody syndrome.

Among vasculitis patients, the number of patients with microscopic polyangiitis (MPA), granulomatous polyangiitis (GPA), anti-glomerular basement membrane (anti-GBM) disease and ANCA negative disease were 12, 8, 2 and 3 respectively. Six patients did not undergo a biopsy and there were no patients with combined ANCA and anti-GBM antibodies. Among LN patients, number of patients with class I, II, III, IV and V disease on histology were 1, 3, 6, 16 and 3 respectively. Five patients did not have a biopsy and two had mixed class III and V disease on histology. The patient characteristics namely age, gender, comorbidities, organ system involvement, eGFR and uPCR at baseline and at the end of follow up, duration of disease and clinic follow up are shown in **Table 4**.

Table 4. Patient characteristics.

	Vasculitis (n = 31)	Lupus nephritis (n = 36)	Miscellaneous (n = 15)
Gender: Male/Female	16/15	8/28	4/11
Age: Median (IQR)	65 (45 - 76)	42 (29 - 55)	60 (39.5 - 64.5)
Comorbidities			
Hypertension	18	25	7
Cardiac Failure	2	4	1
Ischemic heart disease	8	5	1
Peripheral Vascular disease	3	0	0
Stroke	1	4	3
Malignancy	4	2	3
Diabetes Mellitus	4	2	1
Liver disease	0	4	2
Organ involvement			
Cutaneous	1	30	5
Oral/nasal ulcers	0	12	0
ENT	3	0	0
Non scarring alopecia	0	6	0
Arthritis/Arthralgia	4	29	3
Serositis	0	14	0
Neurological	4	7	3
Hematological	0	20	2
Pulmonary	8	3	3
eGFR (ml/mt/1.73m^2) **Baseline** Median (IQR) **End of study** Median (IQR)	18 (9 - 41) 50 (24 - 68)	67.5 (43.5 - 90) 81.5 (44 - 90)	54 (29.5 - 64.5) 61.5 (40.5 - 85.5)
Urine protein/creatinine ratio **Baseline** Median (IQR) **End of study** Median (IQR)	197 (87 - 420) 54 (15 - 147)	85 (29 - 462) 29 (15 - 177)	82 (23.5 - 183.5) 43.5 (20.5 - 146.5)
Number of patients on dialysis **Baseline** **End of study**	6 1	2 2	1 0
Number of renal transplants during course of study	0	3	1
Time since diagnosis (months) Median (IQR) **Duration of follow up (months)** Median (IQR)	24 (15 - 51) 21 (14 - 45)	52 (31 - 62) 45 (23 - 50)	36 (22 - 46) 25 (14 - 41)

IQR, Inter-quartile range; eGFR, estimated glomerular filtration rate.

6. Results

We analyzed data from patients with renal vasculitis and LN separately. During follow up in the vasculitis patients the mean eGFR improved from 32.06 to 45.82 ml/min/1.73m^2 (**Figure 1(a)**). The mean uPCR declined from 420 to 85 (**Figure 1(b)**). There were no deaths while one patient required maintenance dialysis.

We conducted a GEE analysis of the trend of eGFR in patients with vasculitis for age, gender, renal histology, and plasmapheresis (**Table 5**). We found a statistically significant increase in mean eGFR in males as compared to females while with ages less than or greater than 60, there was no difference. During follow up, compared to patients MPA, patients with GPA and anti-GBM disease had a statistically significant increase in mean eGFR and patients with ANCA negative vasculitis did not show a significant change. Among patients requiring plasmapheresis the mean improvement in eGFR was significantly less as compared to patents who did not receive plasmapheresis.

In the LN group the mean eGFR improved from 62.42 to 65.53 ml/min/1.73m^2 (**Figure 1(c)**) and the mean uPCR from 406 to 70 (**Figure 1(d)**). There were no deaths, but 5 patients lost kidney function with 3 receiving renal transplantation and 2, maintenance dialysis.

A GEE analysis was conducted with regards to variables including, age gender, and histology. In LN group there was no statistically significant difference in the trend in eGFR based on age less than or greater than 60 or sex (**Table 5**). As compared to class V LN, class I LN had a mean improvement of 19.80 ml/min/1.73m^2 (P value 0.072) during follow up, not reaching statistical significance. Similarly there was no statistically significant difference in mean improvement in eGFR among other classes of LN.

7. Discussion

We compared results of our study with published data on patient survival and surrogate markers including renal

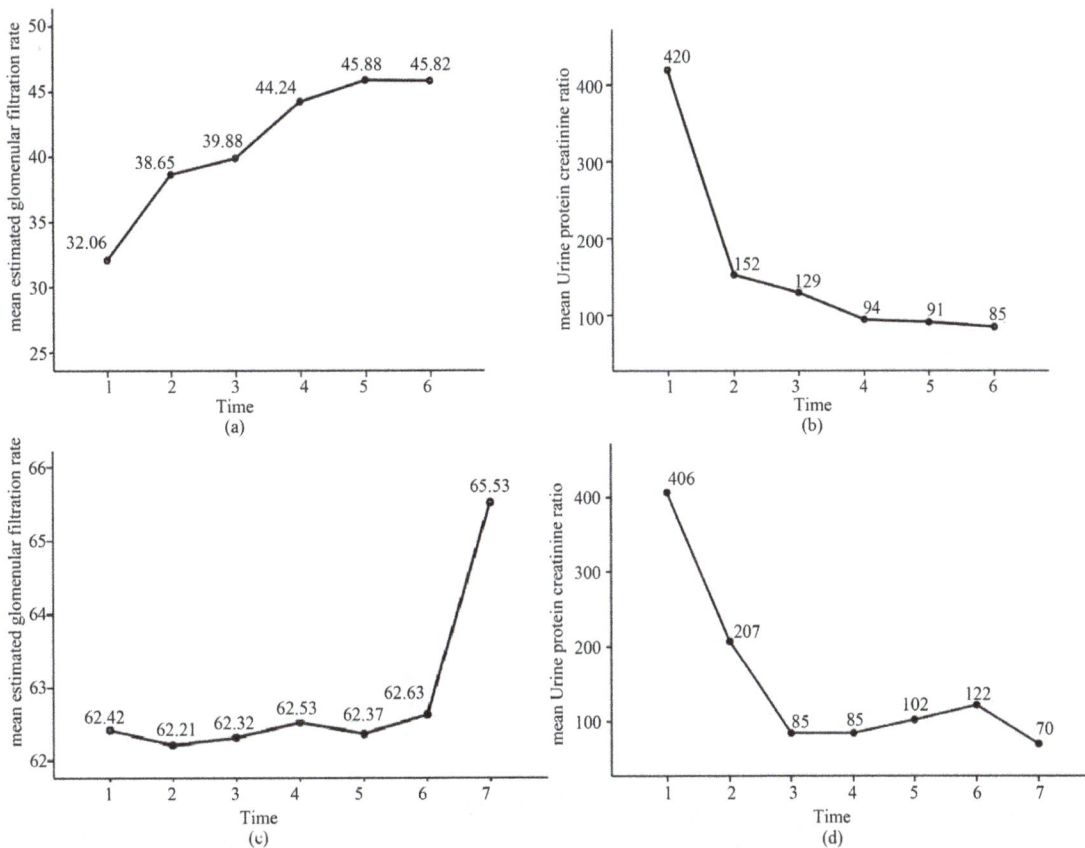

Figure 1. Profile plots for mean estimated glomerular filtration rate and mean urine protein creatinine ratio during follow up in vasculitis (a) and (b) and Lupus Nephritis (c) and (d). Time measured in 6 month intervals.

Table 5. GEE analysis for vasculitis and LN group of Patients eGFR over a time (0^a used for comparison variable).

Variables	Coefficient	95% Wald Confidence Interval		P value
		Lower	Upper	
Vasculitis group of patients				
Age				
≤60	7.03	−6.02	20.07	0.291
>60	0^a			
Gender				
Male	15.53	2.45	28.62	0.020
Female	0^a			
Histology				
No Biopsy	5.01	−11.61	21.63	0.555
Anti GBM	32.96	0.40	65.51	0.047
GPA	18.93	1.65	36.22	0.032
ANCA Negative	−2.28	−14.25	9.68	0.708
MPA	0^a			
Plasmapheresis				
Yes	−16.61	−31.13	−2.10	0.025
No	0^a			
Time	0.38	−1.42	2.19	0.677
LN group of patients				
Age				
≤60	5.51	−20.46	31.49	0.677
>60	0^a			
Gender				
Male	4.47	−16.21	25.15	0.672
Female	0^a			
Histology				
Class 1	19.80	−1.81	41.40	0.072
Class 2	−5.09	−43.07	32.90	0.793
Class 3	2.65	−24.07	29.36	0.846
Class 4	−9.96	−33.76	13.84	0.412
Class 5	0^a			
Dialysis				
Yes	−29.61	−46.70	−12.53	0.001
No	0^a			
Time	0.27	−1.88	2.42	0.807

LN, Lupus Nephritis; eGFR, Estimated glomerular filtration rate; Anti GBM, Anti glomerular basement membrane disease; GPA, Granulomatosis with Polyangitis; ANCA, Antineutophil Cytoplamic Antibody; MPA, Microscopic Polyangitis.

survival, trend in eGFR and uPCR for vasculitis and LN patients respectively.

In a study of 273 ANCA vasculitis patients, survival rates at 1, 5 and 10 years were 90%, 83% and 74% respectively, similar to results from previous studies [2] [19]. At presentation 48% required dialysis, and among those who were independent of dialysis 7% developed ESRD [2]. In our clinic during 4 years of follow up, one patient with vasculitis required maintenance dialysis while none died.

In a study involving 491 patients with LN, the overall cumulative probability of survival at 1, 5, 10 and 20 years was 98%, 88%, 77% and 45% respectively [20]. There were no deaths in our LN group and all patients had preserved renal function at 12 months and 86% at 51 months of follow up.

Studies have shown a declining eGFR is a risk factor for poor outcome of systemic disease related nephropathy [2] [21]. We have shown a clear trend of improvement in eGFR in vasculitis patients which correlates with a better renal and overall survival. Compared to results on LN from a single center cohort that showed a progressive decline in eGFR over a long term follow up of 25 years, our study showed a trend to improvement in eGFR in LN patients [22]. This could however be attributed to a shorter period of observation in our study.

The level of proteinuria is associated with the degree of renal scarring and poor long term renal outcome [23]. Reduction in proteinuria is an important measure of favorable response to treatment, particularly in LN [24] [25]. There was a decline in uPCR, a surrogate marker of renal improvement in patients with LN and vasculitis.

During our observation, there were no deaths in either vasculitis or LN groups. This could be attributable to a few factors. First, the period of follow up of 4 years is relatively short as compared to most published studies on patient survival in LN or renal vasculitis [2] [20]-[22] [26]. Second, the numbers of patients were relatively small in both groups. Third in our study observations dated from the first visit to our clinic rather than from the time of diagnosis while most of our comparator groups have studied outcomes from the date of diagnosis.

In summary, our results show better patient renal survival, improvement in eGFR and reduction in uPCR compared to the published studies. Our findings from four years of observation support advocating combined renal rheumatology clinics in managing renal disease from systemic connective tissue disorders.

References

[1]   Willcocks, L., Jones, R. and Jayne, D. (2011) Lupus Nephropathy and Vasculitis. *Medicine*, **39**, 468-491.
        http://dx.doi.org/10.1016/j.mpmed.2011.05.014

[2]   de Joode, A.A., Sanders, J.S. and Stegeman, C.A. (2013) Renal Survival in Proteinase 3 and Myeloperoxidase ANCA-Associated Systemic Vasculitis. *Clinical Journal of the American Society of Nephrology: CJASN*, **8**, 1709-1717.
        http://dx.doi.org/10.2215/CJN.01020113

[3]   Moroni, G., Quaglini, S., Gallelli, B., Banfi, G., Messa, P. and Ponticelli, C. (2013) Progressive Improvement of Patient and Renal Survival and Reduction of Morbidity over Time in Patients with Lupus Nephritis (LN) Followed for 20 Years. *Lupus*, **22**, 810-818. http://dx.doi.org/10.1177/0961203313492576

[4]   Langford, C.A. (2010) Vasculitis. *The Journal of Allergy and Clinical Immunology*, **125**, S216-S225.
        http://dx.doi.org/10.1016/j.jaci.2009.07.002

[5]   Saxena, R., Mahajan, T. and Mohan, C. (2011) Lupus Nephritis: Current Update. *Arthritis Research & Therapy*, **13**, 240. http://dx.doi.org/10.1186/ar3378

[6]   Vasculitis and Lupus Service, Addenbrooke's Hospital, UK.
        http://www.cuh.org.uk/addenbrookes/services/clinical/vasculitis/vasculitis_lupus_index.html

[7]   Ohio State Lupus Clinic, Davis Medical Research Centre, Ohio, USA.
        http://internalmedicine.osu.edu/rheumatology/patient-care/lupusclinic/

[8]   Paediatric Vasculitis Clinic, Monash Children's Hospital, Australia.
        https://www.monashchildrenshospital.org/page/About_Us/Monash_Childrens_Services/Paediatric_Renal__Continence_Service/

[9]   Kidney International (2012) KDIGO Clinical Practice Guideline for Glomerulonephritis—Chapter 13: Pauci-Immune Focal and Segmental Necrotizing Glomerulonephritis. *Kidney Inter*, **2**, 233-239.

[10]   Kidney International (2012) KDIGO Clinical Practice Guideline for Glomerulonephritis—Chapter 12: Lupus Nephritis. *Kidney Inter*, **2**, 221-232.

[11]   Bertsias, G.K., Tektonidou, M., Amoura, Z., Aringer, M., Bajema, I., Berden, J.H.M., *et al.* (2012) Joint European League against Rheumatism and European Renal Association-European Dialysis and Transplant Association (EULAR/ERA-EDTA) Recommendations for the Management of Adult and Paediatric Lupus Nephritis. *Annals of the Rheumatic Diseases*, **71**, 1771-1782. http://dx.doi.org/10.1136/annrheumdis-2012-201940

[12]   Hahn, B.H., McMahon, M.A., Wilkinson, A., Wallace, W.D., Daikh, D.I., FitzGerald, J.D., *et al.* (2012) American College of Rheumatology Guidelines for Screening, Treatment, and Management of Lupus Nephritis. *Arthritis Care & Research*, **64**, 797-808. http://dx.doi.org/10.1002/acr.21664

[13]   Hiemstra, T.F., Walsh, M., Mahr, A., Savage, C.O., de Groot, K., Harper, L., *et al.* (2010) Mycophenolate Mofetil vs. Azathioprine for Remission Maintenance in Antineutrophil Cytoplasmic Antibody-Associated Vasculitis: A Randomized Controlled Trial. *JAMA: The Journal of the American Medical Association*, **304**, 2381-2388.
        http://dx.doi.org/10.1001/jama.2010.1658

[14]   Jones, R.B., Tervaert, J.W., Hauser, T., Luqmani, R., Morgan, M.D., Au Peh, C., *et al.* (2010) Rituximab versus Cyclophosphamide in ANCA-Associated Renal Vasculitis. *The New England Journal of Medicine*, **363**, 211-220.

http://dx.doi.org/10.1056/NEJMoa0909169

[15] Stone, J.H., Merkel, P.A., Spiera, R., Seo, P., Langford, C.A., Hoffman, G.S., *et al.* (2010) Rituximab versus Cyclophosphamide for ANCA-Associated Vasculitis. *The New England Journal of Medicine*, **363**, 221-232. http://dx.doi.org/10.1056/NEJMoa0909905

[16] Wall, N. and Harper, L. (2012) Complications of Long-Term Therapy for ANCA-Associated Systemic Vasculitis. *Nature Reviews Nephrology*, **8**, 523-532. http://dx.doi.org/10.1038/nrneph.2012.107

[17] Hahn, B.H., McMahon, M., Wilkinson, A., Dean Wallace, W., Daikh, D.I., FitzGerald, J.D., *et al.* (2012) American College of Rheumatology Guidelines for Screening, Case Definition, Treatment and Management of Lupus Nephritis. *Arthritis Care & Research*, **64**, 797-808. http://dx.doi.org/10.1002/acr.21664

[18] Walsh, M., Merkel, P.A., Peh, C.A., Szpirt, W., Guillevin, L., Pusey, C.D., *et al.* (2013) Plasma Exchange and Glucocorticoid Dosing in the Treatment of Anti-Neutrophil Cytoplasm Antibody Associated Vasculitis (PEXIVAS): Protocol for a Randomized Controlled Trial. *Trials*, **14**, 73. http://dx.doi.org/10.1186/1745-6215-14-73

[19] Flossmann, O., Berden, A., de Groot, K., Hagen, C., Harper, L., Heijl, C., *et al.* (2011) Long-Term Patient Survival in ANCA-Associated Vasculitis. *Annals of the Rheumatic Diseases*, **70**, 488-494. http://dx.doi.org/10.1136/ard.2010.137778

[20] Zheng, Z., Zhang, L., Liu, W., Lei, Y., Xing, G., Zhang, J., *et al.* (2012) Predictors of Survival in Chinese Patients with Lupus Nephritis. *Lupus*, **21**, 1049-1056. http://dx.doi.org/10.1177/0961203312445230

[21] Weng, S.C., Tarng, D.C., Chen, C.M., Cheng, C.H., Wu, M.J., Chen, C.H., *et al.* (2014) Estimated Glomerular Filtration Rate Decline Is a Better Risk Factor for Outcomes of Systemic Disease-Related Nephropathy Than for Outcomes of Primary Renal Diseases. *PloS ONE*, **9**, e92881. http://dx.doi.org/10.1371/journal.pone.0092881

[22] Pokroy-Shapira, E., Gelernter, I. and Molad, Y. (2014) Evolution of Chronic Kidney Disease in Patients with Systemic Lupus Erythematosus over a Long-Period Follow-Up: A Single-Center Inception Cohort Study. *Clinical Rheumatology*, **33**, 649-657. http://dx.doi.org/10.1007/s10067-014-2527-0

[23] Cravedi, P. and Remuzzi, G. (2013) Pathophysiology of Proteinuria and Its Value as an Outcome Measure in Chronic Kidney Disease. *British Journal of Clinical Pharmacology*, **76**, 516-523.

[24] Inker, L.A., Levey, A.S., Pandya, K., Stoycheff, N., Okparavero, A. and Greene, T. (2014) Early Change in Proteinuria as a Surrogate End Point for Kidney Disease Progression: An Individual Patient Meta-Analysis. *American Journal of Kidney Diseases: The Official Journal of the National Kidney Foundation*, **64**, 74-85. http://dx.doi.org/10.1053/j.ajkd.2014.02.020

[25] Korbet, S.M., Lewis, E.J., Schwartz, M.M., Reichlin, M., Evans, J. and Rohde, R.D., Lupus Nephritis Collaborative Study Group (2000) Factors Predictive of Outcome in Severe Lupus Nephritis. *American Journal of Kidney Diseases: The Official Journal of the National Kidney Foundation*, **35**, 904-914. http://dx.doi.org/10.1016/S0272-6386(00)70262-9

[26] Mok, C.C., Kwok, R.C. and Yip, P.S. (2013) Effect of Renal Disease on the Standardized Mortality Ratio and Life Expectancy of Patients with Systemic Lupus Erythematosus. *Arthritis and Rheumatism*, **65**, 2154-2160. http://dx.doi.org/10.1002/art.38006

31

Chronic Kidney Failure: Knowledge of Kidney Disease, Perception of Causes and Symptomatology in Uyo, Nigeria

Effiong Ekong Akpan, Udeme E. Ekrikpo

University of Uyo, Uyo, Nigeria
Email: ffngakpan@yahoo.com, udekrikpo@yahoo.com

Abstract

Background: Chronic kidney disease (CKD) is now regarded as a global public health epidemic. Management of chronic kidney disease is often beyond the reach of some patients especially in resource-poor countries of sub-Saharan Africa where patients have to bear the funding. Many Nigerians do not know the functions of the kidney, the symptoms of kidney diseases and the causes of kidney failure. Aims: This study was designed to assess the awareness and knowledge of the kidney and kidney diseases among the people of Akwa Ibom State of Nigeria and their perception of the causes of kidney failure. Method: This was a cross-sectional survey of the Uyo residents in Akwa Ibom State for their knowledge, awareness and perception of CKD. A well structured but simple questionnaire was administered on all medically naïve participants by trained personnel. Data were analyzed using STATA 10, StataCorp, Texas, USA. Categorical data were presented as frequencies and percentages. A p-value of <0.05 was considered statistically significant. Results: A total of 500 questionnaires were distributed, but 410 were returned. There were 214 (52.2%) females and 196 (47.8%) males with an age range of 18 to 60 years and a mean age of 25.97 ± 8.60 years. About ninety five percent (95.1%) of respondents had heard about CKD with their major source of knowledge being from doctors (29.4%) and media (28.9%). Only 43.3% of respondents knew the correct location of the kidneys. With regards to the knowledge and perception of the causes of kidney failure and body swelling, (11%) agreed that it was because of patient's wrongdoing, Hypertension (38.9%), False oath taking (20.8%), Witchcraft (12.7%), Diabetes (46.9%), Parent's wrongdoing (6.4%), Sickle cell disease (47.3%), Familial (19.8%), Herbal medicine (27.9%), Drug abuse (38.9%) and Fake drugs (42.1%). The well educated had better knowledge of hypertension and diabetes as the causes of kidney failure. In conclusion, knowledge of kidney disease is still poor among our populace and more education and public enlightenment is therefore needed.

Keywords

Awareness, Perception, Chronic Kidney Failure, Nigeria

1. Introduction

Kidney disease is now regarded as a global public health epidemic. According to the Global Burden of Disease (GBD) 2010, CKD now ranks as the 9th cause of death, 16th cause of year of life lost from premature death, and 22nd cause of year lived with disability and adjusted life year (DALYs) in the United States [1]. This picture may be worse in resource-poor countries like ours. Management of CKD is often beyond the reach of some patients especially in resource-poor countries of sub-Saharan Africa where patients and their relatives have to bear the funding [2]. Many Nigerians do not know the functions of the kidney, the symptoms of kidney disease and the causes of kidney failure [3]. Many people among the Efik, Ibibio and Annang ethnic groups of Cross River and Akwa Ibom states of Nigeria believe that some of the symptoms of kidney failure especially body swelling is due to evil spirit. It is either because of the patient's wrongdoing or the patient is a thief.

In some instances, the families of deceased patients have been known to conduct certain rituals to appease the local deity as well as mutilate the corpse before burial in-order to prevent other family members from coming down with similar ailments. Because of these beliefs and relatively cheaper cost of treatment by tradomedical practitioners is often first preferred. The few that seek medical treatment often present late in the hospital with a number of them presenting in either stage 4 or 5 CKD [4].

This study was designed to assess the awareness and knowledge of the kidney and Chronic Kidney Disease among the people of Akwa Ibom and their perception of the cause kidney failure.

2. Methodology

This was a cross-sectional survey of Uyo residents for the knowledge, awareness and perception of kidney disease. Uyo is the capital of Akwa Ibom State of Nigeria. The state is named after the great Qua-Iboe River. Being the state capital, it receives people from all the 31 local government areas of the state. Medically-naïve members of the population cutting across different types of occupation and all levels of education were recruited for the study. A convenience sampling of medically naïve respondents was performed. The medically-naïve respondents refers to those who had never worked in a hospital setting before, either as health service providers or health management and support staffs. A well-structured but simple questionnaire was administered on all participants by trained personnel. Both English and Ibibio languages were used. Ibibio language is well understood by the three major ethnic groups in Akwa Ibom State. Their knowledge of the location and functions of the kidneys were assessed. Their knowledge of symptoms of kidney failure as well as beliefs on the causes of kidney failure was also assessed.

2.1. Data Handling

Data was entered and analyzed using STATA 10, StataCorp, Texas, USA. Categorical data was presented as frequencies and percentages. Chi-square was employed in comparing the proportions of the various responses between individuals with less than a secondary school education and those with at least a secondary school education. A p-value of <0.05 was considered statistically significant.

2.2. Exclusion Criteria

All health personnel as well as medical and paramedical students were excluded from the study.

3. Results

A total of 500 questionnaires were distributed, but 410 were returned giving a response rate of 82%. There were 214 (52.2%) females and 196 (47.8%) males with an age range of 18 to 60 years and a mean age of 25.97 ± 8.60 years. Only 352 respondents indicated their marital status of which 121 (34.4%) were married while 231 (65.6%) were single. 22.2% had no formal education while 1.0%, 27.07%, 49.8% had primary, secondary and post secondary education respectively. Majority of respondents were Christians 88.3% (**Table 1**).

We examined knowledge of kidney diseases, number of kidneys, location and functions. Out of 407 who responded to this question, 387 (95.1%) had knowledge of kidney diseases. Of those who had knowledge 113 (29.4%), 39 (10.2%), 56 (14.6%), 111 (28.9%), 50 (13.0%) and 15 (3.9%) had their source of information from doctors, nurses, friends, media, relatives and school respectively. On the outcome of the patient they knew, 68 (24.03%) said the patient had died while 215 (76.0%) said the patient is still alive. On the location of the kidneys, surprisingly 211 (52.2%) said the kidneys are located in the chest, 175 (43.3%) and 1 (0.3%) said the kidneys are located in the abdomen and head respectively. While 17 (4.20%) had no idea. With regards to their knowledge of kidney functions, 384 (94.6%) said yes to urine formation, 369 (90.4%) to waste excretion, 287 (79.5%) to calcium and phosphate regulation, and on the kidney's ability to aid blood production, 281 (70.1%) said yes (**Table 2**).

Knowledge of the symptoms of kidney failure is as shown in **Figure 1**.

Knowledge and perception of causes of kidney failure and body swelling were as follows: Eleven (11%) agreed that it is because of patient's wrongdoing while 53.8% and 35.2% disagreed and had no idea respectively; Hypertension; agree (38.9%), disagree (35.5%), no idea (27.6%). False oath taking agree (20.9%), disagree (36.2%), no idea (43.0%). Stole something; agree (9.3%), disagree (56.2%), no idea (34.5%). Witchcraft; agree (12.7%), disagree (54.8%), no idea (32.5%). Diabetes; agree (46.9%), disagree (34.5%), no idea (18.6%). Parent's wrongdoing; agree (6.4%), disagree (67.5%), no idea (26.2%). Sickle cell disease; agree (47.3%), disagree (20.06%), no idea (30.6%). Familial; agree (19.8%), disagree (44.0%), no idea (36.2%). Herbal medicine; agree (27.9%), disagree (35.3%), no idea (36.8%). Drug abuse (38.9%), disagree (27.9%), no idea (33.3%). Diarrhoea; agree (38.9%), disagree (36.4%), no idea (24.7%). Blood loss; agree (42.8%), disagree (31.3%), no idea (25.9%). Fake drugs; Agree (42.1%), disagree (22.7%), no idea (35.2%) (**Figure 2**).

We analyzed the effect of educational status on perception of kidney failure. Surprisingly more of the well educated believed that kidney disease can be caused by the patient's wrongdoing (p = 0.03). More of the well educated also believed that hypertension (p ≤ 0.001) and diabetes (p = 0.002), familial causes (p ≤ 0.0001), diarrhoea (p = 0.01) and fake drugs (p = 0.01) are causes of kidney failure. While the less educated and no formally educated believed that it is as a result a curse placed on a thief following an act of stealing (P ≤ 0.0001) is a more likely cause of kidney failure (**Table 3**).

African traditional methods were preferred for treatment of kidney failure among 11.3% of the less educated compared to 7.4% of the well educated (p = 0.14).

4. Discussion

The overall awareness of the kidney disease was good among the respondents as only about 5% did not hear about kidney disease. This may be because we study the urban dwellers with more educated respondents. It may also be attributed to the intensive enlightenment of the populace on kidney diseases. Same study was conducted by Okaka and Ojogwu [5] although mainly among undergraduate. Doctors topped the source of knowledge of kidney diseases with 29.4%, followed by the media (28.9%) while schools had the least (3.9%) as shown in **Table 2**. A lot still needs to be done on health education especially in the schools, which may require a revision of their curriculum. Both health workers and the media need to do more in bringing information of kidney disease to the populace. Of those who knew a patient with kidney disease, 24% of them acknowledged that the patient died of kidney disease. This shows a high mortality rate associated with kidney disease among our patients [2] [6]. A greater percentage of the respondents did not know the location of the kidneys. Only 43.3% knew that the

Table 1. Socio-demographic characteristics of respondents.

	Variables	Frequency	Percentage %
Sex	Male	214	52.2
	Female	196	47.8
Marital status	Married	121	34.4
	Single	231	65.6
Educational status	No formal education	91	22.2
	Primary education	4	1.0
	Secondary education	111	27.1
	Post secondary education	204	49.8
Religion	Christianity	362	88.3
	Islam	9	2.2
	Others	39	9.5

Table 2. Knowledge of kidney disease; number, location and functions of the kidneys.

Variable		Frequency	Percentage %
Knowledge of kidney disease	Yes	387	95.1
Source of knowledge	Doctors	113	29.4
	Nurse	39	10.2
	Friends	56	14.6
	Media	111	28.9
	Relatives	50	13.0
	School	15	3.9
Know patient with kidney disease	Yes	283	69.0
Outcome of the patient	Dead	68	24.0
	Alive	215	76.0
Location of kidneys	No idea	17	4.2
	Abdomen	175	43.3
	Head	1	0.3
	Chest	211	52.2
	No idea	1	0.3
No of kidneys	One	8	2.0
	Two	382	97.2
	Three	2	0.5
Functions of kidney	Urine formation	384	94.6
	Waste excretion	369	90.4
	Calcium and phosphate regulation	287	79.5
	Aid blood production	281	70.1

Table 3. Comparison of perception indices by educational status.

Perception indices	Post secondary school education. N (%)	Secondary school and below. N (%)	p value
Patient's wrongdoing	24 (21.8)	21 (13.6)	0.03
Hypertension	104 (51.2)	55 (26.7)	<0.001
Took oath falsely	41 (20.2)	44 (21.4)	0.77
Stole something	11 (5.4)	27 (13.1)	<0.0001
Witchcraft	24 (11.8)	28 (13.6)	0.59
Parent's wrongdoing	11 (5.4)	15 (7.3)	0.44
Diabetes mellitus	114 (56.2)	78 (37.9)	0.002
Sickle cell disease	105 (52.0)	88 (44.7)	0.06
Familial	57 (28.1)	24 (11.7)	<0.0001
Herbal drugs	55 (27.1)	59 (28.9)	0.70
Drug abuse	77 (35.5)	89 (42.2)	0.16
Diarrhoea	92 (45.3)	64 (32.5)	0.01
Excessive blood loss	96 (47.3)	79 (38.4)	0.07
Fake drugs	98 (48.3)	74 (35.9)	0.01

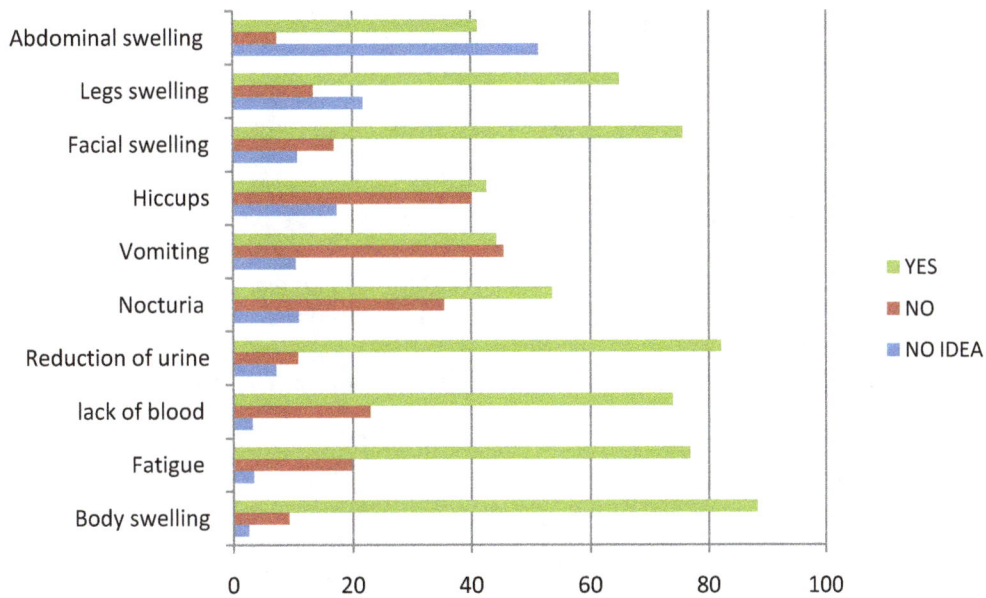

Figure 1. Histogram showing the knowledge of symptoms of kidney failure.

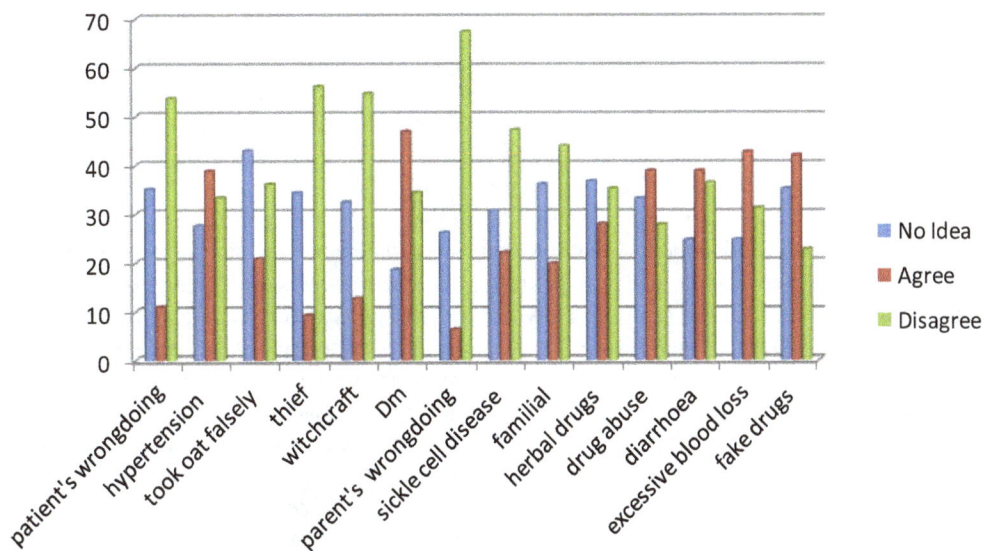

Figure 2. Histogram showing knowledge and perception of causes of kidney failure.

kidneys are located in the abdomen. This was comparable with 44% reported by Okwuonu *et al.* [3]. Fifty two percent of respondents, compared with 43.2% reported by Okwuonu, said the kidneys are located in the chest. This was surprising because we studied the mainly urban population with more educated respondents while theirs was on semi-urban population. The study by Okaka and Ojukwu revealed good knowledge of location of kidney and functions [5]. This may be because their respondents were mainly undergraduates whereas we included both educated and uneducated subjects. However, the knowledge of the number of kidneys by our respondents was very good. Only 2.8% did not know the total number of kidneys per individual compared with 5% by Okaka and Ojugwu [5] and 9.9% by Alebiosu [7]. This may be unconnected with their level of education because there were more people with higher levels of education in Alebiosu's study (68.9%) compared with 49.8% in our study (Table 1). Our study was however different from that of Alebiosu because we excluded hospital administrative and support staff who may have little medical knowledge from their day to day contact with patients. This is however surprising considering the fact that 52.2% said that the kidneys were located in the chest except if they wrongly thought that the lungs and the kidneys are synonymous. However, this is difficult to sustain because the meaning of kidney was interpreted to all respondents in vernacular. Respondents had good knowledge of kidney functions except functions relating to blood production. Ninety five percent and 90.4% agreed that kidney functions in urine formation and excretion of waste from the body respectively. This was higher than that of 65.8% in Alebiosu's study.

Knowledge of symptoms of kidney failure was fair as 88.3%, 76.8%, 82.5% and 75.6% believed that body swelling, fatigue, reduction in urinary output, and facial swellings are symptoms of kidney failure. This showed an improvement when compared with 23.9%, 13.5% and 0.7% of body swelling, body weakness and facial swelling respectively, reported by Alebiosu. Okaka and Ojugwu also reported a lower percentage of 61%, 68.1% and 49.2% corresponding to body swelling, inability to pass urine and fatigue respectively. This showed a marked improvement especially on the knowledge of body swelling which is the commonest symptom of kidney failure [6]. However knowledge of nocturia, lack of blood, vomiting and hiccups are still poor and needs more enlightenment.

Knowledge of the causes of kidney failure was very poor. Eleven percent (11%) of respondents believed that kidney disease is caused by a patient's wrongdoing. Surprisingly, this belief was common among those with higher levels of education than those with a secondary level of education and below. It was difficult to explain this statistical difference as we expected the reverse. We observed that certain beliefs are still very strong among the studied population. 20.9% of respondents believed that kidney disease is as a result of having sworn to an oath falsely for an offence the patient had committed while 6.36% believed that it is because of the parent's wrongdoing. These beliefs were not influenced by level of education as there was no statistically significant difference between those with higher education and those with secondary school education and below. Less number of highly educated respondents compared with those with secondary school education and below did not believe that kidney disease is as a result of thief ($p \leq 0.0001$). Those who attributed kidney failure to witchcraft were 12.7% (**Figure 2**). These beliefs may impact negatively on the willingness of the populace in seeking proper medical treatment on time and may be one of the main reasons for their late presentation in the hospitals. These types of belief are well established in patients suffering from epilepsy [8]. More enlightenment needs to be carried out to dissuade our people from these Stone Age beliefs.

Only 38.88% and 46.94% of respondents believed that hypertension and diabetes are causes of kidney disease. This is appalling considering the fact that hypertension and diabetes remain the leading causes of chronic kidney disease the world over including Nigeria [9] [10]. Also the prevalence of hypertension is on the increase in our rural and urban communities [11] [12]. However the well educated respondents had better knowledge of both hypertension and diabetes as possible causes than the less educated ($p < 0.001$ and 0.002 respectively).

Adult polycystic kidney disease and sickle cell disease are known familial causes of kidney disease. However , more than 50% of respondents did not believe that sickle cell anaemia is a cause of CKD and only 19.8% believed that CKD could be hereditary [13] [14]. More of the well-educated believed that CKD may be inherited when compared with the less educated respondents ($p < 0.0001$).

On drugs as a cause of CKD, only about a quarter (27.9%) of the respondents believed that herbal drugs can be a cause, while less than half believed that drugs abuse and fake drugs can cause kidney disease (**Table 3**). This is lower than 30.6% of Okwuonu et al. [3], but slightly higher than Okaka and Ojukwu [5] despite the facts their study population was mainly students. Herbal medications/concoctions are known causes of kidney failure in Nigeria [4] [15]. This is alarming considering the proliferation of herbal medicine vendors in all nooks and crannies of our communities. All efforts must be on deck in disseminating information to the gullible public on the dangers posed by some of these drugs. Knowledge of excessive blood loss and diarrhoea as a cause of kidney failure was also poor.

5. Conclusion

Although there is little improvement in the knowledge of the kidney and its diseases, the knowledge of causes of kidney failure is still very poor. There is therefore an urgent need for health practitioners, the media and schools to increase their level of information on kidney disease, causes and prevention to general public.

Limitation

This study was done among the urban dwellers and there were more educated respondents. Same study need to be replicated in the rural communities.

Conflict of Interest

We declare no conflict of interest.

References

[1]   Murray, C.J.I., Ezzati, M., Flaxman, A.D., *et al.* (2012) GBD 2010: Design, Definition and Metrics. *Lancet*, **380**, 2063-2066. http://dx.doi.org/10.1016/S0140-6736(12)61899-6

[2]   Ijoma, C.K., Ulasi, I.I. and Kalu, A.O. (1998) Cost Implications of Treatment of End Stage Renal Disease in Nigeria. *Nigerian Journal of College of Medicine*, **3**, 95-96.

[3]   Okwuonu, C.G., Chukwuonye, I.I., Ogah, S.O., Abali, C., Adejumo, O.A. and Oviasu, E. (2015) Awareness of Level of Kidney Functions and Disease among Adult in a Nigerian Population. *Indian Journal of Nephrology*, **25**, 158-163. http://dx.doi.org/10.4103/0971-4065.139096

[4]   Kadiri, S., Arije, A. and Salako, B.L. (1999) Traditional Herbal Preparations and Acute Renal Failure in South West Nigeria. *Tropical Doctor*, **22**, 224-226.

[5]   Okaka, E.L. and Ojogwu, L.I. (2012) Aweareness Level of Kidney Disease among Non-Medical Students in Benin City, Nigeria. *JMBR*, **11**, 29-34.

[6]   Arogundade, F.A., Sanusi, A.A., Hassan, M.O. and Akinsola, A. (2011) The Pattern, Clinical Characteristics and Outcome of ESRD in Ile-Ife, Nigeria: Is There a Change in Trend? *African Health Sciences*, **11**, 594-601.

[7]   Alebiosu, C.O. (2002) Awareness of Kidney Disorders in Nigeria. *African Journal of Health Sciences*, **9**, 165-168.

[8]   Sanya, E.O., Salami, T.A.T., Goodman, O.O., Buhari, O.I.N. and Araoye, M.O. (2005) Perception and Attitude to Epilepsy among Teachers in Primary, Secondary and Tertiary Educational Institutions in Middle Belt Nigeria. *Tropical Doctor*, **35**, 153-156. http://dx.doi.org/10.1258/0049475054620905

[9]   Alebiosu, C.O., Ayodele, O.O., Abbas, A. and Olutoyin, I.A. (2006) Chronic Renal Failure at Olabisi Onabanjo University Teaching Hospital, Sagamu, Nigeria. *African Journal of Health Sciences*, **6**, 132-138.

[10] US Renal Data System (2011) USRDS 2011 Annual Data Report: Atlas of Chronic Kidney Disease and End-Stage Renal Disease in the United States. National Institutes of Health, National Institute of Diabetes and Digestive and Kidney Disease. Bethesda.

[11] Ulasi, I.I., Ijoma, C.K., Onwubere, B.J.C., Arodiwe, E., Onodugo, O. and Okafor, C. (2011) High Prevalence and Low Awareness of Hypertension in a Market Population in Enugu, Nigeria. *International Journal of Hypertension*, **2011**, Article ID: 869675.

[12] Akpan, E.E., Ekrikpo, U.E., Udo, A.I.A. and Bassey, B.E. (2015) Prevalence of Hypertension in Akwa Ibom State South-South Nigeria: Rural versus Urban Communities Study. *International Journal of Hypertension*, **2015**, Article ID: 975819. http://dx.doi.org/10.1155/2015/975819

[13] Dana, V.R. and Arlene, B.C. (2014) Polycystic and Other Cystic Kidney Disease. In: Scott, J.G., Daniel, E.W., Debbie, S.G., Mark, A.P., Marcello, T., Eds., *Primer of Nephrology*, 6th Edition, Elsevier Saunders, Philadelphia, 362-370.

[14] Vimal, K.D. (2014) Sickle Cell Nephropathy. In: Scott, J.G., Daniel, E.W., Debbie, S.G., Mark, A.P. and Marcello, T., Eds., *Primer of Nephrology*, 6th Edition, Elsevier Saunders, Philadelphia, 357-361.

[15] Akpan, E.E. and Ekrikpo, U.E. (2015) Acute Renal Failure Induced by Chiene Herbal Medication in Nigeria. *Case Reports in Medicine*, **2015**, Article ID: 150204.

32

Physician's Awareness of Home Blood Pressure in the Treatment of Hypertensive Patients with Chronic Kidney Disease

Naoki Sugano, Satoru Kuriyama*, Yoichiro Hara, Koki Takane, Yasuhito Takahashi, Yasuko Suetsugu, Takashi Yokoo

Division of Kidney and Hypertension, Department of Internal Medicine, The Jikei University School of Medicine, Tokyo, Japan
Email: *kuriyamas218@yahoo.co.jp

Abstract

Aim: The majority of guidelines recommended the significance of home-based blood pressure (home-BP) measurement. The present study explored that to what extent, general practitioners (GPs) were aware of the importance of home-BP in the daily clinical practice. Method: We sent out questionnaires to GPs who had been specialized in nephrology and hypertension. The questions focused on the awareness of home-BP and the selections of antihypertensive agents for refractory hypertension in chronic kidney disease (CKD) patients. Results: 1) The majority (95.9%) of the responding GPs had utilized home-BP in their clinical practice. 2) When prescribing a single agent for hypertensive CKD patients, the majority of GPs (87.3%) chose ARB for the first line drug, and Ca channel blockers (CCB) were the second. 3) As an add-on drug to the pre-treatment with an angiotensin receptor blocker (ARB), the majority preferred CCB (82.7%) to diuretics (21.8%). In addition, a fixed combination formula of antihypertensive medication consisting of ARB plus diuretic was accepted by the majority of GPs (78.7%). 4) To improve morning hypertension in patients treated with two or more drugs, 87.8% of the doctors agreed that additional night-time dosing could be useful. The choices of the agents given at night-time varied, mainly with $\alpha 1$-blockers (40.6%), followed by α-blockers (30.5%) and α-methyldopa (19.8%). Conclusion: The majority of GPs in Japan are aware of the importance of the home-BP-based management of CKD. They mainly chose ARB as a first line drug, and ARB plus CCB as an add-on therapy.

Keywords

Home Blood Pressure; Chronic Kidney Disease; Guideline for High Blood Pressure; Antihypertensive Agents

---

*Corresponding author.

1. Introduction

Three different methods of BP measurement are office BP, home-BP measured at any given time of the day (home-BP) and 24-hours ambulatory BP (ABP) monitoring. The two latter methods are home-based BP, which give lots of advantages including; 1) it provides multiple measurement of BP in any occasion by days, weeks, months or years; 2) it is obtained in a usual environment for each individual which can avoid white-coat effect; 3) it can detect the white-coat, masked and morning hypertension; and 4) it is closely related to target organ damage and predicts the risk of cardiovascular events.

In cross-sectional studies, ABP values are correlated with the organ damage accompanying hypertension and diabetes mellitus more closely than office BP values [1]-[4]. Similarly, in longitudinal studies, BP values of home-based BP predict the progression of organ damage and the risk of cardiovascular disease more accurately than office BP [5]-[10]. Unquestionably, these data support the notion that home-based BP is a highly valuable tool in the management of hypertension [11]-[15]. Despite very few head-to-head comparisons between home-BP and ABP, the results constantly showed that both were equally reliable in predicting the target-organ damage in hypertensive patients [16]-[19].

However, clinical indications for these home-based BP are substantially different. Compared with ABP, home-BP provides measurement over a much longer period of time, and is cheaper, more widely available, thus more convenient and acceptable for patients [4] [20]-[22]. Based on the European Society of Hypertension/Cardiology recommendations, ABP is advantageous if there is a considerable variability in the clinic BP of the patients' regular visits, and if there is a marked discrepancy between home-BP and office BP. On the other hand, home-BP provides more information on the antihypertensive effect of the treatment by comparing the trough and the peak BP values [22]-[25]. Recently, after several years being exposed to the guidelines published by the Japanese Society of Hypertension, the GPs' recognition and awareness of home-BP-based clinical practice has been surveyed in Japan [26] [27]. These studies showed a high awareness of home-BP among GPs, though they are still confused with how to apply it for patients.

On achieving adequate BP goals, lots of studies showed that more than one antihypertensive agent was needed to reach the target goal [28]. Like many other countries such as the US and Europe [29], Japan has witnessed a substantial influx of fixed formulation tablet of combination medicines consisting of ARB plus diuretic or ARB plus CCB. As a result, in the past several years, several different analogous fixed formulations of two antihypertensive agents combined have come into use. As a result of this trend, some GPs are not sure about how to use and choose these fixed formulation tablets, and others are even perplexed about how to use them.

In this communication, we investigated that to what extent GPs are aware of the importance of home-BP in the clinical practice of CKD as well as their decisions in choosing the antihypertensive drugs. In order to pursue this objective, GPs were asked via questionnaires about the awareness of home-BP, how to prescribe multiple antihypertensive drugs for morning hypertension. The present study is the first to highlight the awareness of home-BP among GPs who are specialized in CKD practice, especially in Japan.

2. Materials and Methods

Materials: During the period between October 2009 and March 2011, we distributed and collected questionnaires to 330 doctors in Tokyo and its vicinity, All participants were general practitioners (GPs) belonging to the department of medicine of the medical universities specialized in nephrology and hypertension. Approximately 80% or more of them had taken educational programs in nephrology and hypertension while they were in the post doctoral training courses, approximately 20% of them were qualified specialists approved by the Japanese society of Nephrology and/or Hypertension. There were some GPs who had their own clinics, not always but often treating CKD patients.

Methods: They were asked about hypertension treatment on the assumption that they had encountered hypertensive CKD patients at their clinics. The questionnaires were on an anonymous basis, and the GPs were requested to answer them with reference to the High Blood Pressure Guideline either by the Japanese Society of Hypertension [30], the 7th Report of the Joint National Committee in the U.S. [31], or the European Society of Hypertension/Cardiology Recommendations [24]. Because of its study protocol using questionnaires in which individual patient's information was no longer revealed, ethical consideration with respect to patient's right was apparently not violated. The questions to the GPs mainly focused on the awareness of home-BP measurement, the expected target BP levels by home-BP (135/85 mmHg), how to select antihypertensive medications, how to prescribe antihypertensive agents, when to measure home-BP and so on. We also asked specifically about the importance of morning BP, how to choose antihypertensive agents including fixed formula of antihypertensive agents; what time is appropriate to take those agents, and then finally to what extent they were aware of the risk factors for hypertension. Questionnaires were delivered, collected and analyzed within a few months. The completion rate of the data available for analyses was 60%.

3. Results

Figure 1 shows that almost all of the GPs (95.9%) utilized home-BP in their daily clinical practice. Nearly three quarter (76.1%) of them answered that home-BP is valuable and that it should be more effectively utilized in clinical practice. In addition, morning BP (39.1%) was regarded as being more important than night time BP (0.5%), and 58.8% answered that both morning and night time home-BP were equally important in the treatment of hypertension.

Figure 2 shows the degree of recognition as to what extent the guideline-recommended definition of hypertension at home (more than 135/85mmHg) was accepted by the GPs. The majority of them approved of the home-BP goal value (86.3%). However, the majority (88.3%) believed that this criterion of home-BP had not yet been scientifically proven, and that more evidence would be needed to scientifically confirm this goal.

Figure 3 depicts the result of the recognition of the progression factors of CKD. They were asked which factors have a strong impact on CKD progression. Hypertension, hyperglycemia, high dietary protein intake, hyperlipidemia, hyperuricemia, anemia were chosen in this order as such factors.

Figure 4 depicts the choice of the antihypertensive agents for CKD when asked to carry out either monotherapy (the upper graph) or dual therapy (the lower graph). More than 80% of the GPs chose an angiotensin type 1 receptor blocker (ARB) as their first choice of medication for hypertensive CKD patients. In contrast, less than 10% chose ACE-I and/or CCB as a first line drug. As to the doctor's preferences for their second choice of an add-on drug to ARB or ACE-I, more than 80% GPs chose CCB as a second line antihypertensive medication. In contrast, less than 20% chose diuretics as a second choice.

Figure 5 shows the responses to the questions about morning hypertension. Almost all of them (99.0%) answered that morning hypertension is a strong risk for cardiovascular diseases, and that control is crucial to achieve better outcomes. For the purpose of reducing the risk of morning hypertension, 87.8% of them agreed that the night time dosing with an additional antihypertensive agent could be effective in lowering morning events. As for the agents to ameliorate morning hypertension, 42.1% of the GPs chose 1-blocker, followed by ARB (27.0%), CCB (15.1%), β-blocker (6.9%) and ACE-I (4.4%).

Figure 6 (upper circle) depicts how to prescribe two drugs when a dual therapy was needed. The responses to this question were diverse. If the two drugs were to be given separately, 46.2% of them would prescribe either ARB or ACE-I at night and CCB or diuretics in the morning. However, 29.9% answered that both ARB/ACE-I and CCB/diuretics should be taken together in the morning.

Figure 6 (lower left circle) describes that 78.7% admitted that a fixed formulation of single tablet with ARB plus diuretic is useful and necessary for their daily clinical practice. Finally, as a third choice for refractory morning hypertension (lower right circle), the majority of the GPs chose α1-blocker (40.6%), followed by α-blocker (30.5%) and α-, plus β-blocker (19.8%).

4. Discussion

We conducted a survey on home-BP among GPs who were specialized in the treatment of CKD in Japan. The use of home-based BP has been recommended in many high blood pressure guidelines. Such guidelines suggested that home-based BP is indicative to all of the patients treated with antihypertensive medications [4] [20]-[22]. As a result of the recently-published hypertension guidelines as well as the penetration of BP measuring device at home, its use has been constantly increased all over the world, and so does in Japan. Compared with ABP which requires 24 monitoring which sometimes bothers patients, home-BP may be more suitable for daily management in the most of hypertensive patients [23]-[25].

First, we were able to confirm a high awareness of home-BP among GPs who deal with hypertensive CKD patients (**Figures 1** and **2**). In addition, the notion that ARB as a first line drug and CCB as an add-on drug was approved by the majority of GPs in Japan (**Figure 4**). Undisputedly, a lot of evidence has confirmed the organ-protective effect of RAS inhibitors, ARB and/or ACE-I. Influenced by these evidences, the majority of GPs

Do you use home BP routinely ?

No 3.0%   Others 1.0%

Yes 95.9%

Is home BP better than office BP for clinical practice ?

Others 8.6%

No 15.2%

Yes 76.1%

Which one is more important, morning or night BP?

Others1.5%

Morning 39.1%

Both 58.8%

Night 0.5%

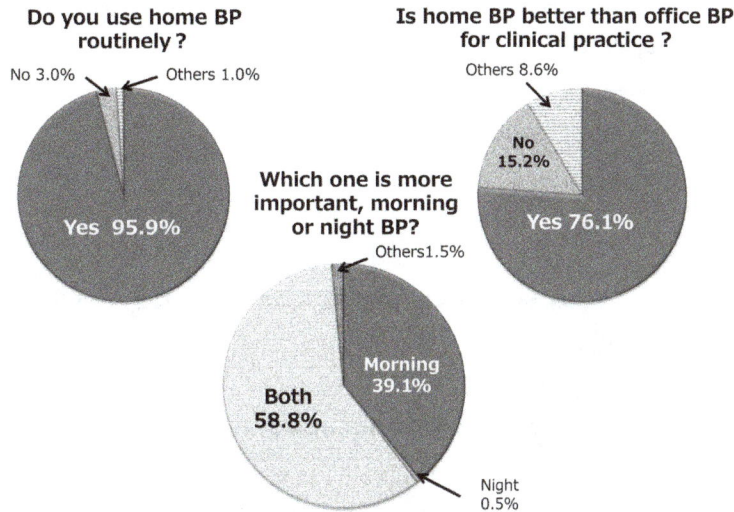

Figure 1. Awareness on the use of home-BP.

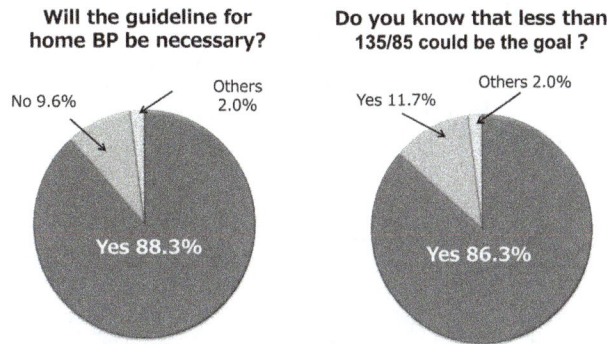

Will the guideline for home BP be necessary?

No 9.6%   Others 2.0%

Yes 88.3%

Do you know that less than 135/85 could be the goal ?

Others 2.0%

Yes 11.7%

Yes 86.3%

Figure 2. Treatment goal for home-BP. The Japanese Society Hypertension (JSH) guideline recommended 135/85 mmHg as the treatment goal of home-BP.

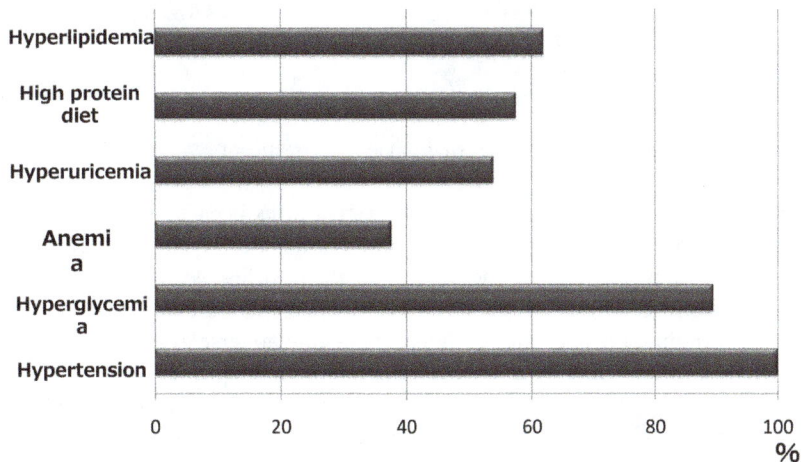

Hyperlipidemia

High protein diet

Hyperuricemia

Anemia

Hyperglycemia

Hypertension

0   20   40   60   80   100
%

Figure 3. Questions on the progression factors for CKD..

have accepted that ARB or ACE-I must be the first-choice agent in patients with CKD.

As to the refractory hypertension which normally needs more than two antihypertensive drugs, the majority of GPs answered that the second choice should be CCB, instead of diuretic. It means that they were reluctant to se

Which one do you think should be the first choice for CKD ?

As an add-on to ARB alone, which one is appropriate ?

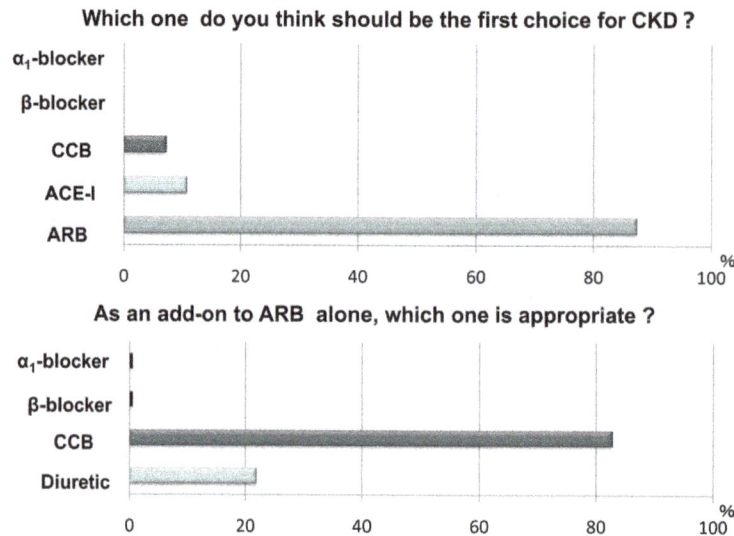

Figure 4. Choices of the antihypertensive agents for CKD.

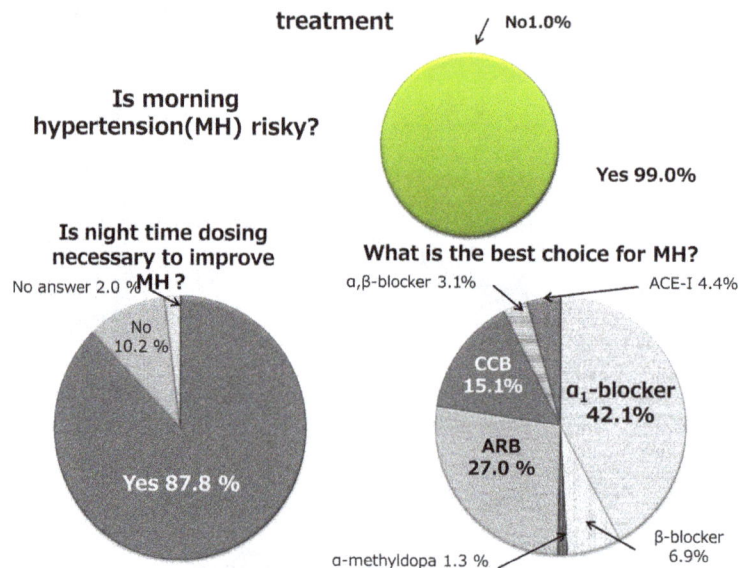

Figure 5. Morning hypertension and the treatment.

lect diuretics even as a second choice. This is surprising to us because before commencing this study, we had anticipated that the majority of GPs would choose diuretic-ridden regimen, as many fixed formulations of combined ARB with diuretics had been on the market for the past few years in Japan. Yet in reality, diuretics were thought to be inferior to CCB [32]. What's behind this? We assume that the GPs believed that CCB is more potent to lower BP than diuretic, and safer with less metabolic adverse effects such as impaired glucose tolerance, hyperlipidemia, hypokalemia and hyperuricemia that diuretics frequently induce [31].

Alleviating morning hypertension was accepted by nearly 90% of the GPs. As CKD progresses into more advanced stage, incidence of morning hypertension increases. In order to reduce the risk of morning hypertension, in addition to the foregoing combination therapy with ARB plus CCB or diuretic for example, night time dosing with a third choice drug could be indispensable. An appropriate chronotherapy in hypertensive patients which concerns administration-time provides a means of accomplishing this purpose. There are several possible agents to ameliorate morning hypertension. Night time dosing with the CCB, $\alpha 1$-blocker, β-blocker, ACE-I and ARB has been proven to be effective [33]-[37]. Among them, $\alpha 1$-blockers appeared to be rational as they have a substantial effect on morning hypertension. Kario et al. addressed whether the night time dosing of $\alpha 1$-blocker alle-

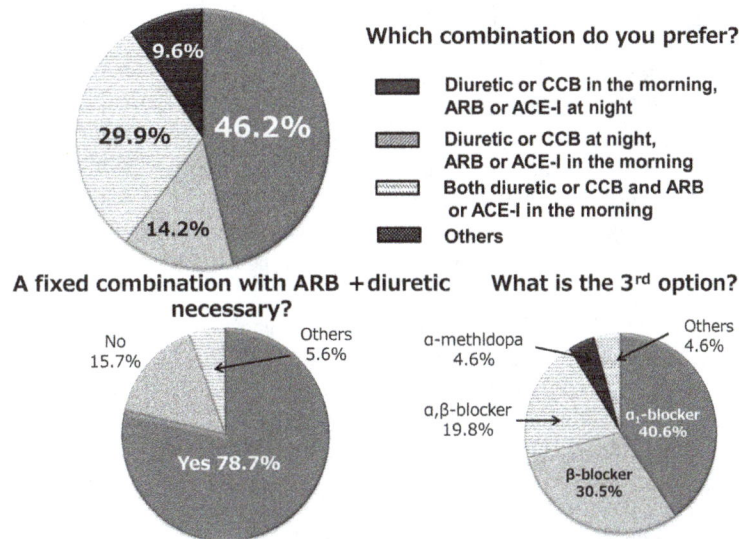

Figure 6. Combined therapies with two drugs and a need for a fixed for- mulation tablet.

viates morning hypertension in patients with hypertension, and found that this agent efficaciously improved morning hypertension [33] [35].

The administration timing of the two drugs if the patients would require dual treatment was quite diverse (**Figure 6**). Administration of a diuretic or CCB in the morning with ARB or ACE-I at night came as the first preference (46.2%). The second preference was an administration of both diuretic or CCB and ARB or ACE-I together in the morning (29.9%). The third preference was an administration of diuretic or CCB at night and ARB or ACE-I in the morning (14.2%). When asked if there was a need to prescribe a fixed formulation with ARB plus diuretic, the majority replied in an affirmative way (78.7%). It implies that a fixed formulation tablet could be prescribed for at least 1/3 of the patients who would be treated with more than two drugs.

To summarize, this present study confirms that the majority of doctors in Japan accepted that home-BP is important. Since little is known about the diagnostic, prognostic and therapeutic values of home-BP, there is an urgent need for clinical studies on how to use home-BP in terms of improving long-term patients' prognostic outcomes.

5. Conclusion

The doctors in clinical practice of CKD in Japan have a high awareness of the importance of home-BP, though choices of antihypertensive agents remain diverse. Since little has been established regarding how to integrate home-BP into clinical practices, it appears imperatively to proceed with further clinical investigations in this field.

Conflict of Interest

No conflict of interest is declared.

References

[1]   Jula, A., Puukka, P. and Karanko, H. (1999) Multiple Clinic and Home Blood Pressure Measurements versus Ambulatory Blood Pressure Monitoring. *Hypertension*, **34**, 261-266. http://dx.doi.org/10.1161/01.HYP.34.2.261

[2]   Mancia, G., Parati, G., Hennig, M., Flatau, B., Omboni, S., Glavina, F., Costa, B., Scherz, R., Bond, G. and Zanchetti, A. (2001) For the ELSA Investigators. Relationship between Blood Pressure Variability and Carotid Artery Damage in Hypertension: Baseline Data from the European Lacidipine Study on Atherosclerosis (ELSA). *Journal of Hypertension*, **19**, 1981-1989. http://dx.doi.org/10.1097/00004872-200111000-00008

[3]   Mancia, G. and Parati, G. (2000) Ambulatory Blood Pressure Monitoring and Organ Damage. *Hypertension*, **36**, 894-900. http://dx.doi.org/10.1161/01.HYP.36.5.894

[4]   Mancia, G., Zanchetti, A., Agabiti-Rosei, E., Benemio, G., De Cesaris, R., Fogari, R., Pessina, A., Porcellati, C., Rap-
      pelli, A., Salvetti, A. and Trimarco, B. (1997) Ambulatory Blood Pressure Is Superior to Clinic Blood Pressure in Pre-
      dicting Treatment Reduced Regression of Left Ventricular Hypertrophy. *Circulation*, **95**, 1464-1470.
      http://dx.doi.org/10.1161/01.CIR.95.6.1464

[5]   Khattar, R.S., Swales, J.D., Banfield, A., Dore, C., Senior, R. and Lahiri, A. (1999) Prediction of Coronary and Cere-
      brovascular Morbidity Blood Pressure Monitoring in Essential Hypertension. *Circulation*, **100**, 1071-1076.
      http://dx.doi.org/10.1161/01.CIR.100.10.1071

[6]   Lurbe, E., Redon, J., Kesani, A., Pascual, J.M., Tacons, J., Alvarez, V. and Batlle, D. (2002) Increase in Nocturnal
      Blood Pressure and Progression to Microalbuminuria in Type I Diabetes. *The New England Journal of Medicine*, **347**,
      797-805. http://dx.doi.org/10.1056/NEJMoa013410

[7]   Perloff, D., Sokolow, M. and Cowan, R. (1983) The Prognostic Value of Ambulatory Bloodpressures. *JAMA*, **249**,
      2793-2798. http://dx.doi.org/10.1001/jama.1983.03330440030027

[8]   Redon, J., Campos, C., Narciso, M.L., Rodicio, J.L., Pascual, J.M. and Ruilope, L.M. (1998) Prognostic Value of Am-
      bulatory Blood Pressure Monitoring in Refractory Hypertension: A Prospective Study. *Hypertension*, **31**, 712-718.
      http://dx.doi.org/10.1161/01.HYP.31.2.712

[9]   Robinson, T.G., Dawson, S.L., Ahmed, U., Manktelow, B., Fotherby, M.D. and Potter, J.F. (2001) Twenty-Four Hour
      Systolic Blood Pressure Predicts Long-Term Mortality Following Acute Stroke. *Journal of Hypertension*, **19**, 2127-
      2134. http://dx.doi.org/10.1097/00004872-200112000-00003

[10] Staessen, J.A., Thijs, L., Fagard, R., O'Brien, E.T., Clement, D., de Leeuw, P.W., Mancia, G., Nachev, C., Palatini, P.,
      Parati, G., Tuomilehto, J. and Webster, J. (1999) Predicting Cardiovascular Risk Using Conventional vs Ambulatory
      Blood Pressure in Older Patients with Systolic Hypertension: Systolic Hypertension in Europe Trial Investigators.
      JAMA, **282**, 539-546. http://dx.doi.org/10.1001/jama.282.6.539

[11] Bjorklund, K., Lind, L., Zethelius, B., Andren, B. and Lithell, H. (2003) Isolated Ambulatory hypertension Predicts
      Cardiovascular Morbidity in Elderly Men. *Circulation*, **107**, 1297-1302.
      http://dx.doi.org/10.1161/01.CIR.0000054622.45012.12

[12] Clement, D.L., De Buyzere, M.L., De Bacquer, D.A., de Leeuw, P.W., Duprez, D.A., Fagard, R.H., Gheeraert, P.J.,
      Missault, L.H., Braun, J.J., Six, R.O., Van Der Niepen, P. and O'Brien, E. (2003) For the Office Versus Ambulatory
      Pressure Study Investigators. Prognostic Value of Ambulatory Blood Pressure in Patients with Treated Hypertension.
      The New England Journal of Medicine, **348**, 2407-2415. http://dx.doi.org/10.1056/NEJMoa022273

[13] Verdecchia, P., Reboldi, G., Porcellati, C., Schillaci, G., Pede, S., Bentivoglio, M., Angeli, F., Norgiolini, S. and Am-
      brosio, G. (2002) Risk of Cardiovascular Disease in Relation to Achieved Office and Ambulatory Blood Pressure Con-
      trol in Treated Hypertensive Subjects. *Journal of the American College of Cardiology*, **39**, 878-885.
      http://dx.doi.org/10.1016/S0735-1097(01)01827-7

[14] Yamamoto, Y., Akiguchi, I., Oiwa, K., Hayashi, M. and Kimura, J. (1998) Adverse Effect of Nighttime Blood Pressure
      on the Outcome of Lacunar Infarct Patients. *Stroke*, **29**, 570-576. http://dx.doi.org/10.1161/01.STR.29.3.570

[15] Zweiker, R., Eber, B., Schumacher, M., Toplak, H. and Klein, W. (1994) "Non-Dipping" Related to Cardiovascular
      Events in Essential Hypertensive Patients. *Acta Medica Austriaca*, **21**, 86-89.

[16] Bobrie, G., Chatellier, G., Genes, N., Clerson, P., Vaur, L., Vaisse, B., Menard, J. and Mallion, J.M. (2004) Cardi-
      ovascular Prognosis of "Masked Hypertension" Detected by Blood Pressure Self-Measurement in Elderly Treated
      Hypertensive Patients. *JAMA*, **291**, 1342-1349. http://dx.doi.org/10.1001/jama.291.11.1342

[17] Kario, K., Pickering, T.G., Matsuo, T., Hoshide, S., Schwartz, J.E. and Shimada, K. (2001) Stroke Prognosis and Ab-
      normal Nocturnal Blood Pressure Falls in Older Hypertensives. *Hypertension*, **38**, 852-857.
      http://dx.doi.org/10.1161/hy1001.092640

[18] Sega, R., Facchetti, R., Bombelli, M., Cesana, G., Corrao, G., Grassi, G. and Mancia, G. (2005) Prognostic Value of
      Ambulatory and Home Blood Pressures Compared with Office Blood Pressure in General Population. *Circulation*, **111**,
      1777-1783. http://dx.doi.org/10.1161/01.CIR.0000160923.04524.5B

[19] Verdecchia, P., Porcellati, C., Schillaci, G., Borgioni, C., Ciucci, A., Battistelli, M., Guerrieri, M., Gatteschi, C., Zampi,
      I. and Santucci, A. (1994) Ambulatory Blood Pressure: An Independent Predictor of Prognosis in Essential Hyperten-
      sion. *Hypertension*, **24**, 793-801. http://dx.doi.org/10.1161/01.HYP.24.6.793

[20] Martinez, M.A., Sancho, T., Garcia, P., Moreno, P., Rubio, J.M., Palau, F.J., Anton, J.L., Cirujano, F.J., Sanz, J., Puig,
      J.G. and MAPA Working Group (2006) Home Blood Pressure in Poorly Controlled Hypertension: Relationship with
      Ambulatory Blood Pressure and Organ Damage. *Blood Pressure Monitoring*, **11**, 207-213.
      http://dx.doi.org/10.1097/01.mbp.0000209073.30708.e1

[21] Mule, G., Caimi, G., Cottone, S., Nardi, E., Andronico, G., Piazza, G., Volpe, V., Federico, M.R. and Cerasola, G.
      (2002) Value of Home Blood Pressures as Predictor of Target Organ Damage in Mild Arterial Hypertension. *Journal*

of Cardiovascular Risk, **9**, 123-129. http://dx.doi.org/10.1097/00043798-200204000-00008

[22] Stergiou, G.S., Argyraki, K.K., Moyssakis, I., Mastorantonakis, S.E., Achimastos, A.D., Karamanos, V.G. and Roussias, L.G. (2007) Home Blood Pressure Is as Reliable as Ambulatory Blood Pressure in Predicting Target-Organ Damage in Hypertension. *American Journal of Hypertension*, **20**, 616-621. http://dx.doi.org/10.1016/j.amjhyper.2006.12.013

[23] Mancia, G., De Backer, G., Dominiczak, A., Cifkova, R., Fagard, R., Germano, G., Grassi, G., Heagerty, A.M., Kjeldsen, S.E., Laurent, S., Narkiewicz, K., Ruilope, L., Rynkiewicz, A., Schmieder, R.E., Boudier, H.A. and Zanchetti, A. (2007) Guidelines for the Management of Arterial Hypertension: The Task Force for the Management of Arterial Hypertension of the European Society of Hypertension (ESH) and of the European Society of Cardiology (ESC). *Journal of Hypertension*, **25**, 1105-1187. http://dx.doi.org/10.1097/HJH.0b013e3281fc975a

[24] Parati, G., Stergiou, G.S., Asmar, R., Bilo G, de Leeuw, P., Imai, Y., Kario, K., Lurbe, E., Manolis, A., Mengden, T., O'Brien, E., Ohkubo, T., Padfield, P., Palatini, P., Pickering, T.G., Redon, J., Revera, M., Ruilope, L.M., Shennan, A., Staessen, J.A., Tisler, A., Waeber, B., Zanchetti, A., Mancia, G. and On Behalf of ESH Working Group on Blood Pressure Monitoring (2010) European Society of Hypertension Practice Guidelines for Home Blood Pressure Monitoring. *Journal of Human Hypertension*, **24**, 779-785. http://dx.doi.org/10.1038/jhh.2010.54

[25] Verdecchia, P., Angeli, F., Mazzatta, G., Gentile, G. and Reboldi, G. (2009) Home Blood Pressure Measurement Will Not Replace 24-Hour Ambulatory Blood Pressure Monitoring. *Hypertension*, **54**, 188-195. http://dx.doi.org/10.1161/HYPERTENSIONAHA.108.122861

[26] Kobayashi, M., Obara, T., Ohkubo, T., Fukunaga, H., Satoh, M., Metoki, H., Asayama, K., Inoue, R., Kikuya, M., Mano, N., Miyakawa, M. and Imai, Y. (2010) Practice and Awareness of Physicians Regarding Casual-Clinic Blood Pressure Measurement in Japan. *Hypertension Research*, **33**, 960-964. http://dx.doi.org/10.1038/hr.2010.89

[27] Obara, T., Ohkubo, T., Fukunaga, H., Kobayashi, M., Satoh, M., Metoki, H., Asayama, K., Inoue, R., Kikuya, M., Mano, N., Miyakawa, M. and Imai, Y. (2010) Practice and Awareness of Physicians Regarding Home Blood Pressure Measurement in Japan. *Hypertension Research*, **33**, 428-434. http://dx.doi.org/10.1038/hr.2010.10

[28] Elliot, W.J. (2002) Is Fixed Combination Therapy Appropriate for Initial Hypertension Treatment? *Current Hypertension Reports*, **4**, 278-285. http://dx.doi.org/10.1007/s11906-996-0005-z

[29] Black, H.R. (2009) Triple Fixed-Dose Combination Therapy. *Hypertension*, **54**, 19-22. http://dx.doi.org/10.1161/HYPERTENSIONAHA.109.132688

[30] Ogihara, T., Kikuchi, K., Matsuoka, H., Fujita, T., Higaki, J., Horiuchi, M., Imai, Y., Imaizumi, T., Ito, S., Iwao, H., Kario, K., Kawano, Y., Kim-Mitsuyama, S., Kimura, G., Matsubara, H., Matsuura, H., Naruse, M., Saito, I., Shimada, K., Shimamoto, K., Suzuki, H., Takishita, S., Tanahashi, N., Tsuchihashi, T., Uchiyama, M., Ueda, S., Ueshima, H., Umemura, S., Ishimitsu, T., Rakugi, H. and Japanese Society of Hypertension Committee. (2009) The Japanese Society of Hypertension Guidelines for the Management of Hypertension (JSH 2009). *Hypertension Research*, **32**, 103-107.

[31] Chobanian, A.V., Bakris, G.L., Black, H.R., Cushman, W.C., Green, L.A., Izzo Jr., J.L., Jones, D.W., Materson, B.J., Oparil, S., Wright Jr., J.T., Roccella, E.J. and Joint National Committee on Prevention, Detection, Evaluation, and Treatment of High Blood Pressure (2003) National Heart, Lung, and Blood Institute; National High Blood Pressure Education Program Coordinating Committee. Seventh Report of the Joint National Committee on Prevention, Detection, Evaluation, and Treatment of High Blood Pressure. *Hypertension*, **42**, 1206-1252. http://dx.doi.org/10.1161/01.HYP.0000107251.49515.c2

[32] Kohro, T., Yamazaki, T., Sato, H., Ohe, K. and Nagai, R. (2013) The Impact of a Change in Hypertension Management Guidelines on Diuretic Use in Japan: Trend in Antihypertensive Drug Prescriptions from 2005 to 2011. *Hypertension Research*, **36**, 559-563. http://dx.doi.org/10.1038/hr.2012.216

[33] Kario, K., Pickering, T.G., Hoshide, S., Eguchi, K., Ishikawa, J., Morinari, M., Hoshide, Y. and Shimada, K. (2004) Morning Blood Pressure Surge and Hypertensive Cerebrovascular Disease. *American Journal of Hypertension*, **17**, 668-675. http://dx.doi.org/10.1016/j.amjhyper.2004.04.001

[34] Kario, K., Schwartz, J.E. and Pickering, T.G. (2000) Changes of Nocturnal Blood Pressure Dipping Status in Hypertensives by Nighttime Dosing of α-Adrenergic Blocker, Doxazosin. Result from HALT Study. *Hypertension*, **35**, 787-794. http://dx.doi.org/10.1161/01.HYP.35.3.787

[35] Hermida, R.C., Ayala, D.E., Fernamdez, J.R. and Calvo, C. (2007) Comparison of the Efficacy of Morning versus Evening Administration of Telmisartan in Essential Hypertension. *Hypertension*, **50**, 715-722. http://dx.doi.org/10.1161/HYPERTENSIONAHA.107.094235

[36] Hermida, R.C., Ayala, D.E., Smolensky, M.H. and Portaluppi, F. (2007) Chronotherapy in Hypertensive Patients: Administration Time Dependent Effects of Treatment on Blood Pressure Regulation. *Expert Review of Cardiovascular Therapy*, **5**, 463-475. http://dx.doi.org/10.1586/14779072.5.3.463

[37] Hermida, R.C. and Ayala, D.E. (2009) Chronotherapy with the Angiotensin-Converting Enzyme Inhibitor Ramipril in Essential Hypertension: Improved Blood Pressure Control with Bedtime Dosing. *Hypertension*, **54**, 40-46.

http://dx.doi.org/10.1161/HYPERTENSIONAHA.109.130203

[38] Hermida, R.C., Ayala, D.E., SCalvo, C., Portaluppi, F. and Smolensky, M.H. (2007) Chronotherpy of Hypertension: Administration-Time-Dependent Effects of Treatment on the Circadian Pattern of Blood Pressure. *Advanced Drug Delivery Review*, **59**, 923-939. http://dx.doi.org/10.1016/j.addr.2006.09.021

33

Association between Chronic Kidney Disease and Depression

Adnan Bashir Bhatti*, Farhan Ali, Siddique A. Satti

Capital Development Authority (CDA) Hospita, Islamabad, Pakistan
Email: *dr.adnanbashir@gmail.com

Abstract

Background: Depression is relatively prevalent in chronic kidney disease (CKD) patients. Knowing the frequency of depression in these patients, the association with variables such as stage of disease, education, and income status may be helpful in devising strategies for better management. Methods: We examined 315 patients diagnosed with CKD presented in the outpatient and emergency department of medicine at Capital Hospital, Islamabad, Pakistan. Depression was diagnosed according to the Hamilton Depression Rating Scale of depressive episode. Results: In the dialysis group, 83.8% were depression positive, while in the pre-dialysis group only 61.3% of patients were given the same diagnosis (P < 0.05). A significant association was moreover found between depression and education status (P < 0.05), but not for income status. Conclusions: Considering the high incidence of depression in CKD patients, screenings should be routinely performed in order to identify and treat depression in its early stages for these patients.

Keywords

Chronic Kidney Disease, Depression, Education Status, Dialysis

1. Introduction

Chronic kidney disease (CKD) is a disease comprising of a wide spectrum of different pathophysiological processes, which is associated with abnormal renal function and a gradual degeneration of the glomerular filtration rate (GFR). The National Kidney Foundation's staging system divides the CKD patients in 5 stages according to GFR. Stage V is usually labelled as end stage renal disease (ESRD) [1].

The worldwide incidence of ESRD is increasing at a rate of about 7% per annum, and the disease has been es-

---

*Corresponding author.

timated to cost approximately 1.1 trillion dollars in medical expenditures worldwide [2]. The high incidence of chronic kidney disease in the Pakistani population is far from surprising, since the prevalence of diabetes and hypertension is very high for this population [3].

Previous studies have reported an overall mortality rate, 83% higher for CDK patients than for the general population, and also found that cardiovascular disease was twice as common in CDK patients, compared to the healthy population. Due to the irreversible nature of this disease and the bleak prognoses associated with it, psychiatric disorders such as depression are commonly observed among CKD patients [4]-[6]. Depression may be triggered by a number of social, biologic, and psychological factors, and this has been reported to occur at any point during the progression of CKD [7]. Factors that affect the risk of depression include socioeconomic factors, and education status, the gender of the patient, and the presence/absence of symptoms such as disturbed liver function due to hepatitis, hypertension or hypoalbuminemia [8].

Although depression is frequently observed among renal dialysis patients, active detection and management (in form of psychotherapy and/or pharmacotherapy) are usually not part of the routine care for these patients [9]. To date, very few data are available regarding the frequency of depression in CKD and dialysis patients in Pakistan, and hence, we aimed to explore this.

2. Materials and Methods

2.1. Overview

A cross-sectional study was conducted in the emergency and outpatient medical department of Capital Hospital, Islamabad, Pakistan from January 1 to December 31, 2010. Permissions were granted from the concerned authorities of Capital Hospital Islamabad (Head of the Department of Medicine, Hospital Ethical Committee) before the initiation of the data collection phase.

2.2. Data Collection

By non-probability convenient sampling, 315 patients with diagnosed CKD (according to K/DQOI of the National Kidney Foundation of USA criteria) were included in the study.

Verbal consent was taken from all the patients after explaining the nature and purpose of the study at the beginning of the study. To minimize bias, all patients were handled by the same physician. After identification of patients with CKD, a detailed history was taken for diagnosis and fulfilment of the required selection criteria.

2.3. Tools

Information was collected using structured proforma. Demographic and clinical data were recorded, including patient history of diabetes mellitus, hypertension, glomerular diseases and interstitial disease. The Kidney Disease Outcome Quality Initiative (K/DOQI) guidelines by the National Kidney Foundation were used to stage CKD into five stages (Pre dialysis-CKD: Stages 2 - 4; Dialysis-CKD: Stage 5) based on the estimated glomerular filtration rate (eGFR). eGFR measurement was done by Cockcroft Gault formula, as follows:

$$\text{Creatinine clearance}\left(C_{Cr}\right) = 140 - \text{AGE} \times \text{weight}\left(\text{kg}\right)\big/\text{Plasma Creatinine}\left(P_{Cr}\right) \times 72.$$

For females, the creatinine clearance was multiplied by 0.85 due to generally lower percentages of muscle mass compared to males. The diagnosis and severity of depression was made according to the Hamilton Depression Rating Scale of depressive episodes. Patients were graded as: no depression (score 0 - 7); mild depression (8 - 17); moderate depression (18 - 25); and severe depression (>25). Each item was read out loud by the physician to the patient, and the symptoms were marked according to the response. To supplement this, the Urdu version of the Hamilton Depression Rating Scale (H.D.R.S) was used.

2.4. Data Analysis

The statistical package for social sciences (SPSS, version 13.0, Chicago, IL) was used to enter and analyse the data. Mean values, standard deviations, frequencies and percentages were calculated. Chi square test was used to compare the frequency of depression between the two groups (Pre-dialysis and dialysis). A P-value <0.05 was considered significant.

2.5. Exclusion Criteria

Patients aged less than 18 years or more than 90 years; patients already receiving treatment for depression; patients with chronic medical illness; patients with somatic symptoms of uraemia; and patients with other psychiatric diseases were excluded from the study.

3. Results

Out of a total of 315 patients enrolled in the study, 204 (64.76%) patients were in dialysis group and 111 (35.24%) were in pre-dialysis group. In the pre-dialysis group, 52 patients were male, with a mean age (±SD) of 56.37 years ± 17.07, and 59 were female, with a mean age (±SD) of 49.36 years ± 19.17. In the dialysis group, there were 106 males and 98 females, with a mean age (±SD) of 49.49 years ± 17.47 and 44.17 years ± 17.83, respectively (**Table 1**).

30.5% of all patients belonged to the low income group; 38.1% of patients belonged to middle income group; and 31.4% of patients belonged to the high income group (**Table 2**). In total, 117 (37.1%) patients had no formal education; 76 (24.1%) had less than, or equal to, eight years of school education; 57 (18.1%) had greater than eight years but less than, or equal to, ten years of education; 52 (16.5%) had greater than ten years education with a less than, or equal to, graduate level education; and 13 (4.1%) had a postgraduate level of school education.

In the dialysis group, depression was present in 171 (83.8%) patients, whereas 33 (16.2%) patients showed no signs of depression. In the pre-dialysis group, depression was present in 68 cases (61.3%; **Table 3**). In the low-income group, 80 patients (83.3%) diagnosed with depression. For the middle-income group, this number was 87 (72.5%), and for the high-income group, 72 patients (72.7%) had depression, as shown in **Table 4**.

Depression was present in 80 (68.4%) patients with no formal education and in 61 (80.3%) of patients belonging to the middle or less education group. The middle to matric education group had 45 (78.9%) cases of depression, whereas the matric to graduation groups had 46 (88.5%) cases of depression. and the post graduation group had 7 (53.8%) cases (**Table 5**).

4. Discussion

There is increasing evidence supporting a role for psychosocial factors such as depression, anxiety, and perceived social support, in the pathophysiology of various chronic diseases, including CKD, where depressive disorders have been found to be associated with an increased risk of mortality, and poor health-related quality of life [10]. We here used the Hamilton Depression Rating Scale to diagnose the different stages of depression. The Hamilton Depression Rating Scale is one of many ways to stage depression, and has recently been shown to be a

Table 1. Gender and age of CKD patients.

	Pre-dialysis (Stage II-IV)	Mean Age ± SD (years)	Dialysis (Stage V)	Mean Age ± SD (years)
Male	52 (46.85%)	56.37 ± 17.07	106 (51.96%)	49.49 ± 17.47
Females	59 (53.15%)	49.36 ± 19.17	98 (48.04%)	44.17 ± 17.83
Total	111 (100%)	52.64 ± 18.86	204 (100%)	47.20 ± 17.74

Table 2. Patients according to income status.

Income	Frequency	Percentage (%)	Valid Percentage (%)	Cumulative Percentage (%)
Low[1]	96	30.5	30.5	30.5
Middle[2]	120	38.1	38.1	68.6
High[3]	99	31.4	31.4	100.0
Total	315	100.0	100.0	

[1]Low income was identified as <10,000 PKR per month; [2]Middle income was identified as 10,000 - 25,000 PKR per month; [3]High income was identified as >25,000 PKR per month.

Table 3. Association of different stages of depression with stages of CKD (dialysis and pre-dialysis groups).

Stages of depression (Hamilton Depression Rating Scale)	Pre Dialysis	Dialysis	P-Value
No depression	43 (38.7%)	33 (16.2%)	
Mild depression	2 (1.8%)	11 (5.4%)	
Moderate depression	6 (5.4%)	20 (9.8%)	<0.001[1]
Severe depression	60 (54.1%)	140 (68.6%)	
Total	111 (100.0%)	204 (100.0%)	

[1]Absent vs. present depression.

Table 4. Association of different stages of depression with different group of income status.

Stages of depression	Low income[1]	Middle income[2]	High income[3]	Total	P-Value
No depression	16 (16.7%)	33 (27.5%)	27 (27.3%)	76 (24.1%)	
Mild depression	10 (10.4%)	5 (4.2%)	2 (2.0%)		
Moderate depression	12 (12.5%)	2 (1.7%)	10 (10.1%)	239 (75.9%)	0.122[4]
Severe depression	58 (60.4%)	80 (66.7%)	60 (60.6%)		
Total	96 (100.0%)	120 (100.0%)	99 (100.0%)	315 (100.0%)	

[1]Low income was identified as <10,000 PKR per month; [2]Middle income was identified as 10,000 - 25,000 PKR per month; [3]High income was identified as >25,000 PKR per month; [4]Absent vs. present depression.

Table 5. Association of different stages of depression with education status.

Stages of depression	No formal education	Middle or less	Middle to matric	Matric to graduation	Post graduation	Total	P-Value
No depression	37 (31.6%)	15 (19.7%)	12 (21.1%)	6 (11.5%)	6 (46.2%)	76 (24.1%)	
Mild depression	5 (4.3%)	1 (1.3%)	3 (5.3%)	2 (3.8%)	1 (7.7%)		
Moderate depression	10 (8.5%)	5 (6.6%)	2 (3.5%)	5 (9.6%)	1 (7.7%)	239 (75.9%)	0.013[1]
Severe depression	65 (55.6 %)	55 (72.4%)	40 (70.2%)	39 (75.0%)	5 (38.5%)		
Total	117 (100.0%)	76 (100.0%)	57 (100.0%)	52 (100.0%)	13 (100.0%)	315 (100.0%)	

[1]Absent vs. present depression.

valid alternative to these other methods [11].

Similar results to what we found in this study have recently been reported by Hung *et al.* (2011), who explored the relationship between depression and demographic, socio-economic and clinical variables in CKD patients [12]. In another study, Wuerth *et al.* (2003) screened chronic peritoneal dialysis (PD) patients from July 1997 to October 2002, using the Beck Depression Inventory questionnaire. Based on the Hamilton Depression Scale and Standard Diagnostic and Statistical Manual of Mental Disorders criteria, 87% (comparable to 83.8% in our study) of their patients were diagnosed as being clinically depressed [13].

Watnick *et al.* (2003) showed that symptoms of depression were frequently observed at the early stages of dialysis treatment. However, they also noted that despite a high prevalence, treatment for the depression was rarely prescribed, even for patients described as having moderate-severe depression [14].

In two studies consisting of 210 and 380 peritoneal dialysis patients, scores consistent with a possible diagnosis of clinical depression were observed in 42% and 49%, respectively. Out of the patients who agreed to further testing, 87% and 84%, respectively, were diagnosed with clinical depression based on standard psychiatric criteria [15] [16].

Hedayatti *et al.* (2009) found in their study that 1 in 5 patients with CKD had experienced at least one major depressive episode, and that, for patient with late-stage CKD, there was an independent association between depression and poor survival outcome [17]. Hence, we suggest, as they also concluded, that, given the high prevalence of depression in CKD patients, routine screenings should be performed.

Lastly, another study also showed that depression correlated with a considerably increased risk of death in CKD patients [18]. However, during the course of our study, no patients died, and we were hence unable to draw any conclusions regarding the correlation between CKD, depression and patient survival.

5. Conclusion

In summary, we here examined 315 Pakistani patients with CKD for signs of depression, and for any associations between depression and education status and income. We found that the frequency of depression was significantly higher in the dialysis group and was significantly associated with education status, with patients with higher levels of education showing a lower frequency of depression ($P < 0.05$). No association was found between depression and income status in this study. We conclude that given the high prevalence of depression in CKD patients, screenings should be routinely performed in order to identify and treat depression in its early stages for these patients.

References

[1] Bargman, J.M. and Skorecki, K. (2008) Chronic Kidney Disease. In: Fauci, A.S., Braunwald, E., Kasper, D.L., Hauser, S.L., Eds., Harrison's Principles of Internal Medicine, Mc Graw Hill, 1761-1771.

[2] Lysaght, M.J. (2002) Maintenance Dialysis Population Dynamics: Current Trends and Long-Term Implications. *Journal of the American Society of Nephrology*, **13**, S37-S40.

[3] Tamizuddin, S. and Ahmed, W. (2010) Knowledge, Attitude and Practices Regarding Chronic Kidney Disease and Estimated GFR in a Tertiary Care Hospital in Pakistan. *Journal Pakistan Medical Association*, **60**, 342-346.

[4] Bossola, M., Ciciarelli, C., Stasio, D., *et al.* (2010) Correlates of Symptoms of Depression and Anxiety in Chronic Hemodialysis Patients. *General Hospital Psychiatry*, **32**, 125-131.
http://dx.doi.org/10.1016/j.genhosppsych.2009.10.009

[5] Chilcot, J., Wellsted, D. and Farrington, K. (2010) Depression in End-Stage Renal Disease: Current Advances and Research. *Seminars in Dialysis*, **23**, 74-82. http://dx.doi.org/10.1111/j.1525-139X.2009.00628.x

[6] Cukor, D., Cohen, S.D., Peterson, R.A., *et al.* (2007) Psychosocial Aspects of Chronic Disease: ESRD as a Paradigmatic Illness. *Journal of the American Society of Nephrology*, **18**, 3042-3055.
http://dx.doi.org/10.1681/ASN.2007030345

[7] Zalai, D.M. and Novak, M. (2008) Depressive Disorders in Patients with Chronic Kidney Disease. *Prim Psychiatry*, **15**, 66-72.

[8] Anees, M., Barki, H., Masood, M., Mumtaz, A. and Kausar, T. (2008) Depression in Hemodialysis Patients. *Pakistan Journal of Medical Sciences*, **24**, 560-565.

[9] Chilcot, J., Wellsted, D. and Farrington, K. (2008) Screening for Depression While Patients Dialyse: An Evaluation. *Nephrology Dialysis Transplantation*, **23**, 2653-2659. http://dx.doi.org/10.1093/ndt/gfn105

[10] McKercher, C., Sanderson, K. and Jose, M.D. (2013) Psychosocial Factors in People with Chronic Kidney Disease Prior to Renal Replacement Therapy. *Nephrology*, **18**, 585-591. http://dx.doi.org/10.1111/nep.12138

[11] Leentjens, A.F.G., Dujardin, K., Marsh, L., *et al.* (2011) Anxiety Rating Scales in Parkinson's Disease: A Validation Study of the Hamilton Anxiety Rating Scale, the Beck Anxiety Inventory, and the Hospital Anxiety and Depression Scale. *Movement Disorders*, **26**, 407-415. http://dx.doi.org/10.1002/mds.23184

[12] Hung, K.C., Wu, C.C. and Chen, H.S. (2001) Serum IL-6, Albumin and Comorbidities Are Closely Correlated with Symptoms of Depression in Patients on Maintenance Haemodialysis. *Nephrology Dialysis Transplantation*, **26**, 658-664. http://dx.doi.org/10.1093/ndt/gfq411

[13] Wuerth, D., Finkelstein, S.H., Kliger, A.S., *et al.* (2003) Chronic Peritoneal Dialysis Patients Diagnosed with Clinical Depression: Results of Pharmacologic Therapy. *Seminars in Dialysis*, **16**, 424-427.
http://dx.doi.org/10.1046/j.1525-139X.2003.16094.x

[14] Watnick, S., Kirwin, P., Mahnensmith, R. and Concato, J. (2003) The Prevalence and Treatment of Depression among Patients Starting Dialysis. *American Journal of Kidney Disease*, **41**, 105-110.
http://dx.doi.org/10.1053/ajkd.2003.50029

[15] Israel, M. (1986) Depression in Dialysis Patients: A Review of Psychological Factors. *Canadian Journal of Psychiatry*, **31**, 445-451.

[16] Wuerth, D., Finkelstein, S.H. and Finkelstein, F.O. (2005) The Identification and Treatment of Depression in Patients Maintained on Dialysis. *Seminars in Dialysis*, **18**, 142-146. http://dx.doi.org/10.1111/j.1525-139X.2005.18213.x

[17] Hedayati, S.S., Minhajuddin, A.T. and Toto, R.D. (2009) Prevalence of Major Depressive Episode in CKD. *American Journal of Kidney Disease*, **54**, 424-432. http://dx.doi.org/10.1053/j.ajkd.2009.03.017

[18] Palmer, S.C., Vecchio, M., Craig, J.C., *et al.* (2013) Association between Depression and Death in People with CKD: A Meta-Analysis of Cohort Studies. *American Journal of Kidney Disease*, **62**, 493-505. http://dx.doi.org/10.1053/j.ajkd.2013.02.369

34

Antiproteinuric Effect of Sulodexide versus Losartan in Primary Glomerulonephritis

Abdul Halim Abdul Gafor[1], Wan Hazlina Wan Mohamad[1], Rozita Mohd[1],
Rizna Abdul Cader[1], Kong Wei Yen[1], Shamsul Azhar Shah[2], Norella C. T. Kong[1]

[1]Nephrology Unit, Department of Medicine, University Kebangsaan Malaysia Medical Centre, Jalan Yaacob Latif, Bandar Tun Razak, Cheras, Kuala Lumpur, Malaysia
[2]Department of Epidemiology and Biostatistics, University Kebangsaan Malaysia Medical Centre, Jalan Yaacob Latif, Bandar Tun Razak, Cheras, Kuala Lumpur, Malaysia
Email: halimgafor@gmail.com

Abstract

Introduction: Limited data are available for the use of sulodexide in primary glomerulonephritis (GN). Objective: We studied the efficacy of sulodexide compared to losartan in patients with primary GN. Design and Method: This was a prospective, open labelled, randomized control trial in patients with stable primary GN. Patients were randomized to receive either sulodexide or losartan to maximum tolerated doses for 12 weeks. Blood and urine investigations were measured at baseline and at 4-weekly intervals. Adverse effects were recorded. Results: 18 patients were recruited (10-sulodexide and 8-losartan). Their baseline characteristics were comparable. At end study, patients in both groups showed no significant reduction in proteinuria and there were no differences between groups at each visit. Nonetheless, there was a trend towards lower protein uria in the losartan but not in sulodexide group. There were no changes in the other parameters of renal function or of coagulation over time. No adverse events in particular clinical bleeding occurred. Conclusion: Sulodexide and losartan did not demonstrate any significant anti-proteinuric effect in primary GN. Nevertheless, there was a trend of better proteinuria reduction in losartan group. Furthermore, other renal parameters were not significantly affected by both drugs.

Keywords

Antiproteinuria, Losartan, Primary Glomerulonephritis, Sulodexide

1. Introduction

Glomerulonephritis (GN) is a renal disease characterized by inflammation of the glomeruli, or small blood vessels in the kidneys. GN is broadly categorized into primary GN and secondary GN. Primary GN is due to intrinsic causes to the kidney while secondary GN is due to infection, drugs, diabetes mellitus or systemic disorders. Primary GN includes minimal change disease (MCN), focal segmental glomerulosclerosis (FSGS), primary membranous GN, immunoglobulin A nephropathy (IgAN) and various proliferative GN.

Little is known about the worldwide variation in incidence of primary GN. A systemic review had shown the incidence of primary GN to vary between 0.2/100,000/year and 2.5/100,000/year worldwide [1]. The commonest primary GN reported by the 3rd report of the Malaysian Registry of Renal Biopsy 2009 was MCN (33.4%), FSGS (29.3%) followed by IgAN (19.6%) and idiopathic membranous nephropathy (9.8%) [2]. GN is the third leading cause of end stage renal disease (ESRD) in United States [3] and fourth in the Malaysian population [4].

Proteinuria is the clinical hallmark of GN and is the most important predictor of outcome. It is also an independent determinant of the progression of chronic kidney disease (CKD)—the greater the proteinuria the more rapid decline of renal function [5]-[7]. These patients also have increased cardiovascular risk which is further aggravated by reduction of the glomerulofiltration rate (GFR) [8]. Hence, therapeutic intervention that reduces the level of proteinuria should impact the progression of proteinuric nephropathies.

As most primary GN is immune mediated, immunosuppressive therapy is an important first line treatment. The next therapeutic approach is the inhibition of the renin-angiotensin-aldosterone system (RAAS) by using angiotensin-converting enzymes inhibitors (ACE-I) and/or angiotensin II receptor blockers (ARBs) and/or aldosterone receptor blockers. These have both antihypertensive and antiproteinuric properties and have been shown to significantly reduce the rate of progression of both diabetic and non diabetic nephropathies [9]-[12].

One of the pathogenic mechanisms leading to proteinuria in GN, involves an alteration in heparin sulfate (HS) expression in glomerular basement membrane (GBM). HS is a member of the family of glycosaminoglycans (GAGs) that is generally bound to a core protein to form a proteoglycan (PG). Alterations in HS expression in the GBM had been reported in many proteinuric renal diseases which include diabetic nephropathy, minimal change nephropathy and membranous GN [13]. The decrease of HS content causes a reduction on the permselectivity to negatively charged macromolecules such as albumin thus allowing protein leak into the urinary space.

Sulodexide is a highly purified mixture of GAGs composed of a fast-moving heparin like substance (80%) and dermatan sulphate (20%), with a low molecular weight, a high oral bioavailability and possesses antithrombotic and profibrinolytic activities [14]. This mixture of GAGs is highly purified from porcine intestinal mucosa by a patented process. It is concentrates in the renal parenchyma for a long time after administration [15]. It was shown to reduce proteinuria in patients with diabetes kidney disease (DKD) and non DKD [16]-[23].

In addition to increasing the permselectivity of the GBM, sulodexide also inhibits mesangial cell proliferation [24] and exerts an antimitogenic effect on glomerular epithelial cells [25]. It reduces transforming growth factor-β expression and has an anti-thrombotic effect which helps to further reduce proteinuria [24] [26] [27].

The fast moving heparin (FMH) and dermatan sulphate (DS) accelerate the inhibition of thrombin by their interaction with ATIII and heparin cofactor II (HCII) and directly inhibit thrombin and thrombin generation by inhibiting the feedback activation of prothrombin. Sulodexide also prolongs the thrombin clotting time and the activated partial thromboplastin time (aPTT) [28] [29]. Several clinical trials have demonstrated the beneficial effect of sulodexide in the treatment of deep vein thrombosis [30] [31], venous leg ulcers [32] and intermittent claudication [33].

Most studies of the antiprotenuric effect of sulodexide have been carried out in patients with type 1 and/or type 2 diabetes mellitus. The antiproteinuric effect of sulodexide in proteinuric chronic primary GN is less well studied [34].

Most studies investigating the use of sulodexide as a novel antiproteinuric agent that works on perm selectivity of the GBM have been performed in patients with DKD and non DKD and many have reported that sulodexide had a significant antiproteinuric effect with or without added RAAS blockade [17] [18] [20]-[22]. However, there are no studies that have directly compared sulodexide and a RAAS blocker (e.g. losartan) as antiproteinuric agents. Hence we would like to perform a head-to-head comparison of this novel GAG with the ARB, losartan to evaluate the efficacy of sulodexide as an alternative antiproteinuric agent in primary GN.

Our primary objective was to evaluate the antiproteinuric effect of sulodexide compared to losartan, an ARB in primary GN. Our secondary objectives were to evaluate the effect of sulodexide compared to losartan on other parameters of renal function and determine the safety of sulodexide on parameters of coagulation.

2. Methodology

2.1. Patients and Method

This was a prospective open labelled randomized control trial involving patients with primary GN on follow up at the Nephrology Unit, Universiti Kebangsaan Malaysia Medical Centre (UKMMC). The study approved by the local Ethics & Research Committee (FF-454-2011).

Only patients with proteinuria of 0.3 g - 3.5 g/day and CKD stages 1 - 3 (eGFR > 30 ml/min/1.73m^2) with the diagnosis of primary GN included in this study. Patients on stable maintenance immunosuppressive therapy were included without altering the immunosuppressive drug. All patients had blood pressure of ≤ 150/90 mmHg and serum potassium of < 5.5 mmol/L at recruitment. Patients with known renal artery stenosis or allergy to study drugs were excluded from this study. Pregnant or lactating patients and patients with childbearing potential without effective method of birth control were also excluded from this study.

2.2. Randomization

Patients who met the eligibility criteria were recruited. Prior to randomization patients who were on RAAS blockers underwent a 4-week washout period. Other antihypertensive medications were continued. The patients were reviewed 2-weekly during the washout period and target systolic BP ≤ 150 mmHg and diastolic BP ≤ 90 mmHg were maintained. Other antihypertensive medications were added and/or dose adjusted until target blood pressure was achieved. Patients naïve to losartan and those who had undergone the RAAS blocker washout period were randomized into the sulodexide or losartan arms. Randomization was done in blocks of four. A short sequence of four probable alphabetical orders of AB combination were put in an envelope and pulled out as patients were recruited.

2.3. Study Protocol

At study entry, full blood count, coagulation profiles and blood samples for renal, liver and lipid profiles were taken. Spot urine sample urine Protein Creatinine Index (uPCI) was also taken. The treatment was for 12 weeks. Patients were reviewed at Weeks 0 (baseline), 2, 4 (V1), 8 (V2) and 12 (V3). At Weeks 4 (V1), 8 (V2) and 12 (V3)-blood pressure, uPCI and blood investigations listed above were taken each visit except for the estimated GFR (eGFR), coagulation and lipid parameters which were evaluated at the beginning (V0) and end of the study-Week 12 (V3). The eGFR was calculated by the Modification of Diet in Renal disease (MDRD) formula.

Losartan and sulodexide doses were titrated up to the maximum tolerated dose as judged by blood pressure. Losartan dosages ranged from 50 - 100 mg daily and those for sulodexide from 100 - 200 mg daily. Patients were strongly advised to adhere to the study drugs given and to report any adverse reactions either by phone or during clinic visits. Patient compliance to study treatment was assessed by pill counts. Compliance was taken as adherence with medications ≥80% of the time.

2.4. Statistical Analysis

All data were recorded and analyzed using the statistical package Statistical Package for the Social Sciences version 20 (IBM SPSS, Armonk, NY: IBM Corp). Our sample size was small and was not normally distributed; hence non-parametric tests were used. Results were expressed as median with interquartile range (IQR). The differences between two groups were analyzed using the Mann-Whitney-U test. Related data across time were analyzed using both the Wilcoxon Rank test and the Friedman's analysis. Nominal and ordinal data were analyzed using Fisher's exact test. A p value of < 0.05 was considered significant.

3. Results

Eighty seven patients were screened and 34 patients were noted to be in complete remission with proteinuria < 0.3 g/day. Ten patients were excluded as they were not on stable immunosuppressive therapies. Eight patients had CKD above stage 3, 7 patients declined, 4 patients were non compliant to medications, 4 females had breast cancer and 2 females were pregnant. Hence only 18 patients were recruited with 10 patients randomized to receive sulodexide and eight patients to losartan.

Baseline demographics and clinical characteristics were tabulated in **Table 1**. Baseline laboratory investigations were tabulated in **Table 2**.

Median dose for sulodexide was 150 (100 - 200) mg daily and losartan was 75 (50 - 100) mg daily. The use of other concurrent medications including antihypertensive, statin, aspirin and immunosuppressive medication were the same between both groups. There was no significant difference of blood pressure across the study duration in both study groups.

Both groups did not show any significant reduction in proteinuria whether intragroup or intergroup and across all visits. Nonetheless, the losartan arm had a trend towards lower proteinuria at end study whilst in the sulodexide group, proteinuria levels remained static (**Figure 1**).

Other renal parameters results were tabulated in **Table 3**. There were no significant differences in all the parameters in between and within both groups.

Over the 12 weeks of treatment, there were no significant changes in the full blood count parameters nor prothrombin time (PT), international normalized ratio (INR) and activated partial thromboplastin time (APTT) in patients in the sulodexide arm. There were also no clinical episodes of bleeding and no other adverse effects occurred.

4. Discussion

Primary GN is one of the common renal diseases that progress to ESRD. Besides immunosuppressive medications, RAAS blockade play an important role in the treatment of primary GN and reduction of proteinuria by reducing the intraglomerular pressure. A few randomized trials have shown that losartan has significant antiproteinuric effect in primary GN [35]-[39].

Table 1. Baseline demographics and clinical characteristics of the study groups.

Parameters	Sulodexide (n = 10)	Losartan (n = 8)	p value
Age (years)	48.5 (39.25 - 53.50)	53.0 (37.75 - 66.25)	0.573
Gender			
Male	1 (10%)	6 (75%)	0.013
Female	9 (90%)	2 (25%)	
Weight (kg)	58.2 (51.85 - 62.15)	66.0 (58.8 - 75.0)	0.460
Height (cm)	156.5 (154.0 - 163.8)	170.0 (155.0 - 175.0)	0.360
Body mass index (kg/m^2)	22.24 (21.40 - 25.85)	25.43 (23.82 - 28.14)	0.203
Blood pressure in mmHg			
Systolic BP	124 (110 - 137)	132 (130 - 143)	0.101
Diastolic BP	70 (70 - 72)	80 (70 - 90)	0.315
Primary Glomerulonephritis			
Ig AN	4 (40%)	4 (50%)	
FSGS	6 (60%)	3 (37.5%)	0.473
Membranous	0 (0%)	1 (12.5%)	
Age at diagnosis (years)	39 (34 - 44)	45 (30 - 51)	0.740
Disease duration (years)	7 (4 - 9)	7 (6 - 10)	0.573
Baseline Co-Morbidities			
Hypertension	4 (40%)	7 (87.5%)	0.066
Dyslipidaemia	6 (60%)	5 (62.5%)	1.000
Smoking	1 (10%)	0 (0%)	1.000

Results in median (IQR), IQR: interquartile range; IgAN: IgA nephropathy; FSGS: Focal segmental glomerulosclerosis; p value < 0.05 is significant.

Table 2. Baseline laboratory parameters of the two study groups.

Parameters	Sulodexide (n = 10)	Losartan (n = 8)	p value
Haemoglobin (g/dl) (NR: 4.0 - 10.0)	12.3 (11.9 - 13.1)	13.5 (12.9 - 13.6)	0.068
Platelets ($\times 10^9$/L) (NR: 150 - 400)	298 (245 - 347)	257 (216 - 332)	0.360
Total white blood cells ($\times 10^9$/L) (NR: 4.0 - 10.0)	7.5 (6.4 - 9.4)	6.9 (4.6 - 9.8)	0.696
Se urea (mmol/L) (NR: 2.5 - 6.4)	4.5 (3.4 - 6.4)	5.1 (3.4 - 5.7)	0.897
Se creatinine (umol/L) (NR: 62 - 106)	67 (54.2 - 100.7)	96 (67.2 - 119.2)	0.101
Se potassium (mmol/l) (NR: 3.5 - 5.0)	4.1 (3.7 - 4.5)	3.8 (3.8 - 4.0)	0.315
Se uric acid (umol/l) (NR: 149 - 450)	353 (303 - 408)	472 (391 - 521)	0.550
Se albumin (g/L) (NR: 35 - 50)	43 (40 - 44)	42 (38 - 45)	0.829
uPCI (g/mmol creat) (NR: <0.02)	0.09 (0.04 - 0.15)	0.07 (0.05 - 0.08)	0.360
CKD			
Stage 1	6 (60%)	2 (25%)	
Stage 2	2 (20%)	4 (50%)	0.343
Stage 3	2 (20%)	2 (25%)	
eGFR (ml/min/1.7m^2)	93 (64 - 104)	63 (55 - 84)	0.203
Total cholesterol (mmol/L) (NR: <5.7)	5.39 (4.62 - 6.37)	5.02 (4.29 - 5.74)	0.370
HDL (mmol/L) (NR: >1.20)	1.75 (1.22 - 1.97)	1.36 (1.10 - 1.65)	0.673
LDL (mmol/L) (NR: <3.80)	3.06 (2.48 - 3.89)	2.83 (2.36 - 2.84)	0.374
Triglyceride (mmol/L) (NR: <1.40)	1.24 (0.85 - 1.74)	1.52 (1.15 - 1.73)	0.606

Results in median (IQR), IQR: interquartile range; uPCI: urine protein index; CKD: Chronic Kidney Disease; eGFR: estimated glomerular filtration rate; HDL: high-density lipoprotein; LDL: low-density lipoprotein; p value < 0.05 is significant.

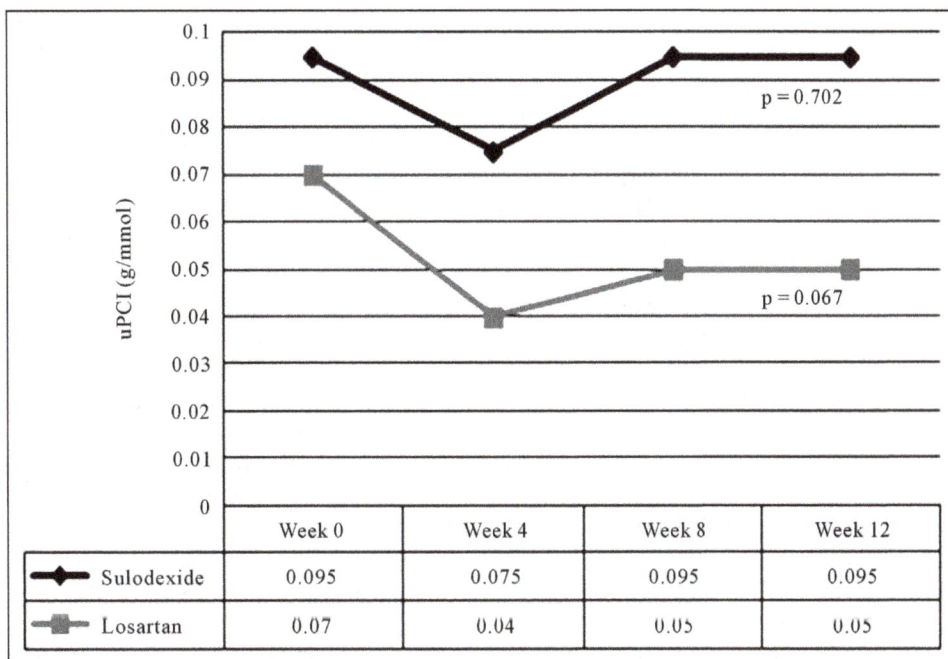

	Week 0	Week 4	Week 8	Week 12
Sulodexide	0.095	0.075	0.095	0.095
Losartan	0.07	0.04	0.05	0.05

Figure 1. uPCI across the study period in both groups.

Table 3. Other renal parameters across the study period and in between the two groups.

		Week 0	Week 4	Week 8	Week 12	p value*
Se creatinine (umol/L)	Sulodexide	67 (54 - 100)	65 (53 - 105)	66 (55 - 114)	56 (46 - 110)	0.200
	Losartan	96 (67 - 119)	93 (71 - 110)	101 (69 - 113)	92 (71 - 99)	0.346
p (inter-Group)		0.101	0.122	0.146	0.101	
eGFR-(ml/min/1.7m²)	Sulodexide	93 (64 - 104)	83 (63 - 110)	93 (52 - 106)	102 (56 - 125)	0.125
	Losartan	63 (55 - 84)	71 (55 - 84)	68 (62 - 84)	74 (64 - 83)	0.672
p (intergroup)		0.203	0.274	0.237	0.246	
Se potassium (mmol/l)	Sulodexide	4.1 (3.7 - 4.5)	4.1 (3.6 - 4.4)	4.1 (3.9 - 4.2)	4.0 (3.0 - 4.3)	0.882
	Losartan	3.8 (3.8 - 4.0)	4.0 (3.8 - 4.3)	4.1 (3.8 - 4.2)	4.2 (3.8 - 4.3)	0.658
p (inter-group)		0.315	1.000	0.768	0.829	
Se Uric acid (umol/l)	Sulodexide	353 (303 - 408)	360 (298 - 470)	367 (303 - 484)	335 (288 - 511)	0.615
	Losartan	472 (391 - 521)	440 (364 - 511)	461 (390 - 477)	408 (365 - 474)	0.700
p (inter-group)		0.055	0.203	0.237	0.408	
Se albumin (g/L)	Sulodexide	43 (42 - 44)	43 (41 - 43)	41 (41 - 44)	43 (42 - 44)	0.887
	Losartan	42 (38 - 46)	44 (41 - 47)	41 (39 - 47)	44 (42 - 46)	0.678
p (inter-group)		0.829	0.146	0.408	0.463	

Results in median (IQR), IQR: interquartile range; eGFR: estimated glomerular filtration rate; p value*: Intra-group analysis using Friedman's analysis; p value: intergroup using Mann-Whitney-U test; p value < 0.05 is significant.

In our study, there was no significant antiproteinuric property in both losartan and sulodexide groups. Nevertheless there was a trend towards significance of proteinuria reduction in the losartan group.

These rather disappointing results in losartan group can be explained by a short study duration of 12 weeks and a the lower median dose of 75 mg daily used due to patient intolerance as manifested by a lowish blood pressure. In DKD, it is a fact that RAAS blockers exert maximal antiproteinuric effects after 6 months of treatment [9] [12] [40] [41]. In several studies using losartan as antiproteinuric agent in non-DKD, losartan even at low doses of 25 - 50 mg were sufficient to significantly reduce proteinuria in primary GN as hypertension is not universal in early non-DKD [38]. Large multicenter trials have also demonstrated the optimum antiproteinuric dose of losartan to be 100 mg daily and that no beneficial effects were seen beyond this dose [42]-[44]. Furthermore, from the extensive experience with the use of RAAS blockers in DKD and more recently in non-DKD, the higher the baseline proteinuria, the greater the proteinuria reduction [5] [9] [11] [12]. Thus, the low baseline proteinuria, low median dose of losartan and short duration of our study may account for the lowered antiproteinuric performance of losartan in our study.

To date, large trials of sulodexide have been conducted only in hypertensive patients with type 2 diabetes mellitus (DM) [20]-[22]. Its use in proteinuric chronic GN is very recent and followed the failure of the SUN-Micro-trial in which sulodexide at the optimal dose of 200 mg daily did not further reduce microalbuminuria [21]. The SUN-Macro-trial which was terminated prematurely by the sponsor had already recruited more than 2000 hypertensive type 2 DM patients with a mean follow-up of 11 months [22].

Several published studies, which included only a small number of patients, had previously investigated the effect of sulodexide on proteinuria in chronic non-DKD [17]-[19] [45]. Almost all these studies on non-DKD involved the use of sulodexide with an ACE-I or ARB. To our knowledge, there has been no head-to-head comparison between sulodexide versus a RAAS blocker in proteinuric renal disease, diabetic or non-diabetic. We believed this was the first study to investigate the antiproteinuric property of sulodexide as a sole antiproteinuric agent in primary GN.

A recent multicenter study by Kitae Bang et al. of sulodexide involved 77 patients with IgA nephropathy who despite RAAS blockade remained proteinuric. They were randomized to receive placebo, sulodexide 75 mg daily or sulodexide 150 mg daily. At the end of 16 weeks only those on sulodexide 150 mg daily had a significant reduction in proteinuria [17].

In a retrospective review, BY Yang *et al.* reported their experience with 20 patients with IgA nephropathy treated with sulodexide 50 mg daily as add-on therapy to optimized RAAS blockade. The investigators found a significant reduction of proteinuria and also noted the higher the baseline levels of proteinuria the greater the reduction [18].

As our study was a head-to-head comparison of sulodexide to losartan, it was not appropriate to compare our results with those of the above studies, which evaluated sulodexide as add-on therapy to RAAS blockade in proteinuric non DKD.

The median dose of sulodexide used was 150 mg daily (100 - 200 mg). In the literature, no previous study had specifically addressed the optimal dose of SDX in primary GN. In earlier study, Gambaro G *et al.* demonstrated a significant reduction of proteinuria with increasing oral doses of sulodexide from 50 mg to 100 mg to 200 mg daily [20]. In a recent study of patients with IgA nephropathy, sulodexide at 150 mg daily had significant anti-proteinuric effects up to 4 months of treatment and maximized at 6 months [17]. Another study by Byeong Yun Yang *et al.* reported that even lower sulodexide doses of 50 mg daily as add-on to ACE-I/ARB resulted in $\geq 50\%$ reduction in IgA nephropthy [18]. The shorter study duration of 12-week could explain the lack of antiproteinuric efficacy of sulodexide in our study.

Serum creatinine and eGFR were stable throughout the study period of 12 weeks and there were no differences seen within or between the two treatment groups. There was even a slight improvement in the serum creatinine and eGFR in both groups. These findings are consistent with other reports of the use of sulodexide in IgA nephropathy [17] [18] as well as in diabetic nephropathy [20]. Studies of losartan in primary GN also reported similar findings to ours [13] [37].

Serum uric acid has emerged as a risk marker for progression of CKD [46]. Hyperuricaemia increases blood pressure, proteinuria, renal dysfunction and renal scarring [46]. The changes of serum uric acid levels in our study patients were not significant in both groups. So far, there have been no reports on changes of serum uric acid in the earlier sulodexide studies [17]-[20]. In contrast, losartan has been proven to reduce serum uric acid and delay renal progression in patients with DKD [47]. There were no changes seen in the serum haemoglobin, platelet count, protrombin time, INR and aPTT after 12 weeks of treatment in our study. This is consistent with findings from numerous trials with sulodexide for renal disease including D.I.N.A.S [20]. No adverse events such as rash, diarrhea, musculoskeletal symptoms, epigastric pain and vomiting were observed in our study.

5. Conclusion

Sulodexide and losartan did not demonstrate any significant anti-proteinuric effect in primary GN. Nevertheless, there was a trend of better proteinuria reduction in losartan group. Furthermore, other renal parameters were not significantly affected by both drugs. These findings may be due to lower dose of study drugs, shorter study duration and low baseline proteinuria in both groups. We found both drugs were safe and well tolerated by patients. A larger and longer study is indicated to confirm our findings.

Acknowledgements

We would like to thank the Dean of the Faculty of Medicine, Universiti Kebangsaan Malaysia, for allowing us to publish these data.

Conflict of Interest

None declared.

References

[1]   Mc Grogan, A.F.C. and de Vries, C.S. (2011) The Incidence of Primary Glomerulonephritis Worldwide: A Systematic Review of the Literature. *Nephrol Dial Transplant*, **26**, 414-430. http://dx.doi.org/10.1093/ndt/gfq665

[2]   Sunita, B. and Lim, S.K. (2009) 3rd Report of the Malaysian Registry of Renal Biopsy 2009. *Primary Glomeruloneph-ritis*, **2**, 24.

[3]   US Renal Data System, USRDS 2012 Annual Data Report (2012) Atlas of Chronic Kidney Disease and End-Stage Re-

nal Disease in the United States. National Institutes of Health, National Institute of Diabetes and Digestive and Kidney Diseases, Bethesda, 226.

[4]   Lim, Y.N., Ong, L.M., Ghazali, A. and Lee, D.G. (2012) Nineteen Report of Malaysian Dialysis and Transplantation Registry 2012: Dialysis in Malaysia. The National Renal Registry, Kuala Lumpur.

[5]   Ruggenenti, P., Perna, A., Mosconi, L., Pisoni, R. and Remuzzi, G. (1998) Urinary Protein Excretion Rate Is the Best Independent Predictor of ESRF in Non-Diabetic Proteinuric Chronic Nephropathies. "Gruppo Italiano di Studi Epidemiologici in Nefrologia" (GISEN). *Kidney International*, **53**, 1209-1216. http://dx.doi.org/10.1046/j.1523-1755.1998.00874.x

[6]   Peterson, J.C., Adler, S., Burkart, J.M., Greene, T., Hebert, L.A., Hunsicker, L.G., *et al.* (1995) Blood Pressure Control, Proteinuria, and the Progression of Renal Disease. The Modification of Diet in Renal Disease Study. *Annals of Internal Medicine*, **123**, 754-762. http://dx.doi.org/10.7326/0003-4819-123-10-199511150-00003

[7]   Lea, J., Greene, T., Hebert, *et al.* (2005) The Relationship between Magnitude of Proteinuria Reduction and Risk of End Stage Renal Disease: Results of the African American Study of Kidney Disease and Hypertension. *Achives of Internal Medicine*, **165**, 2254-2261.

[8]   So, W.Y.K.K., Iseki, C., *et al.* (2006) Glomerular Filtration Rate, Cardiorenal End Points, and All Cause Mortality in Type 2 Diabetic Patients. *Diabetes Care*, **29**, 2046-2052.

[9]   Lewis, E.J.H.L., Clarke, W.R., Berl, T., Pohl, M.A., Lewis, J.B., *et al.* (2001) Renoprotective Effect of the Angiotensin-Receptor Antagonist Irbesartan in Patients with Nephropathy Due to Type 2 Diabetes. *New England Journal of Medicine*, **345**, 851-860. http://dx.doi.org/10.1056/NEJMoa011303

[10]   Maschio, G.A.D., Janin, G., Locatelli, F., Mann, J.F., Motolese, M., *et al.* (1996) Effect of the Angiotensin-Converting-Enzyme Inhibitor Benazepril on the Progression of Chronic Renal Insufficiency. The Angiotensin-Converting-Enzyme Inhibition in Progressive Renal Insufficiency Study Group. *New England Journal of Medicine*, **334**, 939-945. http://dx.doi.org/10.1056/NEJM199604113341502

[11]   Group, T.G. (1997) Randomised Placebo Control Trial of Effect of Ramipril on Decline in Glomerular Filtration Rate and Risk of Terminal Renal Failure in Proteinuric, Non Diabetic Nephropathy. *Lancet*, **349**, 1857-1863. http://dx.doi.org/10.1016/S0140-6736(96)11445-8

[12]   Brenner, B.M.C.M., de Zeeuw, D., Keane, W.F., Mitch, W.E., Parving, H.H., *et al.* (2001) Effects of Losartan on Renal and Cardiovascular Outcomes in Patients with Type 2 Diabetes and Nephropathy. *New England Journal of Medicine*, **345**, 861-869. http://dx.doi.org/10.1056/NEJMoa011161

[13]   Jacob Van Den Born, L.W.J.V., Marinka, H.B., Jacquesh, V., Karel, J.M.A., Jan, J.W. and Jo, H.M.B. (1993) Distribution of GBM Heparan Sulfate Proteoglycan Core Protein and Side Chains in Human Glomerular Diseases. *Kidney Intenational*, **43**, 454-463. http://dx.doi.org/10.1038/ki.1993.67

[14]   Harenberg, J. (1998) Review of Pharmacodynamics, Pharmacokinetics, and Therapeutic Properties of Sulodexide. *Medicinal Research Reviews*, **18**, 1-20. http://dx.doi.org/10.1002/(SICI)1098-1128(199801)18:1<1::AID-MED1>3.0.CO;2-4

[15]   Ruggeri, A., Guizzardi, S., Franchi, M., Morocutti, M. and Mastacchi, R. (1985) Pharmacokinetics and Distribution of a Fluoresceinated Glycosaminoglycan, Sulodexide, in Rats. Part II: Organ Distribution in Rats. *Arzneimittelforschung*, **35**, 1517-1519.

[16]   Dedov, I., Shestakova, M., Vorontzov, A. and Palazzini, E. (1997) A Randomized, Controlled Study of Sulodexide Therapy for the Treatment of Diabetic Nephropathy. *Nephrology Dialysis Transplantation*, **12**, 2295-2300. http://dx.doi.org/10.1093/ndt/12.11.2295

[17]   Bang, K., Chin, H.J., Chae, D.W., Joo, K.W., Kim, Y.S., Kim, S., *et al.* (2011) Anti-Proteinuric Effect of Sulodexide in Immunoglobulin A Nephropathy. *Yonsei Medical Journal*, **52**, 588-594. http://dx.doi.org/10.3349/ymj.2011.52.4.588

[18]   Yang, B.Y., Lee, H.S., Song, S.H., Kwak, I.S., Lee, S.B., Lee, D.W., *et al.* (2012) Use of Low-Dose Sulodexide in IgA Nephropathy Patients on Renin-Angiotensin System Blockades. *Kidney Research and Clinical Practice*, **31**, 163-169. http://dx.doi.org/10.1016/j.krcp.2012.06.006

[19]   Rozita, M., Loo, C.Y., *et al.* (2008) Glycosaminoglycans (Sulodexide) for Resistant Heavy Proteinuria of Chronic Glomerulonephritides (Abstract). 11*th Asian Pacific Congress of Nephrology*, Kuala Lumpur, 5-8 May 2008.

[20]   Gambaro, G., Kinalska, I., Oksa, A., Pont'uch, P., Hertlová, M., Olsovsky, J., *et al.* (2002) Oral Sulodexide Reduces Albuminuria in Microalbuminuric and Macroalbuminuric Type 1 and Type 2 Diabetic Patients: The Di.N.A.S. Randomized Trial. *Journal of the American Society of Nephrology*, **13**, 1615-1625. http://dx.doi.org/10.1097/01.ASN.0000014254.87188.E5

[21]   Lewis, E.J., Lewis, J.B., Greene, T., Hunsicker, L.G., Berl, T., Pohl, M.A., *et al.* (2011) Sulodexide for Kidney Protection in Type 2 Diabetes Patients with Microalbuminuria: A Randomized Controlled Trial. *American Journal of Kidney Diseases*, **58**, 729-736. http://dx.doi.org/10.1053/j.ajkd.2011.06.020

[22] Packham, D.K., Wolfe, R., Reutens, A.T., Berl, T., Heerspink, H.L., Rohde, R., *et al.* (2012) Sulodexide Fails to Demonstrate Renoprotection in Overt Type 2 Diabetic Nephropathy. *Journal of the American Society of Nephrology*, **23**, 123-130.

[23] Gambaro, G., Venturini, A.P., Noonan, D.M., Fries, W., Re, G., Garbisa, S., *et al.* (1994) Treatment with a Glycosaminoglycan Formulation Ameliorates Experimental Diabetic Nephropathy. *Kidney International*, **46**, 797-806. http://dx.doi.org/10.1038/ki.1994.335

[24] Caenazzo, C., Garbisa, S., Ceol, M., Baggio, B., Borsatti, A., Marchi, E., *et al.* (1995) Heparin Modulates Proliferation and Proteoglycan Biosynthesis in Murine Mesangial Cells: Molecular Clues for Its Activity in Nephropathy. *Nephrology Dialysis Transplantation*, **10**, 175-184.

[25] Ceol, M., Gambaro, G., Sauer, U., Baggio, B., Anglani, F., Forino, M., *et al.* (2000) Glycosaminoglycan Therapy Prevents TGF-Beta1 Overexpression and Pathologic Changes in Renal Tissue of Long-Term Diabetic Rats. *Journal of the American Society of Nephrology*, **11**, 2324-2336.

[26] Lewis, E.J. and Xu, X. (2008) Abnormal Glomerular Permeability Characteristics in Diabetic Nephropathy: Implications for the Therapeutic Use of Low-Molecular Weight Heparin. *Diabetes Care*, **31**, S202-S207. http://dx.doi.org/10.2337/dc08-s251

[27] Gambaro, G. and Kong, N.C. (2010) Glycosaminoglycan Treatment in Glomerulonephritis? An Interesting Option to Investigate. *Journal of Nephrology*, **23**, 244-252.

[28] Linhardt, R.J., Al-Hakim, A., Liu, J.A., Hoppensteadt, D., Mascellani, G., Bianchini, P., *et al.* (1991) Structural Features of Dermatan Sulfates and Their Relationship to Anticoagulant and Antithrombotic Activities. *Biochemical Pharmacology*, **42**, 1609-1619. http://dx.doi.org/10.1016/0006-2952(91)90431-4

[29] Furie, B. and Furie, B.C. (1992) Molecular and Cellular Biology of Blood Coagulation. *The New England Journal of Medicine*, **326**, 800-806. http://dx.doi.org/10.1056/NEJM199203193261205

[30] Cirujeda, J.L. and Granado, P.C. (2006) A Study on the Safety, Efficacy, and Efficiency of Sulodexide Compared with Acenocoumarol in Secondary Prophylaxis in Patients with Deep Venous Thrombosis. *Angiology*, **57**, 53-64. http://dx.doi.org/10.1177/000331970605700108

[31] Errichi, B.M., Cesarone, M.R., Belcaro, G., Marinucci, R., Ricci, A., Ippolito, A., *et al.* (2004) Prevention of Recurrent Deep Venous Thrombosis with Sulodexide: The SanVal Registry. *Angiology*, **55**, 243-249. http://dx.doi.org/10.1177/000331970405500302

[32] Coccheri, S., Scondotto, G., Agnelli, G., Aloisi, D., Palazzini, E., Zamboni, V., *et al.* (2002) Randomised, Double Blind, Multicentre, Placebo Controlled Study of Sulodexide in the Treatment of Venous Leg Ulcers. *Thrombosis and Haemostasis*, **87**, 947-952.

[33] Coccheri, S., Scondotto, G., Agnelli, G., Palazzini, E. and Zamboni, V. (2002) Sulodexide in the Treatment of Intermittent Claudication. Results of a Randomized, Double-Blind, Multicentre, Placebo-Controlled Study. *European Heart Journal*, **23**, 1057-1065. http://dx.doi.org/10.1053/euhj.2001.3033

[34] Gluhovschi, G.B.G., Petrica, L., *et al.* (2006) Nephroprotection, Part of Multi-Organprotection. *Temporomandibular Joint Disorders*, **56**, 2-3.

[35] Rutkowski, P., Tylicki, L., Renke, M., Korejwo, G., Zdrojewski, Z. and Rutkowski, B. (2004) Low-Dose Dual Blockade of the Renin-Angiotensin System in Patients with Primary Glomerulonephritis. *American Journal of Kidney Diseases*, **43**, 260-268. http://dx.doi.org/10.1053/j.ajkd.2003.10.032

[36] Renke, M., Tylicki, L., Rutkowski, P. and Rutkowski, B. (2004) Low-Dose Angiotensin II Receptor Antagonists and Angiotensin II-Converting Enzyme Inhibitors Alone or in Combination for Treatment of Primary Glomerulonephritis. *Scandinavian Journal of Urology and Nephrology*, **38**, 427-433. http://dx.doi.org/10.1080/00365590410015687

[37] Praga, M., Andrade, C.F., Luño, J., Arias, M., Poveda, R., Mora, J., *et al.* (2003) Antiproteinuric Efficacy of Losartan in Comparison with Amlodipine in Non-Diabetic Proteinuric Renal Diseases: A Double-Blind, Randomized Clinical Trial. *Nephrology Dialysis Transplantation*, **18**, 1806-1813. http://dx.doi.org/10.1093/ndt/gfg284

[38] Tylicki, L., Rutkowski, P., Renke, M. and Rutkowski, B. (2002) Renoprotective Effect of Small Doses of Losartan and Enalapril in Patients with Primary Glomerulonephritis. Short-Term Observation. *American Journal of Nephrology*, **22**, 356-362. http://dx.doi.org/10.1159/000065227

[39] Tylicki, L., Renke, M., Rutkowski, P., Rutkowski, B. and Lysiak-Szydlowska, W. (2005) Randomized, Controlled Study of the Effects of Losartan versus Enalapril in Small Doses on Proteinuria and Tubular Injury in Primary Glomerulonephritis. *Medical Science Monitor*, **11**, 131-137.

[40] Hou, F.F., Xie, D., Zhang, X., Chen, P.Y., Zhang, W.R., Liang, M., Guo, Z.J. and Jiang, J.P. (2007) Renoprotective of Optimal Antiproteinuric Doses (ROAD) Study: A Randomized Controlled Study of Benazepril and Losartan in Chronic Renal Insufficiency. *Journal of the American Society of Nephrology*, **18**, 1889-1898. http://dx.doi.org/10.1681/ASN.2006121372

[41] Mogensen, C.E., Neldam, S., Tikkanen, I., Oren, S., Viskoper, R., *et al.* (2000) Randomised Controlled Trial of Dual Blockade of Renin-Angiotensin System in Patients with Hypertension, Microalbuminuria, and Non-Insulin Dependent Diabetes: The Candesartan and Lisinopril Microalbuminuria (CALM) Study. *BMJ*, **321**, 1440-1444.

[42] Wright Jr., J.T., Bakris, G., Greene, T., Agodoa, L.Y., Appel, L.J., Charleston, J., *et al.* (2002) Effect of Blood Pressure Lowering and Antihypertensive Drug Class on Progression of Hypertensive Kidney Disease: Results from the AASK Trial. *JAMA*, **288**, 2421-2431.

[43] Arguedas, J.A., Perez, M.I. and Wright, J.M. (2009) Treatment Blood Pressure Targets for Hypertension. *Cochrane Database of Systematic Reviews*, Article ID: CD004349.

[44] Andersen, S., Rossing, P., Juhl, T.R., Deinum, J. and Parving, H.H. (2002) Optimal Dose of Losartan for Renoprotection in Diabetic Nephropathy. *Nephrology Dialysis Transplantation*, **17**, 1413-1418.
http://dx.doi.org/10.1093/ndt/17.8.1413

[45] Gluhovschi, A.S.G., Raica, M., Petrica, L., Trandafirescu, V., Velciov, S., Bozdog, G., Patrascu, C. and Gluhovschi, C. (2001) The Effects of the Therapy with Natural Glycosaminoglycans (Sulodexide) on Proteinuria in Different Types of Glomerulonephritis. *Medicine and Biology*, **8**, 26-30.

[46] Kang, D.H., Nakagawa, T., Feng, L., Watanabe, S., Han, L., Mazzali, M., *et al.* (2002) A Role for Uric Acid in the Progression of Renal Disease. *Journal of the American Society of Nephrology*, **13**, 2888-2897.
http://dx.doi.org/10.1097/01.ASN.0000034910.58454.FD

[47] Miao, Y., Ottenbros, S.A., Laverman, G.D., Brenner, B.M., Cooper, M.E., Parving, H.H., *et al.* (2011) Effect of a Reduction in Uric Acid on Renal Outcomes during Losartan Treatment: A Post Hoc Analysis of the Reduction of Endpoints in Non-Insulin-Dependent Diabetes Mellitus with the Angiotensin II Antagonist Losartan Trial. *Hypertension*, **58**, 2-7. http://dx.doi.org/10.1161/HYPERTENSIONAHA.111.171488

35

Is the Distribution of Microorganisms and Peritonitis Affected by Seasonality in Peritoneal Dialysis?

Ana Elizabeth Figueiredo[1], Ana Carolina Gonçalves Kehl[2], Stephanie Thomaz Bottin[2], Wilem Gomes Daminelli[2]

[1]School of Nursing, Nutrition and Physiotherapy (FAENFI), Pontifícia Universidade Católica do Rio Grande do Sul (PUCRS), PUCRS, Porto Alegre, Brazil
[2]Hospital São Lucas da Pontifícia, Universidade Católica do Rio Grande do Sul, Porto Alegre, Brazil
Email: anaef@pucrs.br

Abstract

Introduction: Peritonitis continues to be the main complication for patients on peritoneal dialysis (PD). Objective: To determine the frequency of peritonitis according to the disease-causing microorganism and its distribution throughout the year, linking to seasonality. Methods: A retrospective study conducted in the Dialysis Unit of the Hospital São Lucas, PUCRS (HSL-PUCRS). Patients undergoing PD between January 1984 and September 2013 were included. Descriptive statistics were used and Fisher's exact test with Monte Carlo simulation for comparison between the categorical variables. Results: Of 415 evaluated patients, 66% had at least one episode of peritonitis with an incidence rate of 0.68 episode/year. There were 601 peritonitis episodes in total. The most common microorganism was coagulase-negative Staphylococcus (26.6%, n = 160), followed by *Staphylococcus aureus* (16.3%, n = 98), with 16.3% of the sample being negative culture. Most episodes occurred in the months of January (10.3%, n = 62) and May (10.1%, n = 61), while June had the lowest occurrence (5.2%, n = 31). The number of episodes observed in January and May were significantly higher when compared to June (p < 0.001). No significant differences were found for the remaining months. There was no association between the microorganisms and months of the year (p = 0.841). Conclusion: The rate of peritonitis is in line with that recommended by the International Society for Peritoneal Dialysis. The distribution of peritonitis-causing germs over the months of the year would seem to be random.

Keywords

Chronic Renal Insufficiency, Peritoneal Dialysis, Peritonitis, Seasonal Variations

1. Introduction

Peritonitis in peritoneal dialysis (PD) continues to be one of the principal complications of this type of dialysis and identification of the modifiable risk factors can contribute to the reduction of morbidity [1]. Among the main causes for interruption of a PD program are: Peritonitis, catheter infection and ultrafiltration failure [2]. Lower rates of peritonitis can be achieved when risk reduction protocols are implemented [3]. The microorganisms that cause peritonitis may be used as an indicator of the route of contamination, the most frequent routes being: Intraluminal through accidental touch contamination of the open access during connection/disconnection of the dialysis bag, periluminal or contamination [4]. Gram-positive bacteria are the main pathogens causing peritonitis [5]. The most common microbial agent in Brazil and in the majority of Latin American countries is *Staphylococcus aureus* and is associated with more severe episodes with a greater risk of hospitalization, catheter removal and death [6]. Historically, the Nephrology Service of the Hospital São Lucas, Pontifical Catholic University of Rio Grande do Sul (HSL-PUCRS) has presented a higher prevalence of Coagulase-Negative Staphylococci (CNS), followed by peritonitis caused by *Staphylococcus aureus* and negative cultures [7] [8].

Peritonitis is mainly caused by CNS and *Staphylococcus aureus*, accounting for 80% of cases associated to intraluminal or periluminal contamination [9]. The presence of *Staphylococcus aureus* nasal carriers among chronic kidney disease patients is common, increasing the chance of skin colonization and leading to infection of the catheter exit-site, and peritonitis as a consequence [3] [10]-[12]. However, there is conflicting information regarding the seasonal distribution of peritonitis.

The aim of this study was to determine the distribution of peritonitis according to the disease-causing microorganisms and time of year.

2. Methods

A retrospective, descriptive and quantitative study was conducted. The sample was composed of patients undergoing PD at the Nephrology Service of the HSL-PUCRS between the years of 1984 and September 2013, during a period equal to or greater than 90 days. The years 1989 to 1992 were excluded due to a lack of complete medical records, and pediatric patients. The data collected included: name, age, gender, birth date, beginning and end of PD, duration of treatment, date of first peritonitis, numbers of peritonitis, month of the year and causing microorganisms.

The results are presented as absolute (n) and relative (%) distributions of categorical variables and mean ± standard deviation for continuous variables. Fisher's exact test with Monte Carlo simulation was used for comparison between the categorical variables.

The software SPSS 20.0 (Statistical Package for Social Sciences for Windows—SPSS Inc., Chicago, IL, USA, 2010) was used for statistical analysis of the data, with a 5% level of significance (α) adopted.

This study was approved by the Research Ethics Committee of PUCRS under protocol number 09/04535. The confidentiality of all data collected from patient-related medical records and databases attended by the Nephrology Service of the HSL-PUCRS was assured.

3. Results

From the 427 patients recorded in the hospital databank from January 1984 until September 2013, 415 met the study inclusion criteria. Sixty-six percent of patients had at least one episode of peritonitis with an incidence rate of 0.68 episode/year. Of these patients, 221 (53.25%) were women with a mean age of 48 ± 19.9 years and a mean time from the start of PD treatment to the first occurrence of peritonitis of 209 ± 68 days; the mean duration for undergoing PD was 545 days with a minimum of 91 days and maximum of 4692 days. During this period, 601 cases of peritonitis were recorded and these were distributed over the months from January to December according to their occurrence.

The distribution of peritonitis cases over the months of the year, have shown that the largest number of cases occurred in the months of January (10.3%, n = 62) and May (10.1%, n = 61), while the month with the least occurrences was June (5.2%, n = 31). A comparison of data verified that the peritonitis episodes recorded in January and May were significantly higher when compared with June (p < 0.001). No significant differences were found in relation to the other months of the year.

It was observed when classifying bacteria by the Gram test that gram-negatives (*Pseudomonas sp.*, *Escheri-*

chia coli, Enterobacter sp., Klebsiella sp.) were more prevalent in the month of February (12.6%, n = 13), as well as in January and December, which presented the same percentage (11.7%, n = 12); the gram-positives (*Staphylococcus coagulase negative, Staphylococcus aureus, Streptococcus sp., Enterococcus sp.*) occurred more in the months of May (10.8%, n = 34) and January (10.1%, n = 32). The distribution throughout the year is presented in **Figure 1**.

Peritonitis with a negative culture had a higher prevalence in August (17.3%, n = 17). Eosinophilic peritonitis and the microorganisms that occurred sporadically were classified as others (*Proteus sp., Coryneumbacterium sp., Acinetobacter sp., Alcaligene sp.*) with the greatest frequency of occurrence being in the months of May, July and December, in the same number of cases for each (16.7%, n = 8). No record of the causative microorganism was found on the peritonitis control sheets for some episodes of the disease (6.8%, n = 41).

Table 1 presents the types of microorganisms involved; cases defined as gram-positive (52.6%, n = 316) were

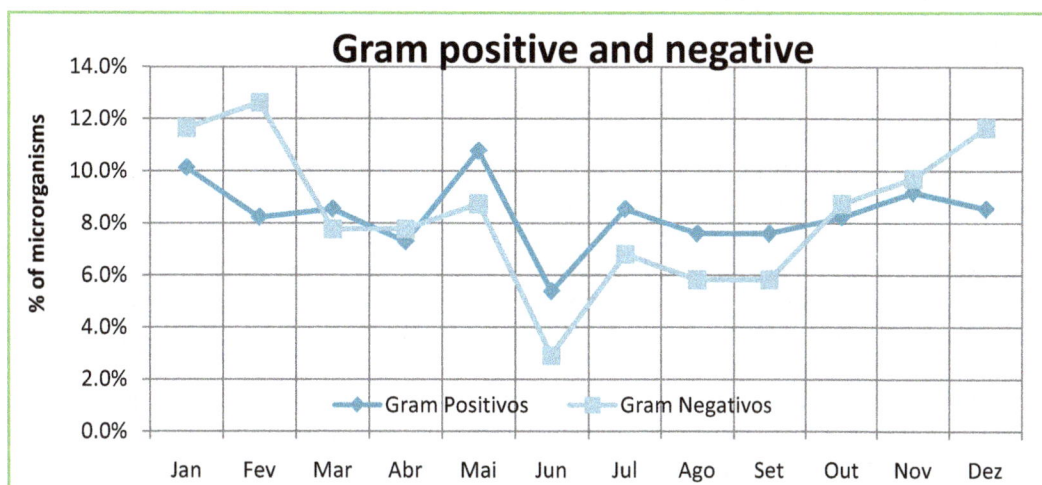

Figure 1. Distribution of microorganisms Gram Positive and Gram Negative during the months of the years.

Table 1. Absolute and relative distribution for the total occurrence of microorganism cases.

Month*	Classification of Microorganisms										Month Total**	
	Gram-Negatives		Gram-Positives		Fungi		Negative Culture		Others			
	N	%	N	%	N	%	N	%	N	%	N	%
Jan	12	11.7	32	10.1	2	12.5	11	11.2	5	7.4	62	10.3
Feb	13	12.6	26	8.2	1	6.3	7	7.1	2	2.9	49	8.2
Mar	8	7.8	27	8.5	2	12.5	6	6.1	6	8.8	49	8.2
Apr	8	7.8	23	7.3	3	18.8	9	9.2	6	8.8	49	8.2
May	9	8.7	34	10.8	2	12.5	8	8.2	8	11.8	61	10.1
Jun	3	2.9	17	5.4		0	5	5.1	6	8.8	31	5.2
Jul	7	6.8	27	8.5	1	6.3	9	9.2	7	10.3	51	8.5
Aug	6	5.8	24	7.6	2	12.5	17	17.3	4	5.9	53	8.8
Sept	6	5.8	24	7.6	1	6.3	7	7.1	6	8.8	44	7.3
Oct	9	8.7	26	8.2	1	6.3	10	10.2	7	10.3	53	8.8
Nov	10	9.7	29	9.2	1	6.3	4	4.1	3	4.4	47	7.8
Dec	12	11.7	27	8.5		0	5	5.1	8	11.8	52	8.7
Total	**103**	**17.1**	**316**	**52.6**	**16**	**2.7**	**98**	**16.3**	**68**	**11.3**	**601**	**100**

*Percentages obtained based on the total of each classification; **Percentages obtained based on the overall total (n = 601).

significantly higher when compared to gram-negative (17.1%, n = 103); negative cultures (16.3%, n = 98); others (11.3%, n = 68); and fungi (2.7%, n = 16) (p < 0.001).

The highest prevalence was of *Staphylococcus epidermidis* or coagulase-negative (26.6%, n = 160), followed by *Staphylococcus aureus* and negative culture, each representing 16.3% (n = 98) of the cases. The proportion of cases of *Staphylococcus epidermidis* or coagulase negative was significantly higher in comparison with the other microorganisms, as was also the case when comparing *Staphylococcus aureus* and negative culture with the other microorganisms.

When considering the most prevalent microorganisms and in accordance with **Table 2**, a statistically significant association (p < 0.0001) was detected in evaluating the relationship between the microorganisms involved and months of the year.

The association between the etiologic agents of peritonitis and months of the year was not confirmed (p = 0.841), indicating that peritonitis was not seasonally dependent for this studied sample; distribution was random.

4. Discussion

Analysis of the dialysis service for peritonitis episodes showed the rate to be within the minimum recommended by the International Society for Peritoneal Dialysis (ISPD), and similar to other Brazilian studies [13] [14].

Census data from the Brazilian Society of Nephrology reported 31.9% of patients receiving renal replacement therapy were greater than or equal to 65 years of age, with a higher incidence of men at 57.7%, whereas the present study presented a younger population with more women [15].

Cho et al. [16] in a study conducted in Australia and Kim et al. [17] in a Korean study demonstrated a higher incidence of peritonitis in the summer months, similar to our findings. Alterations in temperature and humidity that accompany seasonal change may potentially be related to patient hygiene behavior, distribution of normal skin flora and the chance of contamination [16].

A Brazilian study involving health professionals in relation to compliance with hand hygiene techniques showed a decrease in compliance in the summer months, which was associated with the Christmas festivity, vacation and summer period [18]. The same can occur with PD patients and may be aggravated by it being a home therapy; the summer could change household conditions and this may contribute to the rise in infections.

The initial hypothesis that there was a decrease in hand hygiene during the winter months with a consequent increase in peritonitis rates was not confirmed; this probably indicates that hand hygiene is not the only factor contributing to infections. No other study with similar results was encountered.

Table 2. Relative distribution of microorganisms according to month.

Microorganism	Period*											
	Jan	Feb	Mar	Apr	May	Jun	Jul	Aug	Sept	Oct	Nov	Dec
Not identified	9.8	4.9	12.2	7.3	7.3	7.3	7.3	9.8	12.2	12.2		9.8
S. epidermidis	11.9	5.6	9.4	6.3	10	5	6.9	6.9	6.3	10	12.5	9.4
S. aureus	8.2	11.2	9.2	8.2	8.2	7.1	11.2	6.1	9.2	6.1	6.1	9.2
Streptococcus sp.	8.1	10.8	8.1	8.1	18.9	2.7	10.8	10.8	10.8	5.4	2.7	2.7
Enterococcus sp.		11.8		11.8	17.6	5.9		17.6	5.9	11.8	5.9	11.8
Pseudomonas sp.	16.7	16.7		11.1	16.7	5.6	11.1		11.1	0	5.6	5.6
Escherichia Coli	3.2	16.1	6.5	6.5	9.7	3.2	6.5	3.2	6.5	12.9	12.9	12.9
Negative culture	11.2	7.1	6.1	9.2	8.2	5.1	9.2	17.3	7.1	10.2	4.1	5.1
Enterobacter		6.7	13.3	6.7	6.7		13.3	6.7		6.7	26.7	13.3
Klebsiella	35.3	5.9	5.9	5.9				17.6	5.9	11.8		11.8
Others	4.2		4.2	12.5	16.7	12.5	16.7		4.2	4.2	8.3	16.7
	9.8	4.9	12.2	7.3	7.3	7.3	7.3	9.8	12.2	12.2		9.8

*Percentages obtained based on the total of each microorganism.

Other studies corroborate our findings of gram-negative germs being significantly higher in the summer months [16] [19] [20]. However, the study by Kim *et al.* [17] stated that gram-negative peritonitis occurred uniformly throughout the year, while the rate of peritonitis caused by gram-positive germs increased in the hot and humid months. A consistency in peritonitis caused by gram-positive germs was observed in our sample throughout the year, with a peak occurring in May and a significant decrease in June.

It was shown in two studies evaluating the existence of seasonal variations and infections that *Staphylococcus epidermidis* and negative cultures were more frequent during the warmer months of the year [20] [21], unlike our findings where this germ was found to be more prevalent in the spring and the negative culture in the winter.

Cho *et al.* [16] demonstrated that there was a tendency for seasonal variations of peritonitis caused by fungi in the summer, with a peak in the fall. Our findings showed a tendency for peritonitis by fungi to occur in more frequently in April (fall). This same study showed there was no seasonal variation for *Streptococcus sp.* and *Enterococcus sp.*, which differs from our results in which *Streptococcus sp.* was more prevalent in May (fall) and *Enterococcus sp.* in the months of May (fall) and August (winter).

Studies by Chan *et al.* [21] and Cho *et al.* [21] observed that the occurrences of peritonitis caused by *Staphylococcus aureus* were uniformly distributed throughout the year, which is consistent with our study. *Staphylococcus aureus* is a microorganism that naturally inhabits the skin, such as on the hands and around the catheter exit-site, and this can therefore justify the uniformity of peritonitis caused by it throughout all the year [21].

Even in hemodialysis patients there is a 46% risk increase for the development of septicemia associated with the central venous catheter in the summer months, which may or may not be related to the susceptibility of chronic kidney patients [20].

The main limitation of this study is in its being retrospective, without records for the temperatures over the years, nor information related to catheter exit-site infections. It is known that despite the south of Brazil having a temperate climate, there is a great variation in temperature within the same season of the year.

This research brings to the spotlight an important issue in peritoneal dialysis, peritonitis that is still cause of mortality in this group of patients. Identifying risk factor such as the influence of season can help health care professional to act upon this and re-train patients beforehand. Further research in this area can improve outcomes in peritoneal dialysis.

5. Conclusions

The rate of peritonitis is in line with that recommended by the ISPD. Gram-positive bacteria caused the majority of episodes with an even distribution over the months of the year, which suggests that seasonality has no impact on the occurrence of peritonitis. The distribution of peritonitis-causing microorganisms over the months of the year would seem to be by chance.

Although no significant incidence was found in respect of microorganisms and the months of the year, it is important to know that there is a higher occurrence in the summer months so that surveillance measures and patient retraining can be established.

References

[1] Cho, Y. and Johnson, D.W. (2014) Peritoneal Dialysis-Related Peritonitis: Towards Improving Evidence, Practices, and Outcomes. *American Journal of Kidney Diseases: The Official Journal of the National Kidney Foundation*, **64**, 278-289. http://dx.doi.org/10.1053/j.ajkd.2014.02.025

[2] Chaudhary, K. (2011) Peritoneal Dialysis Drop-Out: Causes and Prevention Strategies. *International Journal of Nephrology*, **2011**, Article ID: 434608. http://dx.doi.org/10.4061/2011/434608

[3] Bender, F.H., Bernardini, J. and Piraino, B. (2006) Prevention of Infectious Complications in Peritoneal Dialysis: Best Demonstrated Practices. *Kidney International Supplement*, **70**, S44-S54. http://dx.doi.org/10.1038/sj.ki.5001915

[4] Figueiredo, A.E., Poli de Figueiredo, C.E. and d'Avila, D.O. (2000) Peritonitis Prevention in CAPD: To Mask or Not? *Peritoneal Dialysis International: Journal of the International Society for Peritoneal Dialysis*, **20**, 354-358.

[5] Wong, C., Luk, I.W., Ip, M. and You, J.H. (2014) Prevention of Gram-Positive Infections in Peritoneal Dialysis Patients in Hong Kong: A Cost-Effectiveness Analysis. *American Journal of Infection Control*, **42**, 412-416. http://dx.doi.org/10.1016/j.ajic.2013.12.008

[6] Barretti, P., Moraes, T.M., Camargo, C.H., Caramori, J.C., Mondelli, A.L., Montelli, A.C., *et al.* (2012) Peritoneal Dialysis-Related Peritonitis Due to *Staphylococcus aureus*: A Single-Center Experience over 15 Years. *PloS ONE*, **7**,

e31780. http://dx.doi.org/10.1371/journal.pone.0031780

[7]   Figueiredo, A.E., Poli de Figueiredo, C.E. and d'Avila, D.O. (2001) Bag Exchange in Continuous Ambulatory Perito-
      neal Dialysis without Use of a Face Mask: Experience of Five Years. *Advances in Peritoneal Dialysis Conferenceon
      Peritoneal Dialysis*, **17**, 98-100.

[8]   Figueiredo, A.E., Poli-de-Figueiredo, C.E., Meneghetti, F., Lise, G.A., Detofoli, C.C. and Silva, L.B. (2013) Peritonitis
      in Patients on Peritoneal Dialysis: Analysis of a Single Brazilian Center Based on the International Society for Perito-
      neal Dialysis. *Jornal brasileiro de nefrologia: Orgao oficial de Sociedades Brasileira e Latino-Americana de Nefro-
      logia*, **35**, 214-219. http://dx.doi.org/10.5935/0101-2800.20130034

[9]   Johnson, D.W., Clark, C., Isbel, N.M., Hawley, C.M., Beller, E., Cass, A., *et al.* (2009) The Honeypot Study Protocol:
      A Randomized Controlled Trial of Exit-Site Application of Medihoney Antibacterial Wound Gel for the Prevention of
      Catheter-Associated Infections in Peritoneal Dialysis Patients. *Peritoneal Dialysis International: Journal of the Inter-
      national Society for Peritoneal Dialysis*, **29**, 303-309.

[10] Al-Hwiesh, A.K. and Abdul Rahman, I.S. (2008) Prevention of Staphylococcal Peritonitis in CAPD Patients Combin-
      ing Ablution and Mupirocin. *Saudi Journal of Kidney Diseases and Transplantation: An Official Publication of the
      Saudi Center for Organ Transplantation, Saudi Arabia*, **19**, 737-745.

[11] Nessim, S.J., Komenda, P., Rigatto, C., Verrelli, M. and Sood, M.M. (2013) Frequency and Microbiology of Peritonitis
      and Exit-Site Infection among Obese Peritoneal Dialysis Patients. *Peritoneal Dialysis International: Journal of the In-
      ternational Society for Peritoneal Dialysis*, **33**, 167-174. http://dx.doi.org/10.3747/pdi.2011.00244

[12] Nouwen, J.L., Fieren, M.W., Snijders, S., Verbrugh, H.A. and van Belkum, A. (2005) Persistent (Not Intermittent) Na-
      sal Carriage of *Staphylococcus aureus* is the Determinant of CPD-Related Infections. *Kidney International*, **67**, 1084-
      1092. http://dx.doi.org/10.1111/j.1523-1755.2005.00174.x

[13] Moraes, T.P., Pecoits-Filho, R., Ribeiro, S.C., Rigo, M., Silva, M.M., Teixeira, P.S., Pasqual, D.D., Fuerbringer, R.
      and Riella, M.C. (2009) Peritoneal Dialysis in Brazil: Twenty-Five Years of Experience in a Single Center. *Peritoneal
      Dialysis International: Journal of the International Society for Peritoneal Dialysis*, **29**, 492-498.

[14] Li, P.K., Szeto, C.C., Piraino, B., Bernardini, J., Figueiredo, A.E., Gupta, A., *et al.* (2010) Peritoneal Dialysis-Related
      Infections Recommendations: 2010 Update. *Peritoneal Dialysis International: Journal of the International Society for
      Peritoneal Dialysis*, **30**, 393-423. http://dx.doi.org/10.3747/pdi.2010.00049

[15] Sesso Rde, C., Lopes, A.A., Thome, F.S., Lugon, J.R., Watanabe, Y. and Santos, D.R. (2012) Chronic Dialysis in Brazil:
      Report of the Brazilian Dialysis Census, 2011. *Jornal brasileiro de nefrologia: Orgao oficial de Sociedades Brasileira
      e Latino-Americana de Nefrologia*, **34**, 272-277. http://dx.doi.org/10.5935/0101-2800.20120009

[16] Cho, Y., Badve, S.V., Hawley, C.M., McDonald, S.P., Brown, F.G., Boudville, N., *et al.* (2012) Seasonal Variation in
      Peritoneal Dialysis-Associated Peritonitis: A Multi-Centre Registry Study. *Nephrology, Dialysis, Transplantation: Of-
      ficial Publication of the European Dialysis and Transplant Association—European Renal Association*, **27**, 2028-2036.
      http://dx.doi.org/10.1093/ndt/gfr582

[17] Kim, M.J., Song, J.H., Park, Y.J., Kim, G.A. and Lee, S.W. (2000) The Influence of Seasonal Factors on the Incidence
      of Peritonitis in Continuous Ambulatory Peritoneal Dialysis in the Temperate Zone. *Advances in Peritoneal Dialysis
      Conference on Peritoneal Dialysis*, **16**, 243-247.

[18] Dos Santos, R.P., Konkewicz, L.R., Nagel, F.M., Lisboa, T., Xavier, R.C., Jacoby, T., *et al.* (2013) Changes in Hand Hy-
      giene Compliance after a Multimodal Intervention and Seasonality Variation. *American Journal of Infection Control*,
      41, 1012-1016. http://dx.doi.org/10.1016/j.ajic.2013.05.020

[19] Szeto, C.C., Chow, K.M., Wong, T.Y., Leung, C.B. and Li, P.K. (2003) Influence of Climate on the Incidence of Peri-
      toneal Dialysis-Related Peritonitis. *Peritoneal Dialysis International: Journal of the International Society for Perito-
      neal Dialysis*, **23**, 580-586.

[20] Lok, C.E., Thumma, J.R., McCullough, K.P., Gillespie, B.W., Fluck, R.J., Marshall, M.R., *et al.* (2014) Catheter-Re-
      lated Infection and Septicemia: Impact of Seasonality and Modifiable Practices from the DOPPS. *Seminars in Dialysis*,
      27, 72-77. http://dx.doi.org/10.1111/sdi.12141

[21] Bernardini, J., Price, V. and Figueiredo, A. (2006) Peritoneal Dialysis Patient Training. *Peritoneal Dialysis Interna-
      tional: Journal of the International Society for Peritoneal Dialysis*, **26**, 625-632.

Permissions

List of Contributors

José Siles-González and Carmen Solano-Ruiz
Nursing Department, University of Alicante, Alicante, Spain

Norio Nakamura
Community Medicine, Hirosaki University Graduate School of Medicine, Japan

Michiko Shimada, Ikuyo Narita, Yuko Shimaya, Takeshi Fujita, Reiichi Murakami, Hideaki Yamabe and Ken Okumura
Department of Cardiology, Respiratory Medicine and Nephrology, Hirosaki University Graduate School of Medicine, Hirosaki, Japan

Hiroshi Osawa
Department of General Medicine, Hirosaki University Hospital, Hirosaki, Japan

Kashif J. Piracha, Edward P. Nord and Nand K. Wadhwa
Division of Nephrology, Department of Medicine, Stony Brook Medicine, Stony Brook, USA

Frank Darras
Transplantation Services, Stony Brook Medicine, Stony Brook, USA

Sun Woo Kang
Department of Nephrology, College of Medicine, Inje University, Busan, Korea

Jean Jacques Sehonou
University Clinic of Internal Medicine of the National Teaching Hospital "Hubert K Maga" (CNHU-HKM), Cotonou, Benin

Jacques Vigan, Bruno Léopold Agboton and Gbètondji Michel Massi
University Clinic of Nephrology and Hemodialysis of the National Teaching Hospital "HKM" of Cotonou, Cotonou, Benin

Mathieu Leblanc
Internal Medecine Residency Program, Faculté de Médecine et des Sciences de la santé, Université de Sherbrooke, Sherbrooke, Canada

Martin Plaisance
Nephrology Division, Department of Medicine, Centre Hospitalier Universitaire de Sherbrooke, Sherbrooke, Canada

Marwa Miftah, Loubna Benamar and Aicha Bezzaz
Department of Nephrology-Dialysis-Kidney Transplants, Rabat Ibn Sina University Hospital, Rabat, Morocco

Mohammed Asseban, Adil Kallat, Ali Iken and Yassine Nouini
Urology A Department, Rabat Ibn Sina University Hospital, Rabat, Morocco

Sayed Husain
Cape Fear Valley Hospital NC, Fayetteville, USA

Hani Judeh
St. Luks/Roosevelet Hospital, New York, USA

Manaf Alroumoh
South Texas Regional Medical Center, San Antonio, USA

Farhana Yousaf, Ahla Husain, Chaim Charytan and Bruce Spinowitz
New York Hospital Queens, New York, USA

Prince Mohan
Columbia Medical University, New York, USA

Karima Boubaker, Madiha Mahfoudhi, Amel Gaieb Battikh, Hayet Kaaroud, Ezzeddine Abderrahim, Taieb Ben Abdallah and Adel Kheder
Department of Internal Medicine A, Charles Nicolle Hospital, Tunis, Tunisia

Hiromichi Suzuki
Department of Nephrology, Saitama Medical University, Moroyama, Japan

Hiroshi Omata
Center for Oriental and Integrated Medicine, Saitama Medical University, Moroyama, Japan

Hiroo Kumagai
Department of Nephrology and Endocrinology, National Defense Medical College, Tokorozawa, Japan

Magda M. Bayoumi
Medical Surgical Nursing, Nursing College, King Khalid University, Abha, Saudi Arabia

Rubina Naqvi, F. Akhtar, E. Ahmed, A. Naqvi and A. Rizvi
Sindh Institute of Urology and Transplantation (SIUT), Karachi, Pakistan

Imen Gorsane, Madiha Mahfoudhi, Fathi Younsi, Imed Helal and Taieb Ben Abdallah
Internal Medicine A Department, Charles Nicolle Hospital, Tunis, Tunisia

Imen Gorsane, Madiha Mahfoudhi, Imed Helal and Taieb Ben Abdallah
Internal Medicine A Department, Charles Nicolle Hospital, Tunis, Tunisia

Ali Absar, Quratulain Khan and Waqar Kashif
Aga Khan University Hospital, Karachi, Pakistan

Naila Asif
Liaquat National Hospital, Karachi, Pakistan

Érida Maria Diniz Leite
Department of Nursing, Hospital Academic Onofre Lopes, Natal, Brasil

Sama Mikaella de Oliveira, Maria Isabel da Conceição Dias Fernandes, Maria das Graças Mariano Nunes, Cyndi Fernandes de Lima and Ana Luisa Brandão de Carvalho Lira
Department of Nursing, University of Rio Grande do Norte, Natal, Brasil

Heo-Yeong Kim, Ji Soo Kim, Seung Eun Suh, Yu Kyung Hyun, Kyeong Mi Park and Hyung-Jong Kim
Department of Internal Medicine, Bundang CHA Medical Center, CHA University, Seongnam, South Korea

Samra Abouchacra, Ahmed Chaaban, Mohammad Budruddin, Mohamad Hakim, Mohamad Ahmed, Farida Marzouki and Faiz Al Abbacheyi
Department of Medicine, Tawam Hospital, Abu Dhabi, UAE

Fares Chedid
Department of Pediatrics, Tawam Hospital, Abu Dhabi, UAE

Nicole Gebran
Department of Pharmacology, Tawam Hospital, Abu Dhabi, UAE

Muhy Eddin Hassan
SEHA Dialysis Services, Tawam Hospital, Abu Dhabi, UAE

Alexandre Fernandes and Laura Marques
Pediatric Infectious Diseases and Immunodeficiency Department, Centro Hospitalar do Porto, Oporto, Portugal

Liliana Rocha, Teresa Costa, Paula Matos, Maria Sameiro Faria and Conceição Mota
Pediatric Nephrology Department, Centro Hospitalar do Porto, Oporto, Portugal

António Castro Henriques
Kidney Transplant Department, Centro Hospitalar do Porto, Oporto, Portugal

Abeer A. Al-Refai and Safaa I. Tayel
Biochemistry Department, Faculty of Medicine, Menofia University, Shibin El Kom, Egypt

Ahmed Ragheb, Ashraf G. Dala and Ahmed Zahran
Internal Medicine Department, Faculty of Medicine, Menofia University, Shibin El Kom, Egypt

Stephen Meyer, Aswin Nukala, Nikita Maniar and Waldo Herrera
Department of Internal Medicine, Mt. Sinai Hospital, Chicago, USA

Karima Boubaker, Madiha Mahfoudhi, Amel Gaieb Battikh and Adel Kheder
Department of Internal Medicine A, Charles Nicolle Hospital, Tunis, Tunisia

Azza Bounemra
Cellular Immunology, Blood Transfusion Center, Tunis, Tunisia

Chokri Maktouf
Nuclear Medicine and Clinical Research Department, Pasteur institute, Tunis, Tunisia

Ankita Patel, Suchita Mehta, Ahmad Waseef and Subodh Saggi
Department of Nephrology, SUNY Downstate Medical Center, New York, USA

Imen Gorsane, Madiha Mahfoudhi, Mondher Ounissi, Fathi Younsi, Imed Helal and Taieb Ben Abdallah
Internal Medicine A Department, Charles Nicolle Hospital, Tunis, Tunisia

Amin S. Banaga
Department of Medicine & Nephrology, University of Medical Sciences and Technology, Academy Charity Teaching Hospital, Khartoum, Sudan

Elaf B. Mohammed, Rania M. Siddig, Diana E. Salama, Sara B. Elbashir and Mohamed O. Khojali
Clinical Research Assistants, Department of Nephrology, Academy Charity Teaching Hospital, Khartoum, Sudan

Rasha A. Babiker
Department of Basic Sciences, Faculty of Medicine, University of Medical Sciences & Technology, Khartoum, Sudan

Khalifa Elmusharaf
Department of Epidemiology & Public Health Medicine, Royal College of Surgeon in Ireland (RCSI), Dublin, Ireland

Mamoun M. Homeida
Department of Medicine, Faculty of Medicine, University of Medical Sciences & Technology, Khartoum, Sudan

Ahmed Tall Lemrabott, Mouhamadou Moustapha Cissé, Elhadji Fary Ka, Maria Faye, Aliou Ndongo, Younoussa Keita, Khodia Fall, Abdou Niang and Boucar Diouf
Department of Nephrology, Aristide Le Dantec University Hospital, Dakar, Senegal

Sidy Mohamed Seck
Faculty of Medicine, Gaston Berger University, Saint-Louis, Senegal

Cherif Dial
Anatomo-Pathology Laboratory, Grand-Yoff General Hospital, Dakar, Senegal

Ahmed Tall Lemrabott, Mouhamadou Moustapha Cisse, Elhadji Fary Ka, Maria Faye, Moussa Sarr, Abdou Niang and Boucar Diouf
Department of Nephrology, Aristide Le Dantec University Hospital, Dakar, Senegal

Sidy Mohamed Seck
Faculty of Medicine, Gaston Berger University, Saint-Louis, Senegal

Ngoné Diaba Gaye, Alassane Mbaye and Abdoul Kane
Department of Cardiology, Grand-Yoff General Hospital, Dakar, Senegal

Gaurav Singh
Department of Internal Medicine, Princess Alexandra Hospital, Brisbane, Australia

Lauren White and Patrick Flynn
Department of Internal Medicine, Royal Brisbane and Women's Hospital, Brisbane, Australia

Sajan Thomas, George John and Dwarakanathan Ranganathan
Department of Nephrology, Royal Brisbane and Women's Hospital, Brisbane, Australia

Lakshmanan Jeyaseelan and Mani Thenmozhi
Department of Biostatistics, Christian Medical College, Vellore, India

Paul Kubler
Department of Rheumatology, Royal Brisbane and Women's Hospital, Brisbane, Australia

Effiong Ekong Akpan and Udeme E. Ekrikpo
University of Uyo, Uyo, Nigeria

Naoki Sugano, Satoru Kuriyama, Yoichiro Hara, Koki Takane, Yasuhito Takahashi, Yasuko Suetsugu and Takashi Yokoo
Division of Kidney and Hypertension, Department of Internal Medicine, The Jikei University School of Medicine, Tokyo, Japan

Adnan Bashir Bhatti, Farhan Ali and Siddique A. Satti
Capital Development Authority (CDA) Hospita, Islamabad, Pakistan

Abdul Halim Abdul Gafor, Wan Hazlina Wan Mohamad, Rozita Mohd, Rizna Abdul Cader, Kong Wei Yen and Norella C. T. Kong
Nephrology Unit, Department of Medicine, University Kebangsaan Malaysia Medical Centre, Jalan Yaacob Latif, Bandar Tun Razak, Cheras, Kuala Lumpur, Malaysia

Shamsul Azhar Shah
Department of Epidemiology and Biostatistics, University Kebangsaan Malaysia Medical Centre, Jalan Yaacob Latif, Bandar Tun Razak, Cheras, Kuala Lumpur, Malaysia

Ana Elizabeth Figueiredo
School of Nursing, Nutrition and Physiotherapy (FAENFI), Pontifícia Universidade Católica do Rio Grande do Sul (PUCRS), PUCRS, Porto Alegre, Brazil

Ana Carolina Gonçalves Kehl, Stephanie Thomaz Bottin and Wilem Gomes Daminelli
Hospital São Lucas da Pontifícia, Universidade Católica do Rio Grande do Sul, Porto Alegre, Brazil